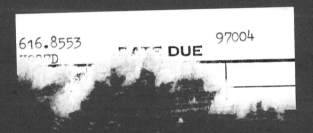

DYSLEXIA

DYSLEXIA
Neuropsychological Theory, Research, and Clinical Differentiation

GEORGE W. HYND

Associate Professor of Educational Psychology
Department of Educational Psychology
University of Georgia
Athens, Georgia

Assistant Clinical Professor of Neurology
Department of Neurology
Medical College of Georgia
Augusta, Georgia

MORRIS COHEN

Assistant Professor of Neurology
Department of Neurology
Medical College of Georgia
Augusta, Georgia

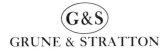

GRUNE & STRATTON

A Subsidiary of Harcourt Brace Jovanovich, Publishers
New York   London
Paris   San Diego   San Francisco   São Paulo
Sydney   Tokyo   Toronto

Library of Congress Cataloging in Publication Data

Hynd, George W.
    Dyslexia: Neuropsychological theory, research,
and clinical differentiation.

    Bibliography: p.
    Includes index.
    1. Dyslexia. I. Cohen, Morris. II. Title.
[DNLM: 1. Dyslexia—In infancy and childhood.
2. Learning disorders. WM 475 H997d]
RC394.W6H95 1983   616.85'53   83-12758
ISBN 0-8089-1584-3

Grune & Stratton, Inc.
111 Fifth Avenue
New York, New York 10003

Distributed in the United Kingdom by
Grune & Stratton, (London) Ltd.
24/28 Oval Road, London NW 1

Library of Congress Catalog Number 83-12758
International Standard Book Number 0-8089-1584-3

Printed in the United States of America

We dedicate our efforts in this volume
to Cyndie and Lisa

CONTENTS

Foreword *by Francis J. Pirozzolo*   **xi**

Preface   **xv**

Acknowledgments   **xix**

PART I: INTRODUCTION

1. *Dyslexia: Definitional Problems, History, and*
    Epidemiology   *3*

    Defining Dyslexia   5
    History of Dyslexia   11
    Epidemiology of Dyslexia   16
    Conclusions   25

2. *Functional Organization of the Brain: An*
    Overview   *26*

    A Little History   27
    Neurological Development   32
    The Brain Stem and Cerebellum   35
    The Functional Organization of the Cerebral Cortex   40
    Conclusions   51

PART II: THEORY AND RESEARCH

3. *Neuropsychology of Language and Reading Failure*   **55**

   Neurological Aspects of Language and Reading   56
   Disordered Brain Function and Cognitive Ability   60
   Neurodevelopmental Asymmetries in Dyslexic
     Brains   82
   EEG Correlates in Dyslexia (BEAM)   86
   Cytoarchitectonic Studies of Dyslexics' Brains   90
   Conclusions   95

4. *Single Factor Research with Dyslexics: The Perceptual-Deficit Hypothesis and Cross-Modal Integration Research*   **97**

   Dysfunction in Visual Perception: The Perceptual-
     Deficit Hypothesis   98
   Dysfunction in Cross-Modal Integration   103
   Conclusions   112

5. *Cerebral Dominance and Dyslexia*   **114**

   Asymmetries in Lateral Preference   115
   Dichotic Listening Research   117
   Tachistoscopic Visual Half-Field Research   127
   Conclusions   134

6. *Subgroups of Dyslexia*   **136**

   Initial Conceptualization   137
   The Contribution of Elena Boder   139
   Articulating the Neuropsychological Characteristics
     of the Dyslexic Subtypes   145
   Conclusions   156

PART III: CLINICAL DIFFERENTIATION AND INTERVENTION

7. *Neuropsychological Assessment of the Dyslexic Child*   **161**

   The Neurologic Examination   162
   Neuropsychological Evaluation: Perspectives   166

Neuropsychological Evaluation: Conceptual
    Framework   170
Neuropsychological Evaluation: Pitfalls   190
Conclusions   192
Case Studies   193

8. *Remedial Approaches to Dyslexia*   *206*

Historical Approaches to Remediation   207
Perceptual Training Approaches   218
The Neuropsychological Approach   222
Conclusions   230

Glossary   **233**

References   **239**

Index   **263**

FOREWORD

Learning disorders, and developmental reading disabilities in particular, are a major public health problem in the United States. The incidence of learning disabilities is alarmingly high. Developmental dyslexia, the syndrome of unexpected reading failure, is probably the most important specific learning disability, both in terms of accounting for the greatest number of children and adults affected and in terms of its devastating effects on those who suffer from it. Simply stated, the effects of developmental dyslexi cannot be measured by reading achievement tests because they fail to examine the personal, social, and other consequences of this disorder. Although dyslexia is well known to cause such problems, it has not been afforded the attention necessary to provide solutions to the difficult questions surrounding it. This is due, in part, to the difficulty all of us have in understanding dyslexia. Why should it be that children have such trouble with this apparently simple cognitive skill? Understanding speech is an extremely crucial cognitive skill that nearly every child develops apparently effortlessly. Why then, several years later, should so many children, indeed normal children as well as disabled readers, have such a terrible time learning a visual code for previously mastered oral language? The answer, of course, lies at the very center of the issue. Reading is not such a simple cognitive skill after all. It is a very complex cognitive process that depends on numerous information processing stages, and all of them must be carried out rapidly and accurately. But even if we acknowledge that reading is difficult and complex, it still does not answer many of dyslexia's innumerable questions.

The specificity and yet sheer mystery of the disorder are striking. I frequently imagine the utter confusion that early researchers must have experienced when they first observed the syndrome of alexia without agraphia. We know the explanation now, of course, but we have the benefit of 100 years of neuropsychological research on written language disturbances.

This is not to say, however, that the specificity of the disorder is no longer alarming. I am reminded of this by my students, who have the remarkable quality of a childlike vivid appreciativeness when they see their first patient with alexia without agraphia. Similarly, they have the capacity for unguarded astonishment when they observe a young child who can carry out binomial expansions, draw precise, articulated designs, and produce the proper memories for cognitive tasks that involve several steps—yet the child cannot read a word beyond monosyllabic length.

Aside from these observational deficiencies, what other deficiencies have affected the understanding of dyslexia? A major deficiency, I believe, and one that happens to be a main theme of this book, is the attempt to find out what is different about dyslexic children other than their inability to read well. This was formally done by taking a large group of dyslexics and comparing them to a large group of normal-reading children. Many things were obscured by this modus operandi, and this in fact has accounted for much of the confusion about developmental dyslexia. The point is, of course, that dyslexia has more than one clinical presentation. In trying to find common deficiencies in dyslexic children, Bronner, in 1917, found "negative" resu lts; in other words, he found some children to have auditory language distu ·bances and others to have quite the opposite pattern of disturbance in the visual modality. These results were largely ignored until recent research provided a better framework for understanding dyslexia. The idea that there may be subtypes of dyslexia got its modern beginning from observations by Joseph Wepman. Wepman noted in his articulation of what he called the "modality concept" that some dyslexic children have auditory disturbances while others have visual disturbances. He thought that this had something to do with the maturation of the neural pathways for audition and vision. The historical precedent for such a suggestion came from Charcot, one of the most influential 19th century neuroscientists. Charcot had made many important contributions to the understanding of neurologic diseases (such as Parkinson's disease) and psychiatric disturbances (he shaped many of the ideas of his famous pupil, Sigmund Freud). He recognized that normal people had learning modality preferences. Nearly all people, he hypothesized, were either "visile" (preferring to learn through the visual modality) or "audile" (preferring to learn through the auditory modality).

By 1963 the secret was out. Kinsbourne and Warrington found two distinct patterns, or subtypes, of developmental dyslexia. Despite the im-

portance of their study, which became part of the public record, their findings were not embraced by all. Several other researchers stumbled onto this
conclusion as well, but little changed in either neuropsychological or educational practice. Elena Boder's work in the mid-1970s did much to advance
the notion of subtypes and in part triggered a considerable amount of research and thinking that continues today.

I have been one of those who has reinvented the wheel. I discovered
subtypes of dyslexia experimentally in 1975. I am sorry to say I had heard
about them before, but perhaps the idea was too arcane for me at the time.
I first heard about dyslexia when I was an undergraduate student. A fellow
student had told me that there were children who read *was* when they saw
saw, and furthermore saw *b* instead of *p*. Curious, I thought, and exhilarat-
ing—all the more so because of the attractive coed who introduced me to
the concept. I went off to graduate school to study neuroscience and spent
long hours in the laboratory trying to learn what the role of the basal gan-
glia was in certain motor functions by making surgical lesions in rats that
would induce akinesia. I was interested in designing a knife and a cannula
that would enable me to completely disconnect the substantia nigra from
the rest of the brain. I thought that this might help to delineate the dopa-
mine system and its role in motor function.

Simultaneously, I was reintroduced to the problem of developmental
dyslexia by Joseph Wepman, who suggested to me that some dyslexia may
involve disturbances in monoamine activity, yet another fascinating suggestion about the enigma of unexpected reading failure. There was more to
think about when he told me about other possible pathophysiologies. Dr.
Wepman was among the first to differentiate between what he called cerebral agenesis (neural underdevelopment) and cerebral damage.

I decided to undertake my first empirical investigation of dyslexia some
time later, but I am sorry to say that I had not learned my lessons well.
Wanting to understand the neuropsychological deficits in dyslexics, I administered the Illinois Test of Psycholinguistic Abilities to a large group of
dyslexics. I expected to find that dyslexics differed from normal readers in
this or that subtest, but I was surprised to find that there were no differences between dyslexics and normal readers. I considered my first attempt
at dyslexia research an utter failure since I learned that diagnostic tests for
learning disabilities did not differentiate at all between the two groups. In
subsequent studies I paid attention to the lessons of Wepman, Kinsbourne,
et al., and distinguished between auditory-linguistic and visual-spatial dyslexics.

Drs. Hynd and Cohen have given us the most up-to-date, authoritative
account of some of the most important issues pertaining to dyslexia. They
provide a sound critical review of previous research on dyslexia and the role
of brain functions in some of the cognitive operations used in reading. They

discuss the most recent research and developments that have given new impetus to dyslexia research. Hynd and Cohen have tackled one of the most difficult topics in science and have produced a remarkably thorough and sound treatment of one of the most important problems in education today.

Francis J. Pirozzolo
Chief, Neuropsychology Service
Baylor College of Medicine
Houston, Texas

PREFACE

This book is for psychologists and reading specialists who work in a clinical setting as well as for researchers in psychology and education who desire a comprehensive and well referenced overview of the neurological and neuropsychological research on dyslexia. Within the past decade, the neuropsychological conceptualization of dyslexia has undergone more extensive evaluation than perhaps any other type of childhood learning disability. Computerized tomographic procedures, refined electrophysiological mapping techniques, postmortem studies, and extensive neuropsychological research have provided convincing evidence that for the dyslexic child, associated neurodevelopmental deficits exist within the functional system of reading.

In response to early uncertainty and controversy regarding the concept of dyslexia, many psychologists and educators rejected the medical model associated with dyslexia. The use of the term "dyslexia" in the title of this volume affirms our conviction that to truly understand the nature of severe reading disabilities, one must be familiar with the research that has provided strong evidence as to the neuropsychology of reading and reading failure. It is for this reason that we feel the term dyslexia and its associated theoretical implications are more appropriate in describing severe reading failure than other terms currently in use.

Unfortunately for the clinician, much of the available research remains unread. For many, a basic knowledge of physiological psychology and neuropsychological theory and research is lacking, making it difficult to conceptualize and place in perspective what is read. Even for those who possess an adequate background in the neurosciences, the literature on dyslexia is so widely distributed that it is nearly impossible to keep current. Finally, there exists a rapidly developing interest in neuropsychology among the professionals who must work with dyslexic children. Whenever a new perspective can be brought to bear on old problems, it is often followed by a too rapid and uncritical acceptance of what the literature appears to offer. It has been our intention in this volume to introduce the reader to neuropsychology and its foundation in behavioral neurology, to discuss critically the current neurological and neuropsychological research, and to suggest how this knowledge might be applied in a clinical setting.

To accomplish these ambitious goals, we organized the book into three parts. The first part provides an introduction to the concept of dyslexia and the functional organization of the brain. Chapter 1 discusses problems associated with defining the concept of dyslexia, provides an overview of the history of knowledge regarding severe reading disorders, and outlines epidemiologic factors associated with dyslexia. It is argued that definitions developed within the past several decades have greatly assisted researchers in articulating the neurological nature of dyslexia. Resolving definitional problems and differentiating dyslexia from other less disabling reading disorders have led to the recognition that dyslexia is a distinct nosologic entity. Chapter 2 was included for those readers needing a fundamental introduction to functional neuroanatomy. Such an understanding is vital to the comprehension of neuropsychological theory and research in dyslexia.

Part II focuses on neuropsychological theory and research on dyslexia. The discussion builds on the perspectives provided in the first two chapters. Chapter 3 addresses the neuropsychology of language and reading disorders. Neurolinguistic theory is related to validating evidence provided by neurodevelopmental studies, research regarding traumatic brain damage, and electrophysiological and cytoarchitectonic studies with dyslexics. The neurological evidence provided in support of a neuropsychological conceptualization of dyslexia serves as a foundation for Chapters 4 through 6, which address the research related to neuropsychological and cognitive processes found in dyslexic children and discuss single-factor theories, cerebral dominance, and subcategorizations of dyslexia, respectively. Central to the focus of this volume is the research in support of differential subgroups of dyslexia, which is important from both a theoretical and clinical perspective.

Part III addresses clinical differentiation in dyslexia and reviews the literature regarding neurologically based intervention programs. Chapter 7 briefly reviews principles of neurological, psychological, and educational assessment, relates clinical appraisal of the dyslexic, and provides several illustrative case reports of differentially diagnosed dyslexic children. Chapter 8 critically reviews the historical approaches to remediation, as well as the admittedly limited literature on neurologically based intervention strategies. Although the success of early intervention programs may have been rare, recent conceptualizations of what constitutes an appropriate focus of intervention may prove more productive than previous approaches.

The material presented in this book is necessarily complex and represents that of multidisciplinary research literature. We have attempted to provide a basic but none-the-less solid overview of the multifaceted advances made in our understanding of dyslexia. We hope that the many figures and tables provided will assist the reader in developing a more thorough and current understanding of what is and is not known about the neuropsychology of dyslexia. If this book serves to help the clinician and researcher to better focus their efforts in working with dyslexic children, then our efforts will have been worthwhile indeed.

George W. Hynd
Morris Cohen

ACKNOWLEDGMENTS

Writing a book on dyslexia has been an exceptional experience, and only those who have undertaken such a venture can appreciate the extent to which many other individuals have contributed to the publication of this volume. Particularly rewarding were the many conversations we were able to have with respected colleagues who have conducted research on the neuropsychology of dyslexia. We have especially appreciated the encouragement and stimulation provided by Dr. Francis Pirozzolo, Head of Neuropsychology at Baylor College of Medicine, whose knowledge regarding the neuropsychology of dyslexia is exceptional. Dr. Walter Isaac, Professor of Psychology at the University of Georgia, and Dr. Jack Obrzut, Professor of Psychology at the University of Northern Colorado, provided many critical and helpful comments on early drafts of these contents. Their efforts are sincerely appreciated. Jo Ann Perrin and Betty Randolph demonstrated tremendous patience with us in typing and retyping our manuscript, and the graphic artists at the Instructional Resource Center at the University of Georgia provided the excellent figures found in this book. We are especially grateful to Dr. Frank Duffy, Department of Neurology, Harvard Medical School, and Director of Developmental Neurophysiology at the Children's Hospital Medical Center in Boston; Dr. Albert Galaburda of the Departments of Neurology, Harvard Medical School, Boston University School of Medicine, and Beth Israel Hospital; and Dr. Daniel Hier, Department of Neurology at Michael Reese Hospital and Medical Center, in Chicago, for allowing us to reprint their figures. Finally, and most importantly, Cyndie and Lisa endured and greatly assisted us during the protracted period of preparation this volume required. Cyndie's expertise in reading education was especially helpful in focusing, challenging, and refining our thoughts.

DYSLEXIA

PART I
Introduction

Chapter 1
Dyslexia: Definitional Problems, History, and Epidemiology

Probably no other term common to educators, physicians, and psychologists is apt to result in so much controversy as dyslexia. Disagreement exists as to whether the disorder of dyslexia actually exists, its nature, how to differentially diagnose the condition, and what to actually do about children identified as dyslexic. The controversy over these important practical and theoretical issues is likely to continue. It is important, however, to fully understand the literature on dyslexia if one is to draw any firm conclusions from which to evaluate the on-going debate over this severe reading disability.

The practical issues can be broadly conceptualized as relating to how one perceives the dyslexic condition, how it is to be treated educationally, and what exactly constitutes the legal responsibility of the public schools in the provision of services for children diagnosed as dyslexic. Several viewpoints exist regarding how one perceives the condition of dyslexia. For instance, there are those who argue that dyslexia represents the bottom end of the distribution of reading abilities. If a child is diagnosed as dyslexic, it is thus assumed that he will not profit substantially from remedial efforts (Snyder, 1979a). As might be expected, there are many who disagree with this position and prefer to think of dyslexia as a delay in cognitive development (Lieberman, 1979; Weinshank, 1979; Wilkie, 1979). This has been called the deficit-delay controversy.

How one views dyslexia has implications for treatment. If one perceives dyslexia as representing one end of the continuum of reading ability and attributes this deficit performance to neurodevelopmental anomalies, then the emphasis in instruction should be shifted away from reading to other avenues of communication (Snyder, 1979b). Support for this notion has been generated from years of experience. There can be no doubt that, for the reading-disabled child who is severely affected, the success of most remedial programs has been dismal (Silberberg, Iversen, & Goins, 1973; Spache, 1976; Tobin & Pumfrey, 1976). This failure of educational practice is despite a long-standing move away from the inadequate visual and neurologic training programs that were once popular (Kaufman & Kaufman, 1983; Zarske, 1982). Promising new techniques designed to replace the early failures in remedial instruction now also seem to be usually recognized as inadequate (Hewison, 1982). The failure of these programs also casts doubt on those who would propose that dyslexia represents developmental delay. If the dyslexic child is delayed, then he should "catch up" eventually. This is an idea not supported by the literature.

Over the past several decades, the courts have affirmed the rights of children regarding appropriate educational practices for those identified as handicapped. In some cases, litigation has led to substantial awards to dyslexic children for the failure of school districts to provide "appropriate" remedial instruction (Angelos, 1982). With the increased demand for remedial educational services in the schools coupled with dwindling fiscal resources, one can but wonder what the future may hold.

Theoretical concerns similarly indicate that important issues are far from resolved. The literature, for example, presents a confusing picture as to whether deficits in cerebral dominance are related to disability in reading and cognitive development (Dean, 1980; Hynd & Obrzut, 1981; Kinsbourne & Hiscock, 1981). Other investigators disagree as to the number and characteristics of differentiated subtypes of dyslexia (Boder, 1971; Pirozzolo, 1979). Still other researchers argue as to whether or not cerebral asymmetries between the brains of dyslexics and the brains of normals are related to the existence of severe reading disability (Haslam, Dalby, Johns, & Rademaker, 1981; Hier, 1979, LeMay, 1981).

These, of course, are only some of the many important concerns related to our efforts to conceptualize dyslexia and our attempts to formulate some reasonably productive efforts to help children so identified. To truly appreciate the many dilemmas facing researchers and practitioners working with dyslexic children, one must have some foundation regarding the various problems associated in defining dyslexia, the history of thought regarding severe reading disability in children, and the factors associated with the prevalence of dyslexia. These important topics constitute the focus of this chapter.

DEFINING DYSLEXIA

Attempting to define dyslexia can be one of the thorniest problems related to the study of this condition. Almost no intelligent professional who interacts with school-age children would deny that a small but significant number of children fail in their attempts to learn to read despite the best of all possible instruction and apparent ability.

Since the condition affects a small percentage of children and is not a life-threatening disorder, the careful articulation of this disorder from a definitional standpoint has not been a high priority for researchers. Investigators within the fields of medicine, education, and psychology have not always communicated well with each other, and, as will be seen, vast philosophical differences contribute significantly to different approaches in examining the nature of the dyslexic child.

Development of the Concept of Dyslexia

Because so many investigators from different professions have taken an interest in children who fail to learn to read, the concept of severe reading failure has often become merely a reflection of the orientation of the investigator. For instance, many of the early researchers published articles in journals for ophthalmologists. Not surprisingly, they favored the term congenital word blindness (Morgan, 1896). Others, favoring this perspective but focusing on the possible genetic link, preferred the term familial congenital word blindness (Drew, 1956). Still other investigators, believing dyslexia to be the result of developmental lags or delays in cortical maturation, preferred the term developmental reading disorders (American Psychiatric Association, 1980).

Seemingly countless terms have been proposed to best describe dyslexia, and a representative few include: amnesia visualis verbalis, analfabetia partialis, bradylexia, congenital alexia, congenital dyslexia, congenital symbolamblyopia, congenital typholexia, constitutional dyslexia, primary reading retardation, specific dyslexia, specific reading disability, and strephosymbolia (Drew, 1956; Pirozzolo, 1979).

While this list is certainly not an exhaustive one, it is at least representative of the many different attempts that have been made to specify the nature of this disorder. Most investigators would probably agree on the basic nature of dyslexia even without an agreed on definition, but the emphasis over the past several decades has been on identifying subtypes of dyslexic children. This shift in focus reflects a recognition that many of the inconsistencies characterizing the early literature were probably due to the inclusion of heterogeneous populations of dyslexics in sample groups. Clinical as well as statistical methods have revealed subtypes of dyslexic children. Similar to the problem once encountered in agreeing on a term to describe severe reading disorders, we now have a state of affairs in which many, and not necessarily comparable, subgroups are being proposed by different investigators.

For example, Pirozzolo (1979) discussed the visual-spatial and auditory-linguistic dyslexic child, and Bannatyne (1971) differentiated between the genetic dyslexic and the minimally neurologically-dysfunctional dyslexic. Other investigators such as Boder (1973a) proposed three subtypes: dysphonetic, dyseidetic, and the combined, or, alexic readers. Mattis, French, and Rapin (1975), whose work has greatly influenced the Task Force on Nosology of Disorders of Higher Cerebral Function in Children for the Child Neurology Society (1981), proposed four discernible subtypes. These subtypes include: the language disorderly dyslexic, the articulatory and graphomotor dyscoordination dyslexic, the visuo-spatial perceptual dyslexic, and the dyslexic with a sequencing disorder syndrome. All of these possible subtypes are discussed later in this volume.

The practical and theoretical implications of differentiating subgroups of dyslexia are indeed important. As Benton (1980) indicates, however, we do not know that the subgroups proposed by different investigators are comparable. As detailed in Chapter 6, the research along these lines offers much promise, but an obvious priority, considering the definitional problems with even the term, dyslexia, should be to develop some commonly agreed-on criteria for conceptualizing subgroups. The efforts of the Child Neurology Society's Task Force (1981) stand out as exemplary in this regard.

Whatever the theoretical perspective of the investigator, it seems obvious that research efforts have been aimed at identifying and understanding the child who is unable to learn to read despite adequate intelligence or conventional or remedial instruction. Most contemporary researchers would probably agree that true dyslexia is a relatively rare disorder affecting 3 to 6 percent of school-age children and may be related to neurodevelopmental deficits. Considerable resistance to these basic notions exists, unfortunately. One must be conversant with the objections to the use of the term dyslexia to adequately understand the schism that exists between medical researchers and many educational and even psychological researchers.

Resistance to the Use of the Term Dyslexia

To those who propose that the term dyslexia has no precise meaning, it would seem that their objections in actuality fall into two rather broad categories. First and foremost, there are those who completely disavow the neurological basis of dyslexia as well as the relevance of dyslexia to reading and reading disabilities. This perspective is best articulated by Ross (1976), who suggested, "The hypothesis that learning disabilities are due to a malformation in the brain has never been proved, and the vagueness of the formulation makes it impossible to disprove" (p. 83).

Drake (1968), however, had previously reported on brain malformations in a learning-disabled child. The statement by Ross demonstrated a neglect of the historical literature in neurology, which associates developmental anomalies with cognitive deficits in learning. Much of this literature is reviewed in Chapters 2 and 3. The attitude of psychologists such as Ross (1976) makes it clear that even if a neural center for reading were identified, it would not have the least impact on their thinking. As Smith (1982), an educator, has said, "I do not believe it would or should make the slightest difference to how reading is taught if it were discovered tomorrow that we all have a critical neural center for reading in the foot (the left foot, for most people)" (p. 78).

He continues to vent his distrust and suspicion of neuropsychological investigations of reading failure based on his reading of seven articles or chapters and concludes that,

> Failure to learn is explained in terms of fad rather than fact, the specialized insights of students of the brain are important in many respects, but they do not yet explain reading or reading problems. The relating of subtle differences in learning, behavior, attitude, and personality to gross differences in the architecture of the brain should not become a new phrenology, as unscientific as making judgments about people's character from the bumps on their skull . . . failure need not be attributed to *dyslexia*, a disease that only strikes children who cannot read, and which is invariably cured when they can read. (Smith, 1982, pp. 68, 188)

Quotes from Smith (1982) were chosen because he is a well-respected theoretician and researcher in the field of reading. This lack of familiarity with research advances in allied fields is unfortunately representative of the current state of affairs. It would seem reasonable to project that this lack of understanding and respect for research from other fields will continue unless attempts are made to bridge this communication gap.

It should be realized that not only is the validity of a neurological conceptualization questioned but also questioned is the very practicality of any such knowledge. Since advances in understanding how the brain functions during reading is perceived as having no direct application in an instructional vein, then that information is deemed meaningless by critics. For investigators in the neurosciences, it must be an eventual priority to provide suggestions as to how medical advances in the study of dyslexia can be translated into practice. For educators still suspicious of neurologically based intervention programs that have not stood the test of time (Zarske,

1982), past failures should not dictate an unwillingness to critically evaluate new perspectives on long-standing educational concerns.

A second source of resistance to the use of the term dyslexia comes from a much broader framework and relates to a disavowment of the usefulness of labels in general. Hobbs (1975), Gaddes (1980), and Wilson (1981) outline a number of arguments against the use of labels with children. Some of these arguments include the following observations. Labels tend to prejudice the responses to a child by teachers, peers and family members. They discourage sensitivity to the child's problems. Labels create a fear of the condition, and placement in special programs may expose the children to potentially damaging effects of treatment (i.e., removal from the regular classroom, inappropriate peer models, etc.). The use of labels focuses on a negative aspect of the child and assumes that the problem is within the child. As Ross (1976) has said regarding such a practice, "it continues to place emphasis on the brain" (p. 63) and by implication, nothing can be done about this negative condition. Labels tend to obscure fundamental individual differences that may have potentially impacted positively on the remedial process. Finally, labels can help generate a negative self-fulfilling prophesy; they contribute to lowered levels of self-esteem and personal expectancy for success.

Gaddes (1980) and Kolstoe (1972) counter these criticisms regarding the use of labels to help children in need of special remedial education. They argue that the negative effects of labeling have not been empirically proven and the entire notion regarding the self-fulfilling prophesy has been seriously challenged since it was first introduced over two decades ago. Also, they believe that labeling has aided society in providing tremendous financial aid, educational facilities, and highly trained professional personnel to deal with problems faced by certain special populations. Finally, they believe that labels and the process of labeling children is not the problem in generating distance between the child and his teachers or peers. The distance exists already whether the child is or is not labeled, simply because the child is not normal. Whether or not the children who cannot read are labeled dyslexic does not alter the fact that they are unlike their peers because of their disability.

It is likely that many within the educational domain will continue to disavow the relevance of advances made in our understanding of the neuropsychological processes involved in reading and reading failure. Perhaps a recognition as to the source of this resistance will eventually give way to increased communication between professionals in all fields concerned with the study of children with reading difficulties. This has, in fact, occurred to some degree in the development of a widely accepted definition of dyslexia. Although many old prejudices still exist depending on one's perspective, excellent progress has been made in defining what is meant by the use of the term dyslexia.

Definitions of Dyslexia

Critchley and Critchley (1978) have likened the debate over the term dyslexia to the situation in the Middle Ages when many ecclesiastics hotly debated the number of angels who could gather on the head of a pin. As long as the debate rages over what dyslexia is, nobody has to do anything about it; therefore, children desperately in need of services might not receive services mandated by law.

The situation today might not be as grim as suggested by Critchley and Critchley (1978), although considering the remarkable variability found in contemporary definitions, one might well argue otherwise. For instance, Kolb and Whishaw (1980) define dyslexia as simply, "a difficulty in reading" (p. 477). *Webster's Third New International Dictionary (Unabridged)* (1966) does little better defining dyslexia as "a disturbance in the ability to read" (p. 712). *Stedman's Medical Dictionary* (1972) is somewhat more precise in defining dyslexia as "incomplete alexia; inability to read more than a few lines with understanding" (p. 385).

In 1968, the World Federation of Neurology published its definition, which has had a significant impact on our thinking during the past decade. As detailed by Critchley (1970), the World Federation of Neurology defined dyslexia as:

> a disorder manifested by difficulty in learning to read despite conventional instruction, adequate intelligence, and socio-cultural opportunity. It is dependent upon fundamental cognitive disabilities which are frequently of constitutional origin. (p. 11)

During the 1960s and early 1970s, parent and teacher organizations placed enormous pressure on Congress to enact laws pertaining to the provision of special education services to all handicapped children. The definition published in the *Federal Register* (1976) for learning disabilities included dyslexia as falling under this broader term. For the first time, school districts in every state in the nation were forced to expand services to children experiencing learning problems, including those who could be diagnosed as dyslexic.

In a more contemporary definition of learning disabilities proposed by the National Joint Committee for Learning Disabilities (NJCLD), it was stated that learning disabilities (including dyslexia), "are intrinsic to the individual and *presumed to be due to central nervous system dysfunction*" [emphasis added] (Hammill, Leigh, McNutt, & Larsen, 1981, p. 336). Since the NJCLD included representatives from the American Speech and Hearing

Association (ASHA), the Association for Children and Adults with Learning Disabilities (ACLD), the Council for Learning Disabilities (CLD), the Division for Children with Communication Disorders (DCCD), the International Reading Association (IRA), and the Orton Dyslexia Society, their proposed definition linking learning disabilities directly to central nervous system dysfunction stands a good chance of becoming the new standard.

Based on the interaction of all of these historical events and trends in defining dyslexia, it would seem that any exemplary definition of dyslexia would require some reference to failure to read as expected despite adequate intelligence, the fact that the deficit must be due to some dysfunction of the central nervous system, and the fact that the disability must be severe, possibly as measured as a discrepancy between expected levels of reading and actual measured performance.

By far the best definition yet advanced was developed by a task force of the IRA (reprinted with permission of the International Reading Association and Harris & Hodges, 1981). Their definition is as follows:

Dyslexia:
1. *n.* A medical term for incomplete alexia; partial but severe, inability to read; historically (but less common in current use), word blindness. *Note:* Dyslexia in this sense applies to persons who ordinarily have adequate vision, hearing, intelligence, and general language functioning. *Dyslexia is a rare but definable and diagnosable form of primary reading retardation with some form of central nervous system dysfunction. It is not attributable to environmental causes or other handicapping conditions.*
2. *n.* A severe reading disability of unexpected origin.
3. *n.* A popular term for any difficulty in reading of any intensity and from any cause(s). *Note:* Dyslexia in this sense is a term which describes a symptom, not a disease. (p. 95)

There can be little doubt that this definition is exemplary. While the definition seems objective and specific enough for general diagnostic purposes, the editorial note appended to this definition steps far beyond the bounds of objectivity that one might expect in a dictionary. It can be seen that assumptions made regarding the effects of labeling have influenced the editors who developed the above definitions.

Due to all the differing assumptions about the process and nature of possible reading problems, dyslexia has come to have so many incompatible connotations that it has lost any real value for educators, except as a fancy word for a reading problem. Consequently, its use may create damaging cause and effect assumptions for student, family and teacher. Thus in referring to a specific student, it is probably better that the teacher describe the actual reading difficulties, and make suggestions for teaching related to the specific difficulties, not apply a label which may create misleading assumptions by all involved. (Reprinted with permission of the International Reading Association and Harris & Hodges, 1981, p. 95)

Editorial comments aside, the IRA definition is an excellent one and defines well the clinical population which is the focus of this volume.

Primary and Secondary Dyslexia

It is not uncommon to read references to primary and secondary dyslexia. Indeed, the IRA definition quoted above makes reference to "primary reading retardation" (Harris & Hodges, 1981, p. 95).

In the most common usage of the terms, primary or developmental dyslexia refers to reading failure of congenital origin. The dysfunction may not be brain damage but relates to neurodevelopmental anomalies that contribute to reading failure. These neurodevelopmental anomalies are discussed in detail in Chapter 3. Frequently, primary reading retardation or developmental dyslexia can be genetically determined. This is in direct contrast to the term alexia, which implies that the reading disability was acquired, usually through trauma of some sort (Benson, 1981; Benson & Geschwind, 1969).

Secondary dyslexia is considered to be the result of other factors, including impoverished home environment, emotional problems, or the direct result of sociocultural or environmental influences. Since most research studies exclude cases of secondary dyslexia, the research discussed in this volume focuses on primary reading failure or developmental dyslexia.

The problems in adequately defining dyslexia have arisen in large part because the history of thought regarding the condition has been so varied. An understanding of this history is needed to place our current conceptualization of this disorder in the proper perspective.

HISTORY OF DYSLEXIA

The history of thought regarding what was first termed congenital word blindness and later dyslexia only dates back approximately 100 years. Since the early reports of Bastian (1898), Hinshelwood (1900, 1902), and Morgan (1896), many theories regarding the neurological and psychological nature of the disorder have been introduced, examined, and, in some cases, rejected. For the sake of organization, we will briefly focus our attention on the literature related to congenital word blindness, laterality and strephosymbolia, and, finally, recent advances in dyslexia research.

Congenital Word Blindness

Long before the disorder that was to become known as congenital word blindness was introduced, it was known that memory loss for words could occur as a result of brain damage. It had also been observed that children suffering no known brain insult evidenced similar patterns of behavior as some brain-damaged adults (Wilde, 1853).

In 1896, Pringle Morgan published his now classic case of developmental dyslexia. The patient he reported was a very intelligent 14-year-old boy who had failed miserably in reading and writing at school. Although he had received many hours of instruction outside of school, knew most of his letters, and could even read some sight words, he could not read phonetically. Morgan's patient did possess adequate and age-appropriate skills in arithmetic and could read numbers well.

Morgan was familiar with Hinshelwood's (1895) report of brain-impaired patients who had lost the ability to read, and he drew a connection between his case and the patients seen by Hinshelwood. Morgan referred to his patient as suffering what he termed as congenital word blindness based on the concept of word blindness as originally applied by Kussmaul (1877).

Both Morgan (1896) and Bastian (1898), who described a similar case, believed the reading disability to be due to developmental deficits in the region of the left angular gyrus. The notion that various functions, such as reading, could be localized was popular at this time and most theorists adhered to this view. A series of papers by Hinshelwood (1900, 1902, 1909) reported on more cases and it soon became an accepted fact that cases of congenital word blindness existed, perhaps in far greater frequency than had even been imagined.

Papers by Hinshelwood (1909) and Nettleship (1901) contributed not only to the growing body of knowledge regarding the clinical manifestations of congenital word blindness but also set the stage for the development of remedial programs (Benton, 1980). For instance, Hinshelwood (1902) suggested that children suffering from congenital word blindness be removed from the regular classroom setting and taught separately using a kinesthetic modality to build a foundation for visual-auditory associations.

The literature on congenital word blindness continued to grow with reports of cases from all over the world (Brunner, 1905; Claiborne, 1906; Foerster, 1905; Jackson, 1906; Peters, 1908; Stephenson, 1907; Thomas, 1905; Variot & Lecomte, 1906). These early papers appeared primarily in medical journals related, not surprisingly, to ophthalmology. Some authors addressed the nature of congenital word blindness and advanced evidence not only as to the preponderance of males being affected but also regarding the fact that the condition could be inherited. Jackson (1906) suggested that the term developmental alexia was more accurate than congenital word blindness. Early estimates as to the incidence of dyslexia ranged from 1:2000 to 1:100 (Fisher, 1905; Warburg, 1911).

As Benton (1980) pointed out, while progress was being made in articulating the factors associated with dyslexia, little conceptual progress was being made. The prevailing view remained that the underlying causative factor in dyslexia was damage or developmental delay of that part of the brain believed to be important in the visual-memory images of words. Since the left hemisphere in the region of the supramarginal gyrus and angular gyrus seemed to be the culprit underlying dyslexia (discussed in detail in Chapter 3), it appeared only reasonable to the theorists of this era that the right hemisphere would assume functions related to reading. For this reason it was logical to suggest that the left hand be used in writing, since it was known to be subserved by the right cerebral hemisphere. The whole word approach, which was thought to rely more on right hemisphere abilities, was also advocated at this time (Fisher, 1905). The idea, of course, was that the right hemisphere could assume the functions subserved by the deficit left hemisphere. These notions are still the source of considerable controversy.

Laterality and Orton's Strephosymbolia

In the United States during the first several decades of the 1900s, the child guidance movement became an established force. The first president of the American Psychological Association, G. Stanley Hall, had a well-known interest in adolescents, and William James (1900) published his book *Talks to Teachers on Psychology*. Based on the clinical model provided by Lightner Witmer in 1896, child guidance clinics grew in number. Mental testing became an established practice in the schools, and the provision of special education services showed remarkable growth such that, by 1953, all 48 states had developed special education programs for children experiencing failure in the schools (Cutts, 1955; Tindall, 1979).

The emphasis on the assessment of cognitive abilities in school-age children affected greatly the research on dyslexia. The medical approach characterized by Hinshelwood (1909) and Morgan (1896) gave way to investigations that were more psychological or educational in nature. As Benton (1980) noted, the theory developed by neurologists and ophthalmologists was considered inadequate.

The investigations that were conducted in the early 1900s centered on differentiating the psychological profile of the dyslexic from that of the reading-retarded child as well as those abilities possessed by normal children. Investigations revealed that dyslexic children suffered deficits in visual discrimination, orientation, memory (Fildes, 1922; Hincks, 1926), written language (Schmitt, 1918), and expressive language (Voss, 1914).

It was Orton (1928), however, who contributed a uniquely different theory regarding the psychological and neurological processes believed to be involved in reading. It had long been recognized that deficient hand preferences were associated with problems in oral language and with reading (Ballard, 1912; Dearborn, 1925). The idea was that left handedness or mixed preferences in laterality was evidence of deficient cerebral dominance. It was believed that one had to be left-hemispheric dominant, and thus strongly right-handed, to be a proficient reader. Dearborn (1925), among others, observed that approximately one-third of nonreaders were left-handed.

Orton (1925, 1928), familiar with this hypothesis, believed that reversals in reading letters or words occurred because the brains of dyslexic children were defective in cerebral dominance. He proposed the term strephosymbolia (twisted symbols) as best describing this symptom of dyslexia. The stimuli, he believed, were represented in the right and left hemispheres, and, because of delayed cerebral dominance, the incorrect or mirror image of the word or letter was read (see Fig. 1-1). What many do not realize is that Orton's hypothesis actually related to the interpretation of the visual memory or image of the written symbols. Orton (1925) suggested that "the process of learning to read entails the elision from the focus of attention of the confusing memory image of the non-dominant hemisphere which are in reversed form and order, and the selection of those which are correctly oriented and in correct sequence" (p. 607).

Orton's ideas offered new insights into the possible psychological and neurological processes involved in the reading process as it related to dyslexics. It offered hope to educators because, if a child was delayed in developing cerebral dominance, then it stood to reason that he could be stimulated in achieving developmental maturity necessary for fluent reading. As will be seen in Chapter 8 on remediation, this idea spawned an incredible number of remedial approaches, all varying on the theme that developmental delay existed in the perceptual or organizational system of the brain.

There can be no doubt that Orton's theory, more than any other, has generated by far the greatest number of investigations on laterality and cerebral dominance in reading-disabled children. Some of this literature is reviewed in Chapter 5. Usually, however, the deficits in peripheral (handedness) and central (auditory or visual) measures of cerebral asymmetry reveal that some dyslexic children may be deficit in the establishment of cerebral dominance. Much of the literature, though, suggests that cerebral dominance does not develop even when measured at infancy (Molfese & Molfese, 1979, 1980) or in the early school years (Bryden & Allard, 1981; Hynd & Obrzut, 1977). There also appears to be no neuroanatomical evidence or neurological rationale acceptable to today's theorists as to the notion that mirror images of a stimuli can be projected to the right or nondominant hemisphere (Corballis, 1980).

It would seem that Orton's contribution can best be described as a milepost in the development of a more refined theory as to why children are dyslexic. His views have provided researchers with a theory to evaluate, and, as reviewed in later chapters in this book, our knowledge base today owes much to him and to other early theorists.

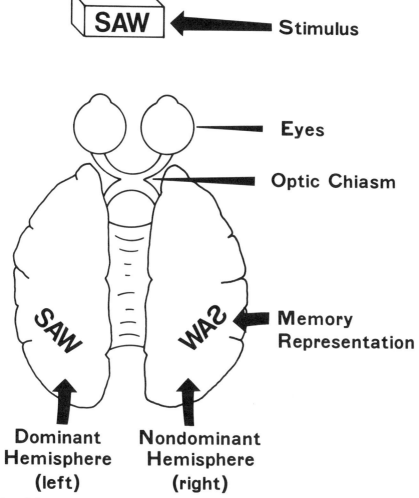

Fig. 1-1. Schematic representation of Orton's theory of perception and storage of visual material. [From Corballis, MC, & Beale, IL. *The psychology of left and right.* Hillsdale, New Jersey: Lawrence Erlbaum Associates, 1976. With permission.]

Recent Advances in Dyslexia Research

Since Orton first introduced his ideas regarding the etiology of dyslexia, the research has headed in four directions. The first, and perhaps the largest group of investigators, sought to evaluate many of the assumptions underlying Orton's theory. These researchers evaluated ideas regarding lateral preferences and cerebral dominance as they related to dyslexia. As had already been suggested, much of the research in this area led to conflicting data, perhaps in large part due to the inclusion of poorly defined clinical populations and inadequate measures of cerebral dominance or asymmetry.

A second large group of researchers focused primarily on psychological processes related to visual and auditory perception in dyslexia (Benton, 1962; Vellutino, 1978; Vellutino, Steger, & Kandel, 1972). The focus of these investigators has been on relating the cognitive processes found deficient in dyslexics to evidence for deficits in basic perceptual abilities. Other investigators in this category have examined deficits in temporal analysis and basic language ability in dyslexic or reading-disabled children who are severely affected (Birch & Belmont, 1964; Zurif & Carson, 1970).

A third group of researchers of major importance to the conceptual framework of this volume have turned their attention toward the identification of dyslexic subtypes. Within each differentially defined subtype of dyslexia are children who may demonstrate deficits in auditory or visual perception, language ability, or cognitive processes (Boder, 1973b; Mattis et al., 1975; Pirozzolo, 1979).

Finally, a last group of researchers have sought to identify specific cortical regions evidencing pathology that may be related to dyslexia. The brain electrical activity mapping (BEAM) techniques of Duffy (1981) and autopsy studies of Galaburda and Kemper (1979) and Galaburda and Eidelberg (1982) have provided us with new insights into the pathology of the brain in dyslexics.

Since these areas of research are the primary focus of this volume, they will not be dealt with here. Suffice it to say, however, that research in the decades since Orton made his studies has taken dramatic new directions, which articulate well the neurological and psychological processes related to dyslexia.

Based on the new directions noted above, it seems likely that computerized brain mapping techniques, as detailed in Chapter 3, will be used in conjunction with neuropsychological assessment procedures to differentially diagnose the various subtypes of dyslexia. Also, the clinical application of measures of brain metabolic activity (^{18}FDG positron emission tomography or regional cerebral blood flow) or even nuclear magnetic resonance imagery of the brain (Oldendorf, 1981) with dyslexics might well provide further insights into the electrical and metabolic factors associated with deficits in the functional system of reading in the brains of dyslexics.

EPIDEMIOLOGY OF DYSLEXIA

Gaddes (1976) noted that, from a medical perspective, epidemiology refers to the study of the distribution, frequency, and causative factors associated with a disease process. In the past several decades, the medical approach to examining diseases has been applied to the more subtle behavioral or psychological disorders. Gaddes suggested that there are a host of problems with applying a medical approach to a behavioral disorder such as dyslexia, since many of the inherent assumptions regarding an epidemiological approach do not necessarily apply.

In fact, of the nine functions of epidemiological studies he lists, only three seem directly applicable to the study of cognitive-behavioral disorders. These include the development of a definition of the disease, specification of the "at risk" population, and articulation of the need for and the focus of preventative programs. Other factors inherent in an epidemiological approach are clearly inappropriate in the study of dyslexia (i.e., calculation of risk factors of infection, study of mortality rates, etc.).

Although some specific behavioral syndromes may be suitable for epidemiological study (e.g., mental retardation) because they have agreed on criteria (e.g., IQ < 70), dyslexia is not as appropriate for study since its definition is variable, depending on the criteria used in defining the population. Gaddes (1976) suggests that it is more appropriate to examine prevalence of learning disorders. While he has an excellent point, there are other factors that need to be discussed in this section; so in a broad sense, we will focus our attention on the factors associated with the occurrence of dyslexia. We will deal with prevalence first, however.

Prevalence Estimates

It has been estimated that between 2 percent and 16 percent of all school-age children are in need of special education services. Estimates vary from country to country. In England, some suggest 14 percent of the students are in need of special services and in Canada between 10 and 16 percent (CELDIC, 1970). In the United States it has been estimated that between 10 and 15 percent should be receiving special services (Myklebust & Boshes, 1969). These figures, of course, include children who could be diagnosed as educable mentally retarded, trainable mentally retarded, emotionally or behaviorally disturbed, and physically handicapped, as well as those children who could be diagnosed as learning disabled or dyslexic.

Clearly, there exists a need to identify those children who might legitimately be diagnosed as dyslexic or at least as developmentally delayed in reading. Yule and Rutter (1976) suggested that the confusion in the literature regarding the nature and prevalence of disabled readers relates to at least one important factor.

They proposed that definitional problems as well as problems associated with estimates of prevalence arise when researchers examine children referred to reading clinics or to a neurologist. There is reason to believe, they proposed, that bias exists in the referral or selection process. While a study of those small and obviously biased populations might be appropriate for developing a working hypothesis of factors associated with severe reading disability, these populations clearly do not provide the source of data that a major epidemiological study would provide.

In the area of reading, only one series of epidemiological studies stands out as exemplary. These investigations were conducted by Yule, Rutter and their co-investigators and are known generally as the Isle of Wight Studies (Rutter, Tizard, & Whitmore, 1970; Yule, 1973). Also, these investigators participated in another significantly large-scale study using inner-city London children (Berger, Yule, & Rutter, 1975). Since a number of important conceptual as well as practical issues are addressed by these investigations, they will be dealt with in some detail.

Isle of Wight Studies

Yule and Rutter were interested in examining the epidemiological factors associated with what they termed "backward readers" and those children who were underachieving in reading, while considering their intellectual level and chronological age. These backward readers were defined as those children who were achieving at the lowest possible level of the distribution of reading abilities, irrespective of ability.

On the Isle of Wight, approximately 3300 children between the ages of 9 and 11 were examined. In addition to tests of general intelligence (nonverbal) and reading achievement, the children received audiometric testing and a neurological examination. The mothers were interviewed regarding their childrens' developmental, social, and behavioral maturation (Rutter, Tizard, et al., 1970; Rutter, Graham, & Yule, 1970).

As Yule and Rutter (1976) point out, the discrepancies between predicted and actual academic attainment should follow a normal distribution. That is to say, a large majority should show little or no discrepancy between actual and predicted achievement. A smaller group should show underachievement or overachievement, based on discrepancies between actual and predicted achievement. The percentage of cases falling into each category should approximate the normal distribution. Defining underachievement in terms of at least two standard errors below traditional achievement levels, these investigators found the rate of severe reading retardation to be greater than expected. The percentage varied above the expected frequency of 2.28 percent. It actually ranged from 3.5 to 6 percent depending on the age level and locale examined. It should be pointed out that the group of backward readers and reading-retarded do not apply to the 32 percent of the children who were diagnostically mixed (Jansky, 1979). Their figures, therefore, are probably very conservative estimates of the prevalence of reading failure. Yule and Rutter (1976) concluded that there are indeed a significant number of children who may be considered specifically as reading-retarded.

It was also of interest to find how the reading-retarded children differed from the backward readers. Not surprisingly, the mean IQ of the reading-retarded group was significantly higher (mean = 102.5) than that of the reading-backward group (mean = 80). Significant differences were also observed between these two groups according to sex, neurological status, motor development, and speech and language abilities. Reading backwardness was found to be associated with neurological disorder, motor delay, and other developmental problems. Reading retardation, on the other hand, seemed to be associated with speech and language problems and had a much higher ratio of male to females (3.3:1).

In addition to validating that a significant number of children were retarded in their development of reading skills despite apparent ability, Yule (1973) found that reading retarded and backward readers had a differential prognosis. Using the Isle of Wight population, Yule (1973) selected 155 backward readers and 86 retarded readers and followed-up four and five years after they had been initially studied. One unfortunate finding that emerged was that if a child was identified at age ten as having a reading problem then the child's academic prognosis was poor. The most significant and intriguing finding to emerge from this study, however, was that the children diagnosed as reading-retarded actually had a poorer academic prognosis than did the backward readers. This finding is despite a significantly higher Full-Scale IQ on The Wechsler Intelligence Scale For Children (WISC) among the reading-retarded children (mean = 98.41; SD = 15.17) as compared with the backward readers (mean = 85.63; SD = 16.15). The reading-retarded children actually made better progress in mathematics than did the backward readers, thus arguing for the highly specific nature of reading retardation (Yule, 1973).

Although Yule and Rutter (1976) argue against the concept of dyslexia, their research stands out as truly important. They document that a significant percentage of school-age children with normal intelligence do, in fact, experience failure in reading attainment.

Factors Associated With Prevalence Estimates

A number of potentially important factors have been identified as possibly contributing to learning and, especially, reading disabilities. These contributing factors include malnutrition (Hallahan & Cruickshank, 1973; Stoch & Smythe, 1968), various emotional problems (Rabinovitch, 1959) such as poor ego development (Kahn, 1963) and psychosexual conflict (Buxbaum, 1964), biochemical disorders (Ross & Ross, 1976), and social-emotional deprivation (Eisenberg, 1966; Walzer & Richmond, 1973).

These factors may produce a condition resembling dyslexia but that does not meet the criteria for primary dyslexia; therefore, most definitions have sought to exclude these potential causative influences in defining the condition (*Federal Register*, 1976; Hammill et al., 1981; Harris & Hodges, 1981). Also, most would agree with the notion that dyslexia is presumed to be of neurologic origin.

Two important aspects of dyslexia that need to be considered in any discussion of prevalence estimators of dyslexia include a possible link to sex and the transmission of this disorder and the possibility that the unique qualities of the language contribute to dyslexia in the general population. Each of these will be considered in some detail.

Effects of Language on Prevalence Estimates

It was proposed by Claiborne (1906) that the unique linguistic characteristics of the English language may contribute greatly to the relatively high incidence of "word amblyopia" in Great Britain. Claiborne suggested that it was the arbitrary pronounciation in English that resulted in difficulties encountered in reading. Children who learned Spanish, Italian, or even German experienced much less difficulty in learning to read since the rules of pronounciation were so regular.

One of the most comprehensive studies to address this concept was conducted by a Japanese investigator (Makita, 1968). Previous to his investigation, only three reports of congenital word blindness in Japanese children had appeared. Makita investigated the incidence of reading disability in Japanese children. He sought to include cases of general reading failure as well as cases of congenital word blindness. He sampled both public and private primary schools in metropolitan Tokyo, resulting in a total population of 9195 students. A 13-item questionnaire was completed by 247 teachers regarding the children in their classes. Based on the results of this survey technique, in which the children were not actually examined, an overall incidence rate of 0.98 percent was obtained.

This rate of reading failure is six to ten times lower than that reported in Western Europe or the United States. As Makita (1968) points out, it is absurd to speculate that maldevelopment of cortical areas important to reading is ten times higher in Western cultures. Also, it is equally inappropriate to think that the brains of Japanese children are organized differently. He proposed that the lowered incidence rate for reading disability may be due to varieties of script used by Japanese.

Japanese script consists of two series of *Kana* script (*Hiragana* and *Katakana*), each consisting of 48 phonetic letters. It also has many ideographs that are called *Kanji* script. Instruction in school begins with the *Kana* script, which is similar to our phonetic system. Unlike English, however, the Japanese phonetic system is constant in usage. Consequently, once the child learns the sounds associated with each *Kana* script or the idea represented by the *Kanji* script, reading becomes an automatic process unencumbered by the ambiguities associated with reading English. Makita (1968) concluded that "theories which ascribe the etiology of reading disability to localized cerebral abnormalities, to laterality conflict, or to emotional pressure may be valid for some instances, but the specificity of the used language . . . is the most potent contributing factor in the formation of reading disability" (p. 613).

There can be no doubt that Makita (1968) has provided some interesting data on the incidence of reading disability in Japanese children and may have even suggested some very basic reasons for his unique findings. His research, however, while offering support to Claiborne's (1906) original idea (which he did not reference), must be faulted and his results considered as only tenuous support for the philological explanation of severe reading disabilities.

First, unlike the Isle of Wight Studies, no actual assessment of the children involved was done. It is impossible, therefore, to state with any certainty that his study represents actual figures of severe reading disability. What the results do indicate is that teacher attitudes regarding the incidence of severe reading disability suggest that the actual rate may be low. What one does not know is how valid the teachers' estimates are. While the argument that it is the unique characteristic of the language that produces reading disorders is an interesting one, the data are only suggestive and the topic in general deserves further study.

Sex and Inheritance of Dyslexia

The fact that more boys seemed to suffer dyslexia was noted early by researchers (Fisher, 1905; Hinshelwood, 1900; Stephenson, 1907; Thomas, 1905). The possibility that dyslexia could be inherited was not, however, the focus of most research despite the fact that any sex link in incidence rates would certainly suggest a link in possible mechanisms of transmission of the disorder. It was not until the 1950s that geneticists took a particular interest in dyslexia and its possible mode of transmission.

Three decades ago it was suggested by Hallgren (1950), the Swedish geneticist, that a single autosomal dominant gene was implicated in the transmission of developmental dyslexia. Sladen (1970) notes that Hallgren (1950) dismissed the idea of the differential effects of genetic transmission and suggested that parents of males worried more about academic performance than if they had a female child experiencing reading problems. He suggested that this factor alone would account for the higher number of males showing up in clinic populations.

There is no doubt that at the time of Hallgren's writing more males were showing up in clinics. Critchley and Critchley (1978) cite evidence for the year 1945 that showed that a total of 1633 children were identified as dyslexic. Of that number 1367 were boys and 266 were girls, giving a sex ratio of 5.1:1. Sladen (1970) reviews Hallgren's (1950) data and, based on

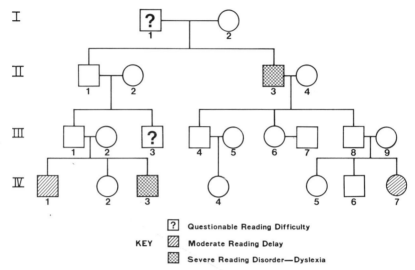

Fig. 1-2. Common family history for severe reading disability.

her own research, concludes that dyslexia is probably a dominant mode of transmission in males while it remains recessive in females (Fig. 1-2).

Going considerably beyond her data, Sladen (1970) proposed that the high male to female ratio may be due to less-than-random mate selection. She also suggested that dyslexia might be considered an example of "genetic polymorphism," which at one time represented optimal survival value (Ford, 1940, 1964). She argued that it is only recently that dyslexia has been identified. This, of course, is due to substantial increase in the worldwide literacy rate. Prior to the demands placed on today's school children in the area of language and reading, the dyslexic would not have been at a disadvantage. She goes even further in proposing that "creative flexibility" and superior "pathfinding ability," as might be found in the dyslexic child, could have been highly-prized skills during food-gathering or hunting eras. Only in the literate world has the emphasis been shifted from spatial reasoning to linguistic competence. Sladen's ideas make interesting reading but remain clearly speculative.

It does seem that a stronger argument can be made as to why boys outnumber girls in diagnosed cases of developmental dyslexia. Hier (1979) has proposed a somewhat more plausible but, nonetheless, controversial explanation.

Recognizing that boys do outnumber girls, Lovell, Shapton and Warren (1964) examined the incidence rate among boys and girls according to IQ level. They categorized the dyslexic subjects into three groups. The first group had IQs less than 90. Lovell et al. (1964) found an incidence rate of 1.2:1 favoring boys. Their second group had IQs ranging from 90 to 99. Boys were again favored, but a 5:1 ratio was found. The third group had IQs in excess of 100. Among this group, boys outnumbered females 10:1.

As Hier (1979) indicated, there is ample evidence that women tend to excell in verbal tasks while men tend to be superior on spatial problem solving (Guilford, 1967; Maccoby & Jacklin, 1974). This seems to be a consistent finding, and it is widely recognized that girls continue to outpace boys on all verbal-linguistic milestones (Hieronymus & Lindquist, 1974; Moore, 1967; Morely, 1965). Hier also cited evidence to suggest that men tend to be more specialized than women in lateralized cerebral function. While language, therefore, seems to be strongly lateralized to the left hemisphere and spatial abilities to the right in men, women on the same tasks show more bilateral cortical distribution.

Hier (1979) proposed that such unique cerebral organization in males may predestine them to be at greater risk for acquiring dyslexia for two reasons. First, he proposed that the strong lateralization to the left hemisphere that men show for language dominance may limit them in overall language capabilities. He recognized that his proposal rests on the "simplistic assumption that two hemispheres are better than one, but it is possible that females derive some benefit from synergistic functioning of both hemispheres in verbal processing that is unavailable to males who depend more fully on the left hemisphere" (p. 78).

His second notion as to why males appear more frequently in groups of dyslexic children relates also to the strong lateralization that males show for verbal abilities. Any one-sided damage to the left hemisphere would obviously affect (under this conceptualization) language more in males than in females, who are more bilaterally organized for linguistic function. Also, he postulated that the strong spatial abilities found in males may inhibit compensation for language abilities affected by left-sided damage. As will be seen in a later section in Chapter 3, Hier did propose that these factors interact with observed cerebral asymmetries as demonstrated on brain scans.

The point to glean from Hier's perspective, however, is that the apparent sex-related link to dyslexia may have more to do with normally predisposed factors related to functional cerebral asymmetry than with any other factor. This is a uniquely different perspective, and, although much of the definitive evidence is lacking, it is based on contemporary research and is an intriguing hypothesis well worth additional research.

While some tempting research exists other than that of Hallgren (1950) and Sladen (1970) on the genetic mode of transmission, no genetic model has yet to gain popularity (Lewitter, DeFries, & Elston, 1980). Decker and DeFries (1981) suggested that this is because dyslexia is now recognized as a heterogeneous disorder, not as the unitary disorder once typically believed. They suggested that subtypes of dyslexia need to be examined from a genetic standpoint if a truly viable model can be articulated.

As part of the Colorado Family Reading Study, 125 reading-disabled children were evaluated by Decker and DeFries (1981) along with their parents and siblings. A matched control group of 125 children and their families were also used, for a total of 1044 subjects. All of the subjects received an extensive battery of tests. Factor analysis of the data on the performance of the reading-disabled children revealed four groups of dyslexics, equivalent to most other studies examining dyslexic subtypes.

Affected parents and siblings of the probands were classified into the subtypes based on their test performance. Forty-one percent of all family members could be classified into one or another subtype. Of special interest, however, it was only the third subtype, characterized by deficits in linguistic processing with strengths on coding/speeded tasks as well as spatial/reasoning tasks, in which a statistically significant number of siblings was found that could be similarly classified. Parents could not be classified into the same dyslexic subtypes as could the proband's siblings.

As Decker and DeFries (1981) note, "The sibling results should be viewed as merely suggestive" (p. 225). The importance of this particular study, however, is that it was the first to examine genetic transmission on such a large scale with well-identified subgroups of dyslexic children.

Based on the often conflicting views regarding the prevalence of severe reading disability or dyslexia, what can one really say about the incidence of this disorder in the general population? Obviously, any estimate of dyslexia will be affected by the criteria employed, the sampling procedures used, by whether or not the children under study are actually assessed for obtained levels of reading skill, by the sex of the subjects, and, quite possibly, by the psycholinguistic characteristics of their native language.

As noted, a variety of studies indicate that it is reasonable to conclude that 10 to 16 percent of the total school population are in need of special education services (e.g., Berger et al., 1975; Kirk, 1972; Mackie, 1969; Myklebust & Boshes, 1969; Rutter Tizard et al., 1970, Yule, 1973). Of this number, and on the basis of large-scale investigations of the population of school-age children, it would be conservative to estimate that the percentage of children who could be classified as dyslexic ranges from a minimum of 3 percent to a maximum of 6 percent. Although it might seem as though this is a small percentage of children on whom to focus our attention, it should be pointed out that this number probably exceeds the combined frequency of children suffering cerebral palsy, epilepsy, and severe mental retardation (Duane, 1979). Practically speaking, this translates into an expected frequency of approximately 15 to 30 dyslexic children per 500 school children.

CONCLUSIONS

The actual concept of dyslexia was first formulated just over 100 years ago. Despite a long-standing history of research during this period by educators, physicians, and psychologists, considerable controversy, however, surrounds the use of the term dyslexia. Early medical views regarding congenital word blindness and the hypothesized neurodevelopmental anomalies associated with dyslexia gave way to investigations focusing on psychological processes and electrophysiological properties of dyslexia. Although debate still exists, the following conclusions seem warranted.

Considerable resistance exists in accepting the very notion that dyslexia is a diagnosable condition or even an appropriate term should the malady exist. The historical antecedents of this resistance may relate to a rejection of the very idea that severe reading disabilities are related to neurodevelopmental factors, and distaste for the application of labels in general. Furthermore, many critics would argue that since neurological knowledge has no immediate practical benefit, it is, therefore, a useless exercise to relate the reading process to cortical functions.

Recent efforts at defining dyslexia have been more productive than past attempts since most well-conceptualized definitions now take into account that dyslexia results from neurodevelopmental factors, dyslexia occurs in children who have adequate or better mental ability, and dyslexic children have a severe reading disability that is not attributable to secondary causes.

The early medical literature concerned primarily with congenital word blindness led to basic understanding as to how brain deficits could be associated with processes important in reading. While some of the speculation was inaccurate, recent research is substantiating many basic neurological concepts regarding the nature of dyslexia.

The conceptualization provided by Orton is now accepted as inaccurate. The importance of his formulation was probably that it gave hope of instructional success with dyslexic children to frustrated educators and provided a springboard for further research into neurological factors associated with severe reading failure.

Concern exists as to the incidence of dyslexia in the general population. Also, such factors as sex, heredity, and the psycholinguistic characteristics of the child's native language may interact with neurological and psychological development. Consequently, incidence rates and estimates as to the prevalence of dyslexia will naturally vary as a function of these important factors. It does seem, however, that the incidence rate in the United States is probably between 3 to 6 percent of the school-age population.

Chapter 2

Functional Organization of the Brain: An Overview

Considering the growing literature from the fields of neurology, neuropsychology, neurochemistry, and the allied medical and psychological sciences regarding the interactive relationship between brain function and its behavioral correlates during reading, it is remarkable how few practicing psychologists or reading specialists can be considered up-to-date in their familiarity with this literature. The objections to the medical model discussed in Chapter 1 have undoubtedly contributed somewhat to this ignorance. It is reasonable to assume, however, that a significant majority of clinical or school psychologists or remedial-reading teachers simply do not have access to much of the literature describing the advances made in our understanding of brain-behavior relationships in dyslexic children. Furthermore, many practicing psychologists may have had either an inadequate background in the physiological basis of behavior through their professional preparation (Hynd, Quackenbush & Obrzut, 1980) or the relevant coursework may have been undertaken in the distant and dim past, and much knowledge may have been forgotten. Among remedial-reading specialists, the situation is probably more grim, as it is highly likely that a significant majority of these professionals have never had a course in which the neurophysiology of brain-behavior relationships was discussed.

It is a disheartening situation that these professionals are either unaware of the recent developments in our conceptualization of dyslexia, based on the neurological literature, or are unable to comprehend it, should it be available because of a different emphasis in training. For example, if a child

26

with neurological deficits should be diagnosed as a developmental dyslexic by some well-intentioned psychologist, and so, staffed for remedial efforts based on building up his areas of deficits, then the intervention strategy probably has a poor potential for success despite appealing remedial approaches based on this notion (Valett, 1980).

If the basis for the dyslexic condition is one of neurological damage, the intervention should center on capitalizing on available strengths, not on teaching to cognitive abilities resistant to the effects of enrichment. A psychologist or remedial specialist trained in brain-behavior relationships and possessing good clinical neuropsychological assessment skills can be expected to differentiate between neurological deficit and developmental delay in diagnosing dyslexia. They will thus be able to actualize the potential for successful intervention based on their familiarity with neuropsychological research and practice.

Since the remainder of this volume concentrates on a neuropsychological model of dyslexia and since so many interested professionals may have had inadequate or dated training in physiological psychology or functional neuroanatomy, the present chapter was included. The goal of this chapter is to cover, in basic terms, enough functional neurology so that the reader is sufficiently prepared to profit from the literature discussed in following chapters. This is especially critical in comprehending the electrophysiological and cytoarchitectonic research presented in Chapter 3. Clinical neuropsychologists or those usually familiar with the principles of brain-behavior relationships may find the following presentation not relevant to their objectives in reading this book. For these readers it might be most appropriate to skip directly to Chapter 3. For those who feel, however, that they would profit from an overview of the functional organization of the brain so that their comprehension of the following chapters is enhanced, this chapter will be of great relevance.*

A LITTLE HISTORY

Certainly one of the most persistent issues that has confronted philosophers since the beginning of time is how to define the mind. In fact, it

---

*It is recognized by the authors that one of the most difficult tasks in learning anything new is becoming familiar with the terminology. For this reason we have provided a glossary of terms at the end of the book. To facilitate the comprehension of the following text, however, the definitions for the terms used most frequently in this chapter are provided in this footnote. *Anterior*, toward the front. *Contralateral*, on the opposite side. *Fissure*, deep fold between two gyri. *Gyri*, raised cortical area or convolution. *Inferior*, below some point of reference. *Lesion*, any tissue that has been damaged or is abnormal due to developmental, congenital, infectious, or other causes. *Posterior*, toward the rear. *Sulci*, usually conceived of as a less pronounced fissure. *Superior*, above some point of reference.

was the conceptualization of mind or soul that forms one of the most basic differences between two of the greatest philosophers of Ancient Greece, Plato and Aristotle. Plato, one of Socrates' students, spoke eloquently of the immortality and preexistence of the soul. Aristotle, on the other hand, thought that like the body, the mind of man perished with death (Stumpf, 1966). In the fifth century BC, Hippocrates of Croton proposed the notion that the brain was the seat of man's intellect, whereas the heart housed the senses. The functional differentiation of cognitive processes was carried a step further approximately 200 years later by Herophilus. He agreed with Hippocrates as to the brain being the seat of intellect and advanced the notion that the middle ventricle housed cognitions while memory was the responsibility of the posterior ventricle. A further refinement in the attempt of early philosophers and scientists to differentiate the functional organization of the brain was made by Galen in the second century BC. Directing critical thought away from the ventricular system, he proposed that cognition occurred in the cortical and subcortical areas of the brain. It was not until some 1800 years later that the brilliant anatomical work of Vesalius confirmed Galen's notions, and that the idea that cognition was the result of cortical and subcortical activity was accepted by the scientific community (Heilman & Valenstein, 1979).

The past three centuries have unquestionably been the most exciting ones in the history of mankind in terms of the explosion of knowledge based on scientific inquiry. Due to the establishment of the medical sciences and their associated clinical and experimental practices, more facts have been generated regarding brain-behavior relationships in the past 100 years than in all of previous history. The foundation for this leap forward in our understanding of the brain and its behavioral correlates can, in large part, be attributed to Gall. After the philosophers had decided that man's intellect was housed in the brain, it remained for individuals such as Gall to suggest differential localization of function. Noting that his brightest and most verbally productive students often had protruding eyes, Gall hypothesized that this was due to the enhanced development of the frontal lobes (Pirozzolo, 1978). Consequently, the area of the brain that was responsible for speech and language functions must, he believed, be found in the cortical mantle of the frontal lobes. Correctly, Gall also suggested that life-sustaining mechanisms must reside in the brain stem, whereas intellectual or cognitive functions were the result of neural activity in the two cerebral hemispheres.

Regrettably, Gall became involved in advancing the notion that discrete variations in skull size could reveal underlying cognitive and moral development. This notion, of course, was based on the idea that protuberances on the skull directly revealed those areas of the brain that were advanced in neural development. It is indeed unfortunate that Gall became so enamored with this hypothesis, since the discredit it brought to all of his work was enormous and clouded the importance of his earlier contributions. Truly worthwhile advances in science seem to endure, however, and, as Heilman and Valenstein (1979) note, his writings and teachings form the foundation for modern neuropsychology.

Contributions by Broca and Wernicke

A proponent of Gall's ideas on functional localization, Jean Baptiste Bouillaud published evidence that suggested that discrete lesions could result in limb paralysis. As Dean of the Medical Faculty in Paris, Bouillaud had considerable influence. Most appropriately perhaps, this influence was greatest on his son-in-law, Ernest Auburtin. In 1861 Auburtin presented an address to the Paris Society of Anthropology arguing Gall's hypothesis and presenting several case studies that suggested that the anterior lobes of the brain were responsible for speech. Pierre Paul Broca attended Auburtin's presentation and asked him to visit with a patient of his who suffered speech arrest coupled with a right-sided paralysis. After Laborgne (called "Tan Tan" because *tan* was the only syllable he could utter) died, Broca examined his brain and found a lesion involving the first temporal gyrus, the insula, the corpus striatum, and parts of the inferior transverse convolution. These findings correlated well with Gall's hypothesis. Later that same year Broca saw a similar patient who could also comprehend speech (as did Laborgne) but who failed to perform in speech or in writing. At postmortem a lesion was observed in the same site as in his first case. History tells us that Broca eventually saw eight such patients who also could not speak and who suffered left-frontal lesions. He termed this loss of speech aphemia (later termed aphasia by Trousseau) and his contribution to neuropsychology is probably unparalleled as he provided the first clear-cut clinical evidence regarding the localization of cerebral function.

As any student of the vast aphasia literature knows, Broca's (1861) publication threw his colleagues into a state of chaos. Some questioned Broca's interpretation of the symptoms of his patients and even questioned whether his patients had the mental capacity required for speech prior to their stroke (Pirozzolo, 1979). Others, best exemplified by Pierre Marie (1906), suggested that the site of the lesions described by Broca were not as localized as he presented in the clinical data. While these antilocalizationists continued to advance the notion of "mass action" or equipotentiality, as being responsible for behavior, important new developments in the localization of cerebral function were soon to be reported. For instance, in 1869 Bastian provided his contribution to the localization literature by suggesting that some of his patients not only were aphasic but also that others had lost the ability to name common objects in their environment (anomia). He further postulated functional cortical centers for visual, auditory, kinesthetic, and tongue functions.

Perhaps the most significant contribution following that of Broca's, however, was made by Wernicke, a 26-year-old who published his doctoral dissertation, "Der Apasische Symptomenkomplex" (1874). Based on Meynert's (1867) hypothesis that sensory nerves traveled to posterior brain regions and that the anterior portion of the brain was responsible for all movement, Wernicke demonstrated that damage to the posterior region of the temporal lobe resulted in comprehension deficits. He believed that this area of the brain was responsible for auditory images as compared with Broca's area, which was preprogrammed for motor images. Furthermore, he hypothesized that the area for auditory images was connected to Broca's area by a neural commissure that could be disconnected from either cortical area by a lesion. These correct and important ideas were further elaborated on by Lichtheim (1885) and Charcot (1889). These notions will be further discussed in Chapter 3 as they relate to reading and dyslexia.

Other Contributions to the Localizationist Theory

While it is popular to think of the localizationist literature in terms of its contributions to our knowledge of language and the process of reading, considerable progress was also made during the late 1800s in understanding the function of the minor cerebral hemisphere. Jackson's (1874) contribution is a good case in point. He was in reality not a localizationist as Broca and Wernicke can be considered. He believed that the brain was organized hierarchically and that brain disease essentially reversed the evolutionary process, allowing more primitive neurological systems to take command (Filskov, Grimm, & Lewis, 1981). Nonetheless, in 1874, Jackson hypothesized that the function of the left hemisphere was to automatically revive images, and that of the right hemisphere was for voluntary image recall and recognition.

In 1876, Jackson reported a case study in support of his notions. A woman with a right-sided cerebral tumor experienced a great deal of difficulty in naming objects presented to her by Jackson. Based on this evidence Jackson (1876) suggested the following, which is presented here as quoted by Joynt and Goldstein in 1975.

> The posterior lobes are the seat of the most intellectual processes. This is in effect saying that they are the seat of visual ideation, for most of our mental operations are carried on in visual ideas. I think too that the right posterior lobe is the 'leading' side, the left the more automatic. This is analogous to the difference I make as regards use of words, the right is the automatic side for words, and the left the side for that use of words which is speech. (Joynt & Goldstein, 1975, p. 148)

Other clinical reports by Pick (1898) and Babinski (1914) added to our knowledge of right-hemispheric functions, in that patients with lesions in the right hemisphere typically seem unaware or unconcerned with the impairment of function. Also, Jackson (1876) demonstrated that patients with right-sided lesions often had great difficulty in dressing themselves correctly (dressing apraxia).

Controversy Becomes Paramount

The heyday of the localizationists continued through World War I, which provided an unparalleled opportunity to study the localized effects of discrete brain insult. Gestalt psychologists became the moving force after the discrediting of Gall and his advocacy of phrenology. Those who contributed greatly to our knowledge of localized brain function (Bastian, 1898; Broca, 1861; Charcot, 1889; Dejerine, 1914; Henschen, 1922; Lichtheim, 1885; Wernicke, 1874) were actively challenged by the proponents of wholistic or equipotential views of brain function. These proponents are best represented through the writings of Head (1926), Isserlin (1929, 1931, 1932) and Wilson (1926). It was the American, Lashley (1938), however, who provided the most compelling evidence against the localizationist arguments. His widely circulated research suggested that the site of a lesion was not so important in functional loss as was the mass of brain tissue involved in the lesion. These ideas, which were based on experiments with animals as opposed to the clinical reports of neurologists of the times, held much credence with the scientific community (Heilman & Valenstein, 1979). Based on Lashley's evidence, the arguments of the mass actionists (Conrad, 1948; Goldstein, 1948; Leischner, 1957; Weisenburg & McBride, 1964) gained much popularity.

Heilman and Valenstein (1979) suggest that a reawakening of the localizationist theory, which has returned to acceptability, is probably due to a number of developments. These developments include that neurologists continued to publish verifiable clinical findings; new and useful electronic experimental methods were devised to study brain-behavior relationships (e.g., electrostimulation, electroencephalograph, dichotic listening and visual half-field paradigms, Wada technique, etc.); anatomical and pathological studies were refined and new techniques and methods enhanced our ability to comprehend functional anatomical organization; and, new clinical discoveries allowed for not only the study of brain-behavior relationships but also behavioral-chemical relationships. Certainly, the experimental and clinical work of Halstead (1947), Reitan (1955, 1956, 1958), Penfield (1959), Geschwind (1962, 1970, 1974a), and Sperry (1964, 1973) must be considered as preeminent in contributing to the factors stimulating the resurgence in interest in the localizationist theory. In fact, the evidence in favor of this conceptualization of brain function has led Luria (1970), long considered an advocate of the mass actionist position, to conclude that *individ-*

ually distinct cortical zones work together to effect each type of mental process; and, each process, or activity, has a unique and distinguishable psychological structure.

While it is tempting to accept the localizationist conceptualization completely, it should be stressed that like all positions in search of scientific truth, the most reasonable approach lies somewhere in between the two extremes. As will be seen in the following sections, many areas of the brain subserve discrete functions. As will be demonstrated in Chapter 3, however, any complex cognitive task, such as reading, or even more simple motor actions, such as catching a ball, require the coordinated interaction of many cortical as well as subcortical structures.

As indicated in the introduction to this chapter, the following overview of functional brain organization is offered so that the material presented in Chapter 3 can be more easily comprehended within a solid framework.

NEUROLOGICAL DEVELOPMENT

Neural differentiation begins at the end of the second week of gestation. Cells at the end of the neural tube in the human embryo begin to accumulate, thus forming the basis for the development of the central nervous system. By the end of the 20th day, two regions can be seen on examining the neural tube. At one end is a tubule that eventually becomes the spinal cord. At the other end is a broader area that eventually develops into the brain. The entire central nervous system thus develops out of the neural tube (the spinal cord, medulla, and pons; the midbrain; and the diencephalon and telencephalon). By ten weeks the telencephalon becomes differentiated and begins its development, eventually leading to its final form, the frontal lobes. Nine weeks later the most prominent sulci appear (Sylvian), and at full-term most of the sulci and gyri are visible to the naked eye (Jacobson, 1972).

At birth the human brain weighs approximately 300–400 g, reaching almost 1000 g by the end of the first year. When fully developed, the brain will weigh approximately 1500 g. It is interesting to note that at birth the human brain is only 40 percent of its eventual adult size whereas in the ape it is nearly 70 percent of its eventual size (Geschwind, 1974a). Some theorists have even gone so far as to suggest that the relative weight of the brain corresponds to intellectual level (Witherspoon, 1960); others have proposed equations to determine this hypothesized relationship (Jerison, 1961).

The "Neurone Doctrone"

Prior to the mid 1800s, many thought that the nervous system operated much like the vascular system, through which electricity or a fluid of some sort flowed. Gardner (1975) notes that even though the cell theory was proposed decades earlier, it was extraordinarily difficult to demonstrate the existence or structure of the neuron. It was finally accomplished, however, by Otto Frederick Karl Deiters (1834–1863), who isolated single cells in hardened brain tissue. His discovery was confirmed and supported by Ramón y Cajal (1852–1934), perhaps the most important of all neuroanatomists. It was Cajal, for instance, who demonstrated the physical properties of neurons, their relationship to other neurons, and the existence of synaptic junctures. It was Waldeyer (1836–1921) who proposed the "neurone doctrone" in which systems were thought to be made up of many nerve cells. He also proposed that nervous impulses were conducted from one cell to another. Although some resisted the ideas of Waldeyer through the 1930s, the notion that the brain and the nervous system are made up of billions of neurons is fully supported by the literature. Not only have the neurons been photographed but they have also been, in some cases, individually recorded as to their contribution to various functional systems (Fuster & Jervey, 1981).

There are an estimated 5 to 25 billion neurons comprising the central nervous system (Jacobson, 1972; Sholl, 1956). While there may be more neurons in larger mammals, they are placed further apart and the proportion of small to large neurons is smaller. While the number of nerve cells may seem astronomic, approximately equal to the number of stars in our galaxy (Filskov et al., 1981), this number is small indeed in comparison to the number of interconnections among these neurons!

Neurons differ considerably in size. Some neurons are 50–100 μm (1 micron = 1/1000 mm) across and are almost visible to the eye. They also may have an axon nearly a meter in length. Most neurons, however, are very small, perhaps 4–5 μm in diameter. The body (soma) of a neuron is distinctly different from other cells in the body in that we are born with the total number allotted us, they cannot repair themselves, and they possess dendrites and axons (Gardner, 1975) (Fig. 2-1).

The neuron consists of the cell body, the dendrites, and the axon. The dendrites are typically covered with synaptic knobs of afferent neurons. The axon conducts impulses away from the neuron to the dendrites of another neuron. The axon may be myelinated by what are sometimes known as satellite cells called neurilemma. These cells coat the axon with a fatty material called myelin. The velocity of the neural impulse is accelerated as it passes through a myelinated axon. Myelin thus acts to ensure not only the integrity of the neural circuitry but also acts to facilitate efficient transmission of neural impulses to the synaptic junction. As will be discussed in a later section in Chapter 3, malnutrition, environmental variables, and a host of other factors can impede the process of myelinization and may very well result in disorders in cognitive functioning, as are often found in dyslexia.

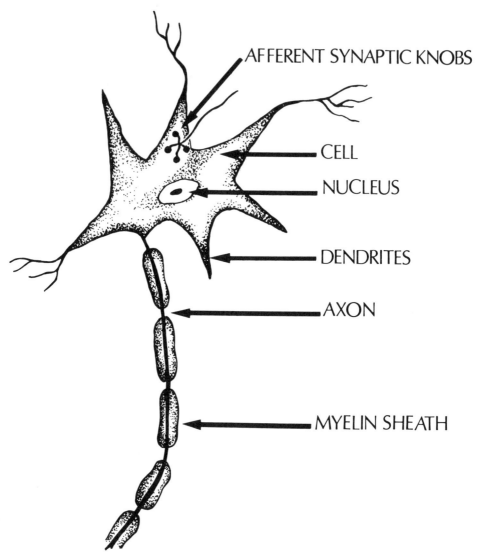

AFFERENT SYNAPTIC KNOBS

CELL

NUCLEUS

DENDRITES

AXON

MYELIN SHEATH

Fig. 2-1.   Schematic representation of a typical neuron.

Based on the notion that function does seem to be localized in various areas of the brain and that all cortical and subcortical areas are primarily comprised of neurons that allow for the "circuitry" of cognition, it is appropriate to briefly examine subcortical and cortical areas that may impact on the reading process. It should be kept in mind that while these various brain regions are discussed in isolation, in reality they function as an integrated whole. While this will become more apparent when the neuropsychology of reading is discussed in the following chapter, it nonetheless should be kept in mind. For the sake of organization, the following discussion will first focus broadly on the brain stem and cerebellum and then on the cerebral cortex.

THE BRAIN STEM AND CEREBELLUM

While some may question why a book on the neuropsychology of dyslexia offers a discussion of the brain stem and cerebellum, such structures have special relevance to any cognitive task and need to be considered if a complete picture of brain-behavior relationships is to be developed (Hynd, 1981; Sandoval & Haapanen, 1981). In fact, there are those who argue that one of the underlying causes in disorders of learning, including dyslexia, is related to subtle neurological deficits in the brain stem region (Dykman, Wallis, Suzuki, Ackerman, & Peters, 1971).

For the purposes of our discussion, the following will focus on three important neuroanatomic subdivisions: the hindbrain, the midbrain, and the forebrain. The reader should refer to Figure 2-2 so that the relationships among these various structures can be understood.

The Hindbrain

Consisting of the lowest clearly identifiable part of the brain, the hindbrain is one of the oldest and most simply organized neural structures. The medulla or bulb, reticular activating system (RAS), and pons are usually associated with the hindbrain.

The medulla is the lowest section of the hindbrain and, with the pons, is responsible for life-maintenance functions. Respiration, maintenance of blood pressure, and regulation of heartbeat are coordinated through the medulla. Neural decussation also occurs at the medulla level. This refers to the crossover of neural tracts and explains why most sensory and motor functions are coordinated by the contralateral (opposite side) cerebral cortex. Needless to say, significant injury to the medulla usually results in death.

Running through the bulb to the diencephalon (including the thalamus and hypothalamus) is the RAS, which in reality is not a single functional unit. Actually, the RAS consists of many nerve centers or nuclei, which are clusters of functionally related cells. These nuclei mediate postural reflexes, the smoothness of muscle activity, and help to maintain muscle tone. The primary function of the RAS, however, is to contribute to wakefulness and to maintain alerting mechanisms. Electrostimulation of the cerebral cor-

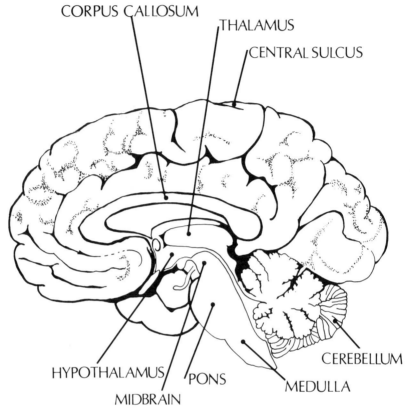

CORPUS CALLOSUM
THALAMUS
CENTRAL SULCUS

CEREBELLUM
HYPOTHALAMUS
PONS
MEDULLA
MIDBRAIN

Fig. 2-2. Diagram showing sectioned brain in the median plane so that brain stem and associated structures are visible.

tex in anesthetized patients will not wake them up (French, 1966). Clearly, activation from the RAS is needed for arousal. It seems, furthermore, that in the absence of the functioning cerebral cortex (e.g., in a newborn baby with a poorly developed cerebral cortex), the RAS coordinates wakefulness so that feeding can occur. This phenomena is also demonstrated in anencephalic babies (children who are literally born without a cerebral cortex but who do possess a brain stem). If these babies survive for any length of time, they can feed, can seem conscious, and may even smile or coo even though such behavior is often inappropriate.

Since disorders in RAS functioning may well result in drowsiness, inattention, hyperactivity, and stupor or coma, it seems theoretically reasonable that neurological deficits in this brain stem region may result in learning deficits. In fact, Dykman and his colleagues (1970, 1971) have proposed just such a theory. A brief review of their proposal is that hyperactive and distractible tendencies noted in dyslexic children may be attributable to damage to this area of the brain stem. Based on Luria's (1980) formulations of the brain, it can also be hypothesized that the reason these attention deficits or hyperactive behaviors disappear during adolescence is that the rapidly developing frontal lobes are finally exerting control over the dysfunctional RAS. Consequently, the distractibility appears to disappear (Golden, 1981). The effects of stimulant medication are also thought to exert effects on the nuclei in the RAS.

Since the pons and cerebellum form an integral functional unit they will be considered together. These two structures work in concert and manifest nearly absolute control over posture, muscle-movement sense (kinesthetic functions), and refined motor movements. The pons contains neural pathways transversing between the cerebral cortex and the cerebellum. The cerebellum consists of three clearly identifiable zones and include the archicerebellum, paleocerebellum, and the neocerebellum. The oldest part of the cerebellum, the archicerebellum, is important in keeping the child spatially oriented. Deficits to this important part of the cerebellum can result in staggering and swaying when walking. The second oldest area of the cerebellum, the paleocerebellum, is responsible for what might be termed "antigravity" posturing. That is to say, this area of the cerebellum is important in keeping us upright, keeping us in our seats, and keeping us from falling over. Finally, the neocerebellum is considered the youngest portion of the cerebellum and acts as a central computer that refines and controls, or regulates, volitional motor movements so that they are coordinated and appropriate for the intended movement (Chusid, 1970).

It is probably incorrect to attribute all the motor deficits occasionally seen in dyslexic children to cerebellum dysfunction. As Hughlings Jackson suggested, "It will not suffice . . . to speak of co-ordination as a separate faculty. Co-ordination is a function of the whole and every part of the nervous system" (quoted by DeMyer, 1974, p. 237). There are, however, four prominent clinical signs that the knowledgeable clinician should be alert to note while examining for a possible neurological basis to dyslexia. These four clinical signs of cerebellar dysfunction include dystaxia (considered to be an incoordination of volitional movements), dysarthria (slurred speech), nystagmus (jerky eye movements), and hypotonia (a floppiness of the extremities); (DeMyer, 1974). More will be said in a following chapter about neurological signs that may be associated with the neuropsychological examination of the dyslexic child.

The Midbrain

The midbrain is forward of the hindbrain and structurally incorporating the area between the thalamus and pons. The major portion of the RAS

Table 2-1
The Cranial Nerves, Their Names, and Their
Related Function

Cranial Nerve Number	Name	Related Function
I	Olfactory	Smell
II	Optic	Vision
III	Oculomotor	Movement of eyes
IV	Trochlear	Movement of eyes
V	Trigeminal	Facial sensory & mastication
VI	Abducens	Movement of eyes
VII	Facial	Facial expression & taste
VIII	Acoustic—vestibular	Audition & balance
IX	Glossopharyngeal	Swallowing & taste
X	Vagus	Reflexes of viscera
XI	Accessory	Movement of head
XII	Hypoglossal	Movement of tongue

For a complete discussion of the cranial nerves and associated disorders the reader is referred to Sears, ES, & Franklin, GM. Diseases of the cranial nerves. In Rosenberg, RN. (Ed.): *Neurology*. New York: Grune & Stratton, 1980.

is situated in the midbrain area, as also are most of the cranial nerves. Reflexes such as the blink, startle, and gag reflexes owe their origins to nuclei in the midbrain region. Neurological dysfunction may result in certain types of tremor and rigidity, as well as in extraneous movements of local muscle groups due to the motor nuclei incorporated in the midbrain region. Table 2-1 notes the cranial nerves associated with the structures of the brain stem region. While the psychologist or remedial-reading specialist need not commit these nerves to memory, they are important and the cranial nerves should be evaluated for possible dysfunction in any dyslexic child referred for a neurological examination. Damage to these nerves, many of which could very well be related to the reading process, will be manifested on tests of motor or cognitive performance.

The Forebrain

Conceptually, the forebrain in man can be subdivided into the diencephalon (between brain) and the telencephalon (the cerebrum or end brain). Broadly, the diencephalon is thought to consist of the thalamus and hypothalamus. Ovoid in shape, the thalamus comprises the largest portion of the diencephalon and acts as a way station for all sensory data transmitted to the cerebral cortex. Only smell does not pass to the cortex by way of the thalamus. For this reason, any thalamic lesion can result in sensory impairment. The thalamus also is connected to the limbic system, which controls emotionality to a large extent. Thalamic lesions or dysfunction can result in a number of symptoms including sensory disturbances, impaired intellectual performance (especially as associated with arousal), gross memory loss, and, in extreme instances, a "withering" of speech leading to mutism (Gardner, 1975; Lezak, 1976).

The hypothalamus is somewhat in front of and below the thalamus and acts as a regulating body influencing appetite, sexual arousal, thirst, and so on. Also, behavior patterns, including rage and fear reactions, can be the direct result of lesions in this subcortical area. Other manifestations of dysfunction to the hypothalamus include obesity; disorders of temperature control; changes in libido, or drive state; and subtle disorders in mood.

The most advanced part of the brain results from the furthest extension of the neural tube: the telencephalon, or cerebrum. Most recently evolved, the cerebrum consists of two nearly alike hemispheres. The internal white matter consists largely of three neural fibers. Association fibers transmit impulses between cortical points within a given hemisphere. Commissural fibers, on the other hand, cross through the corpus callosum and transmit neural impulses between the two cerebral hemispheres. Lastly, projection fibers are responsible for the transmission of impulses between the cerebral cortex and the lower neural centers (Lezak, 1976).

The outer convoluted layer is called the cortex and, interestingly, at full term almost 70 percent of the cortical surface is hidden from view and lies deep within the sulci (Jacobson, 1972). Nature and its handmaiden seem to have a purpose for everything and the wrinkled appearance of the cerebral cortex is no exception. It appears that the primary reason the cerebral cortex is so wrinkled is to gain precious surface area in the limited allotment of space provided by the skull. It has been estimated that if the brain were not so convoluted then we would have a brain the size of a basketball in order to obtain equal surface area (Gaddes, 1980)!

Children with dyslexia probably have a dysfunction at the cortical level. In fact, when we consider the cytoarchitectonic studies reported in Chapter 3, we will find that both of the postmortem case studies reported involving dyslexic subjects revealed cortical abnormalities. The electrophysiological investigation, furthermore, provide supportive data to the notion that cortical abnormalities are responsible for dyslexia. For these reasons, the functional organization of the cerebral cortex will be considered in significantly more detail.

THE FUNCTIONAL ORGANIZATION OF THE
CEREBRAL CORTEX

On gross inspection it would appear to the casual observer that the two cerebral hemispheres were symmetrical. Closer inspection, however, would reveal that in most brains the left cerebral hemisphere is somewhat larger than the right. As our brief review of neurological history has demonstrated, the localization of function has produced considerable knowledge regarding which areas of the cerebral cortex typically subserve various sensory, motor, and cognitive abilities. The early localizationists attempted to develop cytoarchitectonic maps in which all known abilities were subserved by specified areas of the cortex. This notion, of course, while exceptionally appealing to those who would like an ordered universe, is usually without foundation. While there seem to be a number of generalizations we can make about the cerebral cortex and its behavioral correlates, there is a significant degree of individual variation in its organization (Whitaker, 1981). In fact, there are in reality only two ways in which we can know for sure what specific functions are subserved by any given cortical area. The first way is to observe the effects of electrostimulation during a craniotomy. The second way is to observe the resulting behavior of an individual who is known to be functioning without a given cortical area as a result of some known brain lesion.

Over the last 100 years enough evidence has accumulated from clinical as well as experimental investigations to support the statement that in approximately 95 percent of the population, the left hemisphere is responsible for linguistic and sequential processing abilities. The right cerebral cortex usually seems to subserve spatial abilities and simultaneous processing functions. Like any area of endeavor, it seems as though a host of investigators are more than ready to attribute almost any conceivable ability or cognitive process to a given hemisphere. While there may be a solid foundation for some generalizations regarding the lateralization of functional processes, the reader is cautioned not to believe all one reads. For instance, dichotomizing language as a left-hemispheric function is a valid generalization. The initiation of its affective nature, however, (intonations, expressions, pitch, etc.) may be a result of input from the right hemisphere (Butler & Norrsell, 1968). In reviewing some of the functions attributed to the right and left hemispheres outlined in Table 2-2, therefore, the reader is urged to recall that the brain does act as a whole unit with various cortical areas simply having more input or influence over a given behavior.

Based primarily on clinical evidence, we know that damage or dysfunction to the left cerebral hemisphere may usually be manifested in language or speech disorders. The musculation of speech, also, although bilaterally represented, seems to be most severely affected by left-hemisphere

Table 2-2
Brain Functions Attributed to the Left and Right Cerebral Hemispheres

Left Cerebral Hemisphere		Right Cerebral Hemisphere	
Function	Source*	Function	Source*
Expressive speech	Broca, 1861	Spatial orientation	Sperry, 1974
Receptive language	Wernicke, 1874	Simple language comprehension	(above)
Language (general)	Sperry, 1974	Nonverbal ideation	(above)
Complex motor functions	Dimond & Beaumont, 1974	Picture & pattern sense	Eccles, 1977
Vigilance	(above)	Performancelike functions	(above)
Paired associate learning	(above)	Spatial integration	Dimond & Beaumont, 1974
Liaison to consciousness	Eccles, 1977	Creative associative thinking	(above)
Ideation	(above)	Facial recognition	Milner, 1967
Conceptual similarities	(above)	Sound (environmental) recognition	(above)
Temporal analysis	(above)	Nonverbal paired associate thinking	Stark, 1961
Analysis of detail	(above)	Tactile perception	Boll, 1974
Arithmetic	(above)	Gestalt perception	Bogen, 1969a, 1969b
Writing	Sperry, 1974	Logographic (pictograph) processing	Hatta, 1977
Calculation	Gerstmann, 1924	Intuitive problem solving	Torrance, Reynolds, Ball & Reigel, 1978
Finger naming	(above)	Psychic	
Right-left orientation	(above)	Produces humorous thoughts	
Sequential processing	Bogen, 1975	Simultaneous processing	Bogen, 1975

Modified from Berent, S. Lateralization of brain function. In Filskov, SB, & Boll, TJ. (Eds.): *Handbook of Clinical Neuropsychology.* New York: John Wiley and Sons, 1981, p. 76. Reprinted by permission of John Wiley and Sons, Inc.
* References do not imply original authorship.

lesions. When a child sustains damage to the left cerebral cortex, an acute anxiety over the loss of function may result; and, in extreme cases it may result in agitation or even catastrophic reactions. In a sense, however, the anxiety produced by the loss of function due to a left-hemisphere lesion may be the lesser of two evils, as psychotherapy can frequently be a beneficial intervention strategy for such children (Lezak, 1976).

Traditionally thought of as the "silent hemisphere" because so little was known about its behavioral correlates, the right hemisphere is especially important in tactile and visual-shape recognition, perception of orientation, processing and storage of visual data, native musical ability, and even some rudimentary verbal abilities. Any of these functions could thus easily be affected through damage or dysfunction to the right hemisphere. Interestingly, children or adults with right-sided lesions may have a lack of self-awareness as to the resulting behavioral or cognitive deficit and, hence, may have a great deal of difficulty in trial-and-error learning. It can usually be said that it would not be unusual to find that the child with a right-sided lesion has a diminished capacity for interpersonal awareness, may set unrealistic goals, and may be more of a behavioral or management problem than a child with left-hemisphere dysfunction. It is important to remember, however, that each child may present unique challenges.

Cortical and Functional Geography

Conceptually, each cerebral hemisphere can be divided into four lobes, named after the bones in the skull under which they lie. There are two fissures of note. The central fissure, or sulcus, is often referred to as the fissure of Rolando and divides the anterior and posterior portions of the brain. The Sylvian fissure runs laterally across the frontal and parietal lobes, forming the superior boundary for the temporal lobe. The occipital lobe is the most posterior part of the brain and borders on both the parietal and temporal lobes.

In terms of function, it helps to think of primary sensory and motor cortical areas and association areas of the cerebral cortex. Running more or less vertically, for instance, is the Rolandic fissure (central sulcus). Posterior (toward the rear) to this fissure is the sensory cortex. All (or nearly all) sensory neurons are organized in this region of the brain and operate on a point-to-point representation basis. That is to say, there is a direct relationship between the amount of cortex devoted to a function and its relative complexity. Much more sensory cortex, for example, is devoted to the tongue than to the small of the back. The result is that the tongue is a much more sensitive area of the body as compared with the small of the back. On the other side (anterior or toward the front) of the Rolandic fissure is the motor strip, which is organized in a similar fashion as the sensory cortex. Visual

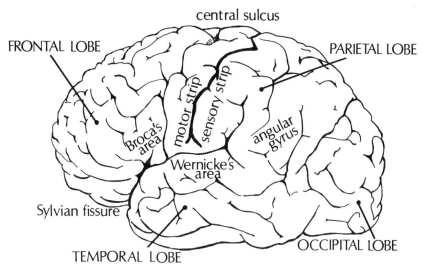

Fig. 2-3. Diagram of the cerebral cortex showing major landmarks and lobes.

perception occurs on the medial portion of the occipital lobes, and audition is subserved by Heschl's gyrus, which is located in the middle and superior portions of the temporal lobe.

The motor and sensory cortical areas, as previously stated, operate on pretty much of a point-to-point basis (i.e., the cortical area devoted to the function is well defined or discrete). If one stimulates the visual cortex, one might perceive flashes of light. There is, however, a significant cortical area not devoted to the primary cortical zones. In fact, in studies examining the comparative amount of cortical area devoted to the association cortex in monkeys, chimpanzees, and man, one finds a progression of ever-increasing cortical commitment (Heilman & Valenstein, 1979). The association areas of the cortex encompass most of the areas not devoted to primary sensory or motor function. It can be said that the role of neurons in the association cortex is to integrate and refine sensory perceptions and to assist in the integration of functions. Neurological dysfunction in the association cortex does not result in motor or sensory loss. Deficits in the comprehension or in the integration of sensory stimulation instead become manifest. This is an important concept, as will be seen in Chapter 4, which examines the single-factor research focusing on the cross-modal integration paradigms. One final point needs to be made prior to examining specific neurological correlates of behavior as they relate to the various lobes. At a cortical level, most right-sided functions are served by the left cerebral hemisphere. The same principle of contralaterality holds true for the right hemisphere, which controls or monitors the left side of space. Consequently, any dysfunction in the left motor cortex will manifest itself in a right-sided paralysis.

The following discussion will be organized according to the lobes of the cerebral cortex for the sake of clarity. Discussing the lobes in isolation could be a task analogous to the fabled blind men in their attempts to describe an elephant by touching various parts of its anatomy. A grossly oversimplistic perception of brain function could be the result of such a fragmented approach. This is probably justified, however, since the comprehension of brain-behavior relationships must begin at some level. As such, the reader is cautioned that the following is but a mere outline of the very basics of functional neuroanatomy of the cortex, which is shown in Figure 2-3.

The Occipital Lobes

The occipital cortex is usually thought of as the visual cortex because all visual perception is registered in the medial aspects of the occipital lobes. Research has demonstrated that the left side of each retina is connected to the left occipital lobe while the right side of the retina is connected to the right occipital lobe. In this fashion, any stimulus presented in the right visual field will project onto the left retina and thus be transmitted to the left occipital visual cortex (Marcus, 1972). While there are some exceptions to this basic conceptualization since some fibers from each side of the retina do go to the opposite visual cortex, it serves our discussion to think in these terms. Immediately anterior to the primary visual cortex are the visual association zones. Any damage or deficit to the primary visual cortex will result in visual-field blind spots. Any deficits in the visual association zones will result in visual incomprehension (visual agnosia). Benton (1979) has provided us with a short history of how the notion of visual association/integration function came about.

In 1876, Hughlings Jackson described a case of a patient with a tumor in the posterior region of the right hemisphere. Jackson noted that the patient suffered what he termed imperception, in that the patient had difficulty in recognizing faces and would get lost. Two years later Munk (1878) advanced the notion of seelenblindheit, or, mindblindness, to describe a condition observed in his dogs. His dogs had received bilateral ablations of the occipital association zones bordering on that of the parietal lobes. Of specific interest was that his dogs upon recovery could run, jump, and play as usual. They seemed, however, to have lost the ability to associate visual stimuli with meaning. Not only did they fail to recognize familiar stimuli (the face of their master), but also even seemed not to react to the presentation of meat. While this may suggest an extreme method in dieting, it also has theoretical implications that are of most interest to us. Munk suggested that the ablations had destroyed the "memory images," in that the stimuli were no longer matched to previously learned associations. The term mindblindness was eventually replaced by agnosia by Freud (1891).

The concept of agnosia is an especially interesting one since the disassociation between stimuli and its associative can occur in any sensory modality (e.g., audition, tactile-kinesthetic). Furthermore, controversy surrounds the issue of exactly what is agnosia (Rubens, 1979). Some have argued, for instance, that agnostic symptoms are the result of mental deficit correlated with an associated primary sensory-processing loss (Bay, 1953; Bender & Feldman, 1972). Luria (1959) has proposed that agnostic symptoms are not specifically due to mental dysfunction per se but, rather, are the manifestation of deficits in perceptual exploration. Presenting an alternative hypothesis, Geschwind (1972) draws question to the very notion of agnosia and proposes that the behavior observed in patients with agnosia-like symptoms are, in reality, confabulations due to disconnected cortical areas. Whatever the case, agnosia does seem to be a common enough clinical manifestation to warrant its brief discussion. For a more complete discussion of the agnosias the reader is referred to Rubens' (1979) excellent chapter.

Lezak (1976) tells us there are several types of agnosia. Apperceptive visual agnosia refers to the inability to recognize familiar objects because they are not perceived correctly. These individuals will not be able to copy correctly even the simplest geometric design or recognize once-familiar shapes. Basically, however, we know they can perceive colors and are able to see. As Rubens (1979) notes, though, these cases are rare and have little bearing on our dyslexic children.

Associative visual agnosia refers to a condition in which the patients are unable to copy or to match objects they are unable to recognize. Interestingly, these patients typically have more difficulty in recognizing pictures of items than the actual objects themselves (Rubens, 1979).

Other forms of agnosia exist that are probably due to occipital association-area dysfunction and include optic agnosia (patient is unable to name a presented object but can use it correctly or point to it when asked), color agnosia (unable to name colors but suffering no deficit in color perception), and prosopagnosia (has difficulty in recognizing familiar faces).

The concept of agnosia is a meaningful one when we discuss the neuropsychology of dyslexia, as it is often the case that the dyslexic child may evidence subtle agnosia-like clinical symptoms. Knowledge as to the various functions subserved by the primary visual cortex and the occipital association zones is important in this regard.

The Parietal Cortex

As previously indicated, one of the important cortical areas of relevance to our discussion is that which lies just posterior to the central fissure. The sensory strip is disproportionate in its representation of sensory areas, with cortex devoted to the face requiring approximately 40 percent of the available space, the hand 40 percent, and the rest of the body receiving the remaining 20 percent (Penfield & Rasmussen, 1955). It is commonly believed that the actual perception of sensation is a function of the thalamus, but it remains the task of the postcentral cortex to locate the sensation and determine its intensity. In this task the association cortex seems to be equally involved (Gardner, 1975). Interestingly, and perhaps of a more theoretical importance, there seems to be evidence to suggest the existence of a secondary somatic-sensory projection zone that is bilaterally represented (Schaltenbrand & Woolsey, 1964). Reports of this finding, although relatively few, indicate that this secondary area is buried deep in the Sylvian fissure close to the end of the central sulcus (Penfield & Jaspar, 1954).

Sensory awareness associated with the postcentral gyrus include positional sense, tactile localization, two-point discrimination, stereognosis (the ability to distinguish the shape of an object by touch alone), haptic recognition, and graphesthesia (the ability to recognize letters or symbols drawn on the hand or fingers). Much of our knowledge regarding parietal lobe functions comes from the clinical work of Benton (1959), Critchley (1953), and Luria (1973).

Lesions acquired to the postcentral gyrus in infancy or early childhood may result in delayed skeletal growth contralateral to the damage. A later neurological examination will reveal not only sensory loss but also relative smallness of contralateral limbs (Marcus, 1972). Deep lesions into the underlying white matter of the inferior parietal and temporal lobe may damage the optic radiations transversing this subcortical region en route to the visual cortex. As Gaddes (1980) notes, dysfunction in this region may, by its proximity to the optic radiations, result in subtle deficits such as disturbances in figure-ground relationships, which are common among certain subtypes of dyslexic children.

When lesions occur in the right and left hemispheres, as expected, there appear to be different symptoms manifested. The syndrome described by Gerstmann (1957) describes a constellation of four symptoms, which more or less tend to appear together with lesions or dysfunction in the left parieto-occipital region. These symptoms include dysgraphia, dyscalculia, left-right confusion, and finger agnosia (inability to identify which fingers have been touched). While some question the validity of the Gerstmann syndrome (Benton, 1961, 1977), it does seem to have clinical validity and often these symptoms are seen in dyslexic children. Also found in patients with left-hemisphere (parietal lobe) lesions is ideomotor apraxia, which is the inability to pretend one is performing some manual task (common examples include waving good-bye, saluting, etc.). Ideational apraxia, on the other hand, is demonstrated by an inability to show how to use some well-known object. The Illinois Test of Psycholinguistic Ability (ITPA) has an excellent test, called "Manual Expression," for this disorder in which the child is shown an object and is asked to demonstrate its use. If a child is deficient in parietal lobe function, the ideational motor skills and ideomotor abilities will undoubtedly be affected.

Nondominant parietal lobe lesions create deficits or abnormalities in body sense/image, in perception of space and drawing, or in constructional ability. Disturbances in body image could easily result in a lack of awareness of the left side of space resulting in left-sided neglect, a denial of illness or dysfunction, and difficulty in interpreting drawings or in reading maps (Marcus, 1972).

The Angular Gyrus

If the reader examines the location of the angular gyrus as presented in Figure 2-3, it can be seen that this cortical area is located most strategically. The angular gyrus is situated such that it comprises a tertiary area bordering on the visual and sensory association zones. It also is on the boundary of the temporal lobe. As Gaddes (1980) has suggested:

> Many writers have considered the angular tyrus and the immediate cortical areas to be vital in mediating these intersensory functions . . . lesions of these areas do not produce disturbances specific to vision, audition, or tactile sensation but do disrupt the integrated reception and analysis of information. Probably the most common behaviors disturbed in this way are reading, writing, and all forms of perception involving spatial imagery. (pp. 109–110)

This, as will be seen in the next chapter as well as Chapter 4, is a critical concept and Gaddes' statement serves well to highlight the important integrative function of the angular gyrus.

The Temporal Lobes

Primarily responsible for speech comprehension and audition, the left temporal lobe in man reaches its greatest differentiation by far when compared with lower animals. Defined as the cortical area below the lateral (Sylvian) fissure and anterior to the occipital lobe, the left temporal lobe has been the source of much controversy. For instance, Geschwind and Levitsky (1968) disagreed with the prevailing notion that the left hemisphere was not structurally asymmetrical for the purpose of subserving speech. Von Bonin (1962) has previously advocated this notion. Geschwind and Levitsky examined 100 brains acquired at postmortem. So that the symmetry of the hemispheres could be measured, they made a cut across the plane of the planum temporale (area directly posterior to Heschl's gyrus, the cortical area on the superior surface of the temporal lobe that is responsible for audition). Based on their study of the cut brains, they found that the planum temporale was enlarged on the left in 65 percent of the cases, and on the right was enlarged only 11 percent. Also, the left planum temporale was, on the average, one-third longer on the left in comparison with the right. It is intriguing to speculate whether an enlarged left temporal lobe is directly related to the development of language functions. Certainly, the notion that there is some correlation is without much support, although Geschwind (1979) does report a case of an exceptionally gifted lawyer whose planum temporale was seven times as large on the left as on the right. The planum temporale is thought to be that area of the brain responsible for auditory associations and comprehension, an ability obviously of relevance to the practice of law. Wernicke's area is usually considered to be in the region of the planum temporale and is specifically important in the comprehension of language.

Lesions to the left temporal lobe can result in damage to Heschl's gyrus, causing cortical deafness. When Wernicke's area is involved the comprehension of speech is affected. Needless to say, if there is early damage or congenital dysfunction in this area affecting a young child, language or speech abilities are sure to be affected as also are auditory associations and many memory functions (Mahl, Rothernberg, Delgado, & Hamlin, 1964; Meyer & Yates, 1955; Penfield & Perot, 1963; Penfield & Roberts, 1959). Damage to the inferior temporal region may cause deficits in visual association since there are a significant number of connections in this region of the cortex to the visual association cortex, which is in turn connected to the limbic system below the temporal lobe (Marcus, 1972). In fact, some recent evidence has even been able to pinpoint neurons in the inferior temporal region that seem to play an important role in retaining the relevant features of visual stimuli, thus supporting the role of this lobe in memory (Fuster & Jervey, 1981).

Dysfunction in the right temporal lobe rarely affects speech, although it may produce deficits in nonverbal sound discrimination. Other functions seemingly impaired by right-sided lesions to the temporal region include primitive musical ability (anterior portion of the right temporal lobe) and picture comprehension (Lezak, 1976; Milner, 1958).

The limbic system lies subcortically and includes the amygdala, the hippocampus, and the uncus, which are closely tied to the expression of emotional states. It is for this reason that temporal lobe epilepsy frequently is associated with abnormal emotional expression. Some psychological manifestations frequently associated with temporal lobe seizures include fear, alterations in perception; hallucinations in visual, auditory, and olfactory senses; confusion often associated with memory problems; and, occasionally, automatisms may result (Marcus, 1972).

It is clear that the left temporal region is of most relevance to our discussion of brain function in dyslexia, and for this reason more will be said in Chapter 3 about the contribution of temporal lobe structures to reading. The only remaining lobe not addressed is the frontal lobe, and our focus on this vital cortical area will conclude this brief overview of the functional organization of the brain.

The Frontal Cortex

When neurologists or neuropsychologists talk about the frontal lobes, they include all of the cortical mantle anterior to the Rolandic (central) fissure, distinguishing man from other animals in the tremendous development of this part of the brain. It can be said that the frontal lobes include approximately 40 percent of the total brain area (Filskov et al., 1981). Gall hypothesized that the frontal lobes were the seat of our intellectual capabilities and, despite a lack of support for this notion, it persists today among certain circles (Pirozzolo, 1979). We owe much of our knowledge regarding the frontal lobes to individuals like Halstead (1947) and his colleagues. Today, however, we operate under a different knowledge base regarding the importance of the frontal lobes.

Directly anterior to the central fissure is the motor strip, which is organized much the same as its sensory analogue on the other side of the fissure. Most importantly, directly below the motor strip in the left hemisphere is Broca's area and, as discussed earlier, this region is critical in expressive speech. It used to be thought that the motor cortex was responsible for initiating movement and that an area directly in front of the motor strip (premotor area) was responsible for inhibiting motor activity (McCulloch, 1944). While this idea has been usually discredited, we now know substantially more about the cortex directly anterior to the motor area. We know now, for instance, that the cortical area directly in front of the motor strip is connected to it by short association fibers and probably acts as a motor association area (Filskov et al., 1981).

The most anterior portion of the frontal lobes is probably the least understood portion of the cortex. Luria (1969, 1980) believed this cortical area to be important in planning behavior, in determining its structure, and in evaluating it. One can often but wonder when observing children who experience great difficulty in carrying out sequential motor movements (e.g., kicking and throwing a ball) or cognitive processes (e.g., subtraction of two-digit numerals) exactly what brain functions may or may not be operating properly.

Early research regarding the effects of experimentally-induced damage on frontal lobe functioning produced some interesting results. Jacobsen (1936) investigated the relationship between the frontal lobes and intelligence in monkeys. To study the effects of frontal ablations, he used a delayed-response task in which the monkey was shown some food; the food was placed under a cup; and, after a delay, the monkey was allowed to choose a cup.

After frontal lobe lesions, the monkey performed calmly and was not the least bit upset by errors as he had been previously. Similar to the temporal lobes, the frontal lobes have many connections to the limbic system. It has been hypothesized that frontal lesions somehow disconnect these two areas of the brain. For this reason frontal lobotomies were often used as a therapeutic tool with severely disturbed and dangerous patients (Hebb, 1945; Rylander, 1939).

More recent research has revealed that the frontal lobes are significantly different from the rest of the cortex. Most lesions in the cortex produce circumscribed effects. Frontal lobe lesions influence complex motivational processes, possibly due to the many acknowledged connections to the subcortical areas involved in motivation (Milner, 1970). Consequently, it seems reasonable that a lesion in the frontal cortex could affect performance on almost any task. As Gross and Weiskrantz (1964) have noted, frontal lobe lesions have thus been associated with deficits or dysfunction in attention, volition, personality, emotion, perception, and motor behavior. While dysfunction may result from such lesions, the most striking finding is that frontal lobe deficits do not seem to automatically lead to significant intellectual impairment (Hebb & Penfield, 1940). What actually may result from lesions to the frontal cortex is a loss of motivation and a higher frustration tolerance, thus leading to delayed and possibly perservative performance. Consequently, the motivation or drive to sequence the behavior Luria speaks of may become impaired, giving way to more primitive patterns of response possibly mediated by lower brain structures. Neurological signs of frontal cortex dysfunction include abnormal reflexes (grasp, sucking, snout, palmomentel, etc.), bradykinesia (slow movements), abnormal gait or posture, changes in the control of eye movements, changes in arousal or the orienting response, or changes in emotionality or cognition (Damasio, 1979).

The remedial specialist or psychologist does need to be cautious, however, about generalizations made regarding the frontal lobe and its function. Some would argue that the frontal lobes do not actually exert any significant control over behavior or cognition until the child is well into puberty. As suggested earlier when discussing attention deficits, the development of frontal lobe functions in some people may well continue into their early 20s. It may be this factor that contributes to the gradual "disappearance" of hyperactivity and other impulse disorders during puberty (Golden, 1981). It should also be obvious that if this assertion regarding the development of frontal lobe function is correct, then tests designed to evaluate frontal lobe functions in adults (e.g., Similarities on the Wechsler Adult Intelligence Scale; the Category Test on the Halstead-Reitan batteries) might be testing functions related to an entirely different area of the cortex in children. This notion awaits the attention of researchers.

CONCLUSIONS

By the very nature of the topic of this chapter, the previous discussion of the functional organization of the brain has been barely adequate in covering in any sufficient detail the enormous complexity of brain-behavior relationships. It should, however, serve to provide the reader with a reasonable foundation so that the ensuing discussion on the neuropsychology of language and reading makes sense.

In summary, this chapter has provided a brief description of the history of thought related to the localization of function. We have seen how neurological development is related to the functional organization of the brain stem, cerebellum, and cerebral cortex. The conclusions, which will serve as the springboard for the remainder of this volume, include the following.

Based on our review of the history of clinical neurology research, there is every reason to believe that structural and functional asymmetries exist within the brain. Attempts to dichotomize brain function as being either highly localized or as "wholistic" is based on a simplistic and uninformed knowledge of the existing literature. For example, the primary motor and sensory cortical areas are very localized. Those cortical areas responsible for higher-order associations and abstractions based on sensory stimulation are, however, more diffuse and interactive.

Perception and cognition do not occur in a vacuum, as most cortical areas (especially the temporal and frontal lobes) have many neural connections to subcortical structures, most notably the limbic system. Communication consequently occurs not only between various cortical regions but also in the vertical plane.

There are cortical areas including the angular gyrus, frontal lobes, and planum temporale that seem particularly well differentiated in man. It seems that this neurological development is of optimal importance on tasks of higher cognitive processing that requires cross-modal integration and the abstraction of language, and in the organizing and sequencing of cognitive behavior.

Damage or dysfunction due to congenital factors may result in very discrete observable neurological signs. For instance, damage to the primary visual cortex will result in visual-field deficits. Dysfunction in the motor cortex will result in a contralateral hemiparalysis. Dysfunction in the more recently evolved cortical areas, however, will result in more subtle deficits such as those manifested in speech, memory, associative learning, or reading.

Consequently, if dysfunctions in these areas are implicated as possible correlates of disabilities in learning, including dyslexia, it should seem that specific neurological correlates should be available to support this tentative conclusion. The purpose of Chapter 3 is to demonstrate that neurological correlates are indeed at the root of dyslexia. It is proposed that once this relationship is demonstrated, the vast and often conflicting research with dyslexics will fall into its proper perspective and appropriate assessment and intervention strategies will readily emerge.

PART II

Theory and Research

Chapter 3
Neuropsychology of Language and Reading Failure

Our knowledge as to how the brain is organized and functions has, in large part, been derived from several sources. First, we can conduct comparative studies in that the brains of animals and man are examined for significant differences in structure and presumed function. Second, it is possible to infer from cases when areas of the brain fail to develop (agenesis) as to the associated cognitive deficit, thus providing some insight as to the relationship between structure and function. Third, an examination of cases when children or adults have sustained brain trauma can reveal important findings as to cortical-functional relationships as well as to the ability of the brain to recover from trauma. Finally, and for obvious reasons an avenue not usually followed, we can alter brain function by systematically impairing cortical areas through surgery. The first three methods have the most meaning for our review of brain-behavior relationships in language and reading failure.

This chapter will review briefly the neuropsychological processes thought to be involved in language and reading. Since Chapter 2 is designed to provide an understanding as to functional neuroanatomy, the focus of the present discussion will be on the development of cortical pathways responsible for language and reading. Second, an examination of the literature concerned with disordered brain function due to agenesis and brain damage will be presented. The intent in this section will be to demonstrate that any alteration in brain structure almost inevitably leads to associated cognitive deficits. In a large part, this section is presented as a response to those who incorrectly would lead one to believe that the brain can endure rather dramatic impairment without associated cognitive difficulties (Sandoval & Haapanen, 1981).

Finally, recent advances in research with developmental dyslexics will be presented. This section will outline several significant advances from a neurological standpoint, thus serving as a conceptual framework for the next three chapters. Chapters 4, 5, and 6 present research more concerned with psychological processes involved in developmental dyslexia. It is believed that only through a perspective emphasizing neurological correlates of reading failure will the confusing state of affairs in the arena of psychological research emerge clearer.

NEUROLOGIC ASPECTS OF LANGUAGE AND READING

Nearly any topic could logically be included in a section dealing with the neurobiologic correlates of language and reading. As Whitaker (1976) notes in his seminal chapter on this important topic, fields of relevant study include neurolinguistics, neuroanatomy, neurophysiology, neurochemistry, and, with more recent advances, perhaps electrophysiology, neuropathology, and neuroradiology. The relevant research in these fields can assist us in developing a conceptual framework that relates brain structure to function. To the reader who may wish to pursue a more complete understanding of these fields of study as they relate to language and reading, the works of Geschwind (1974a, 1974b, 1979), Lenneberg (1967), Meader and Muyskens (1962), and Whitaker (1976) are strongly recommended.

It will be recalled that, in Chapter 2, evidence was presented suggesting a structural asymmetry in the brain of man. Geschwind and Levitsky (1968) demonstrated that in a majority of cases the left temporal lobe was enlarged, presumably for language and speech functions. Other studies suggest that the right Sylvian fissure is angled more upward than on the left and that the left parietal operculum is more developed than the right (Lemay & Culebras, 1972). The question arises: are these differences in any way related to the unique difference in language abilities between man and other primates?

Von Bonin and Bailey (1961) addressed this question and found that historically the uniqueness of the brain of man was focused in the temporal lobe, in the inferior parietal lobe, and in the frontal lobe just anterior to Broca's area. The difference in the brain of man when compared with the brain of a chimpanzee is found primarily in those areas subserving language and speech function. As Whitaker (1976) notes:

The picture that begins to emerge is one of a clearly distinct speech vocalization system in man based on a species-specific neural structure (Broca's area)
and anatomic structure (the vocal tract), coupled with a significant increase in
the quantity of and the information processing capacity of the homologous
cerebral cortex (inferior parietal and superior temporal lobes). (p. 127)

We know from our previous discussions that the cortical area known
as Broca's area is responsible for speech production. The superior temporal
lobe is responsible for language and much of language comprehension. This
area is usually referred to as Wernicke's region. Broca's area and Wernicke's
region are connected by the arcuate fasciculus, and it is believed that were
it not for this major pathway both regions would be disconnected. While
other pathways between these two regions have been postulated (Penfield
& Roberts, 1959), most would agree that the arcuate fasciculus is vital to
speech production (Whitaker, 1976).

While the comprehension of language may take place in large part in
the area of Wernicke's region, what anatomical structure underlies reading?
It was suggested in Chapter 2 that the angular gyrus could very well be of
critical importance in reading. Although some authors (Von Bonin & Bailey, 1961) deny the uniqueness of this region in man, most researchers in
neurophysiology and neuropsychology stress this posterioinferior parietal
region in conceptual models of reading and cognitive functioning (Geschwind, 1962, 1974a, 1979; Goldstein, 1927; Pirozzolo, 1979).

The Angular Gyrus and the Reading Process

From a neurodevelopmental standpoint, various regions in the cerebral
cortex mature at differential rates. It can usually be stated that the primary
projection zones mature first, with the secondary association cortex matur-
ing last. While there is a tendency for the motor cortex to lead the sensory
cortex, both are the most mature areas of the cortex up through five to six
years of age. The primary visual and auditory cortex mature at a slightly
slower rate. Full maturation of the cerebral cortex probably proceeds through
puberty and may not be complete until some people are in their early 20s
(Whitaker, 1976). Figure 3-1 presents a simplified representation of the maturational sequence.

In comparing this representation of cortical maturation with Figure 2-
3, it can be seen that one of the last regions to reach neuronal maturation
in that area typically associated with language abilities is the temporal lobe.
It is also interesting to note that the area (known as the angular gyrus)
bordering on the temporal lobe is one of the regions associated with late
maturation. It is of critical importance that language functions and an area
thought to relate to reading processes are late in the maturational sequence.

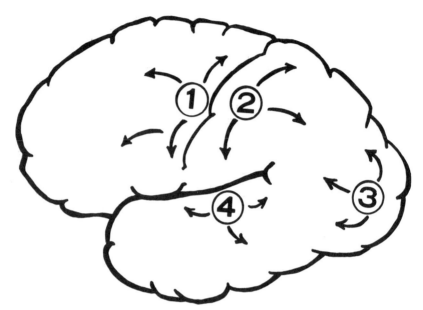

Fig. 3-1. Sequence of cortical maturation. [From Whitaker, HA. Neurobiology of language. In Carterette, ER, & Friedman, MP (Eds.), *Handbook of perception* (Vol. 7). New York: Academic Press, 1976, p. 133. With permission.]

It may be this factor that accounts in large part for so many children having language-related learning disabilities, including reading. As most clinicians know, the vast majority of children evidencing language or reading disorders are rarely identified until they experience failure on the higher-order tasks usually required of them in the primary grades. Any late maturation in these regions will not be noticed unless there exists a requirement for higher-order cognitive processes for which only a delayed substrata or no substrata exists. It is proposed that reading disorders due to trauma and those due to developmental delay mimic one another (Aaron, Baxter, & Lucenti, 1980). In support of this notion, it should be emphasized that there has never been a documented case in which slowed neuronal maturation has been shown to have "caught up."

It is logical from a neurodevelopmental standpoint that there would exist more natural variation in abilities associated with a more phylogenetically advanced cortical area (Geschwind, 1979). During the evolutionary process, sensory and motor abilities have most likely developed to a relatively stable level of function, whereas greater differences in levels of individual performance probably exist on almost any higher-order cognitive skill such as reading. Whether neurological deficit or developmental delay is at play if an area of the cortex associated with reading is affected, it thus seems reasonable to assume that reading failure will result.

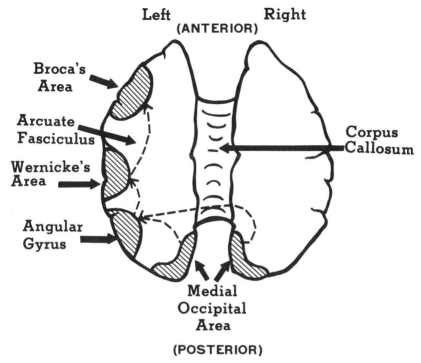

Fig. 3-2. The brain as viewed in horizontal section. The major pathways and cortical areas thought to be involved in reading are shown.

One may well ask exactly how the cortical area known as the angular gyrus is involved in reading. Geschwind (1974a) has argued that the uniqueness of the angular gyrus is that it lies between the association cortexes of vision, audition, and somesthesis. It is strategically placed, as such, to serve the vital function of acting as a center for cross-modal associations. Geschwind (1974a) has even suggested that "this area may well be termed 'the association cortex' of the association cortexes" (p. 99). A simplistic example of this process may serve to illustrate how reading for meaning may occur. Suppose a child reads the sentence, "the top of the large round table felt rough and looked unfinished." The perception of these words occurs in the medial aspects of the occipital lobes. Short association fibers transmit the perception to the association areas immediately adjacent to the primary visual projection zone, where meaning is attached to the visual stimulus. It may well be here that the words take on some rudimentary meaning. Connecting fibers running to the angular gyrus make the associations available for integration with other cross-modal precepts. The word *rough*, for instance, may take on new meaning as associations are formed with fibers in the sensory cortex. Similar associations may be made with the word *round*, originating from the parietal cortex. So, as Geschwind (1979) suggests, the angular gyrus allows for not only naming but also for cross-modal associations to occur. Comprehension of the written material probably occurs in the cortical region incorporating Wernicke's area and the angular gyrus. If the passage were to be read aloud, Broca's area would become involved with the arcuate fasciculus connecting the area for spoken language with that region responsible for its comprehension (Fig. 3-2). This example is too simplistic, perhaps, since it ignores the potential contribution of the limbic system, among others. As an example, however, it is presented to demonstrate a conceptual paradigm for understanding what we believe may occur during oral or silent reading. From this paradigm it can be easily understood why a deficit anywhere in the functional system of reading may well result in dyslexia. In large part, conceptualizing the psychological research from this perspective explains why some studies show intra-modal, cross-modal, or even perceptual deficits as the foundation for dyslexia.

As shall be seen in the final section of this chapter, discrete neuropathological findings in children who suffered dyslexia, as well as electrophysiological evidence using dyslexics and matched controls, support this conclusion. Prior to examining this evidence, we need to consider the literature associated with disordered brain function due to either neurodevelopmental anomalies or brain damage. Only through an understanding of how the brain can and cannot function with neuroanatomical deficits can we truly understand the context of research with dyslexics. Furthermore, such an understanding can provide a benchmark for our developing reasonable expectations regarding the prognosis of a child identified as dyslexic.

DISORDERED BRAIN FUNCTION AND COGNITIVE ABILITY

Agenesis and localized brain trauma provide unique opportunities to determine how a child will behave without the input from a given cortical or subcortical region. As has been noted by many writers, cases of documented brain damage or agenesis do not provide a model of how the brain functions due to the damage. Rather they provide good examples as to how the person functions in the absence of cortical structures. In this sense, the behavioral result of brain damage is how the organism acts without tissue. Since there is a considerable literature both in the area of agenesis and brain damage, each will be dealt with separately.

Agenesis

Agenesis is the failure of a particular region or structure in the brain to develop as it should. When considering possible mechanisms related to neural plasticity, the concept of agenesis needs to be given careful consideration. If a region of the brain that we know subserves a given function fails to develop, what then of the ability? Does the ability also fail to manifest itself, thus forever handicapping the child? We know that in most cases the ability subserved by an area of the brain that has not matured as it should is not lost. Rather, the ability seems to be coordinated by some other available cortical structure not originally programmed to subserve that function.

There seems to be some confusion as to the nature of agenesis. Some (Sandoval & Haapanen, 1981) suggest that plasticity and the equipotential nature of the brain account for the lack of split-brain characteristics found in children with agenesis of the corpus callosum. Based on their limited purview of the literature, they (Sandoval et al., 1981) conclude that "obviously the brain has amazing healing and compensatory properties" (p. 383). Of course, the brain has amazing properties and does seem to be able to withstand considerable developmental anomalies. Anyone truly familiar with the literature, however, would know that in-depth studies of children or adults with agenesis of a brain region usually present with other severe neurologic problems. When they do not evidence such obviously handicapping conditions as hypertelorism or hydrocephalus, the cases deserve special attention and some rather extraordinary cases are available for study. The important point to realize, however, is that when a region predestined to subserve a given function fails to develop, either gross or at best subtle neurological or psychological deficits can be identified.

Most of the research regarding agenesis has been conducted on patients presenting with agenesis of the corpus callosum (Chiarello, 1980). Relatively few cases are reported regarding other important brain structures. The corpus callosum at one time or another was thought to be responsible for forming the internal structure of the brain, for keeping the two cerebral hemispheres connected, and for being responsible for the imagination (Clarke & O'Malley, 1968). Others have suggested that it is not related to any identifiable function and thus, by implication, deserves little attention (Tomasch, 1954). Since most current theories regarding the function of the corpus callosum correlate it to the establishment of language and learning abilities, it is important to consider cases in which this interhemispheric commissure has failed to develop.

Agenesis of the Corpus Callosum

The corpus callosum is a thick bundle of nerve fibers that link homologous regions of the cortex. By referring back to Figure 2-2 the reader can see that, by its strategic location, the corpus callosum is in an excellent position to link the two hemispheres. The corpus callosum is found only in mammals and is conceptually divided into important regions. The most anterior portion of the corpus callosum is called the rostrum while the thinner main body of the corpus callosum is referred to as the truncus. The curved, larger region at the most posterior part of the corpus callosum is called the splenium (Selnes, 1974). These landmarks are important because different cortical regions seem to be connected to each other through fibers transversing different regions of the corpus callosum.

Nerve fibers from the two cerebral hemispheres radiate through the corpus callosum, connecting both hemispheres. Estimates vary as to the actual number of fibers, but it seems safe to say that somewhere between 1 million (Bonin, 1961) and 7 million fibers (Spitzka, 1905) exist here. Other estimates are even higher (Blinkov & Glezer, 1968; Tomasch, 1954). The development of the corpus callosum begins at approximately 12 weeks after gestation (Rakic & Yakovlev, 1968) and achieves nearly complete function at birth (Hewitt, 1962). Importantly, and this may be critical when considering the effects of malnutrition or poor environmental stimulation on later learning abilities, full myelinization of fibers in the corpus callosum takes place at a later time than other fibers (Villaverde, 1931). Estimates regarding the complete myelinization of the corpus callosum range from 20 months (Mingazzini, 1922) to 6 years (Yakovlev & Lecours, 1967). Whatever the actual case, myelinization of callosal fibers seems to be delayed when considering other cortical areas. This delayed process may in some way be related to our notions as to the age at which plasticity ends.

As near as can be determined, there is no direct evidence as to why this seemingly vital commissure would fail to develop. Recent speculation has suggested the cytomegalovirus (CMV) may be responsible for various unexplained brain malformations and some neurodegenerative disorders seen in young infants (Bray, Bale, Anderson, & Kern, 1981). Bray et al. hypothesized that CMV can be transmitted to the fetus transplacentally where it acts like a "slow" virus, resulting in brain malformations in seemingly normal-appearing postnatal infants. The malformations they suggest (polymicrogyria) may be the result of CMV, and it is of interest to note that this neurologic anomaly will turn up later in a postmortem of a dyslexic child. While this is certainly an appealing idea, there is no direct evidence that this may be the case in agenesis of the corpus callosum. Evidence also exists that agenesis of the corpus callosum may be transmitted through autosomal dominant inheritance (Lynn, Buchanan, Fenichel, & Freeman, 1980). In this particular case both a father and a son presented with agenesis of the corpus callosum. Only a few other cases of this nature have been reported in the literature (Dogan, Dogan, & Lovrencic, 1967; Menkes, Philippart, & Clark, 1964; Sauerwein, Lassonde, Cardu, & Geoffroy, 1981) and considering the rather large number of cases reported with no evidence of transmission, it seems that inheritance alone cannot account for the high incidence of this neurodevelopmental disorder.

The case study literature. Contrary to the early ideas regarding the functions of the corpus callosum, recent ideas center on the notion that the corpus callosum is important in interhemispheric sharing of information. Based on the split-brain research (Bogen & Vogel, 1962; Sperry, 1961, 1964, 1970), it seems as though the role of the corpus callosum on a cognitive level serves to integrate two unique modes of information processing (Zaidel, 1979). As was noted in Chapter 2, the left hemisphere seems to facilitate logical-sequential processing while the right cerebral hemisphere seems more facilitative of wholistic or gestalt processing. At a more basic level, the corpus callosum also seems important in mediating interhemispheric transfer of sensory information. This was first rather dramatically illustrated by Bykov and Speransky (1924) when a dog with a severed corpus callosum failed to transfer a conditioned reflex from one forepaw to another. The dog with the corpus callosum could easily accomplish this transfer.

Over 50 cases of agenesis of the corpus callosum exist in the literature and most relate to cases in which the diagnosis has been made in adults. A relatively few studies relate cases of school-age children with agenesis of the corpus callosum (Ettlinger, Blakemore, Milner, & Wilson, 1972, 1974; Gott & Saul, 1978; Lassonde, Lortie, Ptito, & Geoffroy, 1981) and even fewer yet exist with preschool children (Hynd & Teeter, 1981; Teeter & Hynd, 1981).

Usually, agenesis of the corpus callosum is accompanied by low-average to below-average intellectual ability. Some have gone so far as to suggest that, based on this observation, the size of the corpus callosum may be related to intellectual level, and indices exist for this hypothesized relationship (Bremer, 1966; Schepers, 1938; Spitzka, 1905). In the 27 cases reviewed by Chiarello (1980) in which IQ levels were available, the mean IQ was 89 (SD = 12.45). For the 25 cases in which verbal and performance IQs were presented, it turns out that no significant ($p > .05$) difference existed between these IQ scores (Mean VSIQ = 88.52, SD = 12.58; Mean PSIQ = 88.76, SD = 15.75). There is some speculation that this lowered IQ level may be due to the reduction of cortical cells found in callosal agenesis patients (Shoumura, Ando, & Kato, 1975). In Chiarello's (1980) cases many other neurological and psychological abnormalities were noted. In order of frequency these included: EEG disturbances (nine cases), hydrocephalus (four cases), epilepsy (four cases), cysts (three cases), and cortical atrophy (three cases). Figures 3-3 and 3-4 demonstrate a typical case of megaloencephalus associated with agenesis of the corpus callosum. Note the expanded and slit-like lateral ventricles and vertically enlarged third ventricular area.

It can be argued that these cases are the result of aberrant history and do not represent those cases in which the "amazing healing and compensa-

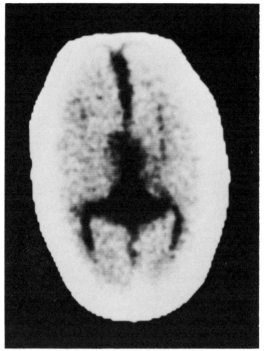

Fig. 3-3. A CT scan showing megaloencephalus with vertically expanded third ventricle. [From Teeter, A, & Hynd,
GW. Agenesis of the corpus callosum: A developmental study
during infancy. *Clinical Neuropsychology*, 1981, *3*, 29–32. With
permission.]

tory properties" (Sandoval, et al., 1981, p. 383) of the brain can be manifested. For this reason the following case will be briefly reviewed since it
represents one of the best and certainly most thorough evaluation of a patient with agenesis who seemed at first glance to be normal.

Dennis (1981) reports a case of a 27-year-old woman who developed
normally until age 11 when two "staring spells" were reported. No EEG
abnormalities or other abnormalities were found and the spells never appeared again. An initial air encephalogram revealed dilated lateral ventricles, which were displaced accompanied by an expanded third ventricle. A
Dandy-Walker syndrome was also apparent (agenesis of the vermis of the
cerebellum). On the Wechsler Adult Intelligence Scale (WAIS) she achieved
a full-scale IQ of 106 with verbal and performance IQs being 96 and 119,
respectively. An exceptionally thorough evaluation of language (phonologi-
cal aspects, naming, fluency, word and sentence comprehension, and so

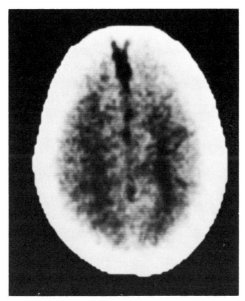

Fig. 3-4. A CT scan showing the agenesis of the corpus callosum. This is the same patient in the CT scan in Figure 3-3. [From Teeter, A, & Hynd, GW. Agenesis of the corpus callosum: A developmental study during infancy. *Clinical Neuropsychology*, 1981, *3*, 29–32. With permission.]

on), visual perception, memory and attention, and cerebral dominance was completed using matched controls.

In general, this patient performed well and in some cases exceptionally well on a limited number of linguistic tasks (e.g., sound blending, fluency, etc.). She also presented no visual deficits. A significant disability, however, was evidenced in the semantic aspect of linguistic performance. For instance, she had great difficulty in establishing the meaning of passive-but-affirmative sentences and was inaccurate in evaluating the representation of negation. She also experienced difficulty in a task requiring a sentence-to-picture match. Finally, in addition to poor performance on a sentence repetition task, she was severely impaired on complex sentence production. Although she was strongly right-handed, she evidenced no ear effect on a task designed to measure cerebral language lateralization.

This is an excellent report because it demonstrates that when an agenesis case is viewed critically and thoroughly, deficits do emerge and, in fact, indices of severe impairment of complex linguistic function may exist. In large part this is consistant with the idea that the corpus callosum is necessary for satisfactory performance of normally lateralized functions

(Chiarello, 1980). The fact of the matter is that patients with agenesis of the corpus callosum do not mimic the split-brain subjects and usually do evidence some interhemispheric transfer abilities (Bryden & Zurif, 1970; Saul & Sperry, 1968). Pirozzolo, Pirozzolo, and Ziman (1979) have suggested a most plausible explanation for this phenomena. They suggest that in patients with callosal agenesis, the commissural fibers may be rerouted either through the still intact anterior or posterior (splenium) pathways or through even more caudal pathways. This notion may have merit, as it is known that a relatively small number of fibers are needed for transcortical transmission (Galambos, Norton, & Frommer, 1967). In another vein, Dennis (1981) has advanced the idea that the variable deficits observed in patients with callosal agenesis may be the result of a whole "constellation of pathological events" (p. 51) associated with the neurodevelopmental anomaly. Whatever the case, it does seem that some compensatory mechanisms are at work to make optimal use of the available commissural or subcortical pathways.

Since the corpus callosum represents a unique commissure, it may not present the best case for what many consider an optimal base for the mechanism of plasticity. What would better represent an optimal agenesis model for the mechanism of plasticity is a case in which one portion of the brain failed to develop but in which there was an intact homologous region ready to subserve the function. While the hemispherectomy literature does provide some insights along this line, trauma associated with surgery and age of trauma cloud the optimal mechanism for plasticity to occur. It is usually believed that the earlier the release from the neural substrata destined originally to subserve the function the better the potential for optimal success in functional and structural representation.

A Unique Case of Left Temporal Lobe Agenesis

As we know from our discussion presented in this chapter as well as in Chapter 2, the left temporal lobe in the vast majority of the population is responsible for speech and language comprehension. Although few cases of temporal lobe agenesis exist, the available cases typically report many neurologic complications, including arachnoid cysts, sixth nerve palsy and exophthalmos, associated asymmetry of the skull, and chronic subdural hematoma (Robinson, 1964). Needless to say, the deficits associated with the left temporal lobe agenesis would be much complicated by these and other anomalies and the correlated cognitive-linguistic impairment would be severe.

Pirozzolo and Horner (in press) present a unique case of left temporal lobe agenesis in which no neurologic complications were present. Their patient was a nine-year-old boy referred for headaches possibly associated with a fall. No seizures were reported. Although somewhat restless on examination, no significant neurologic findings were reported other than that

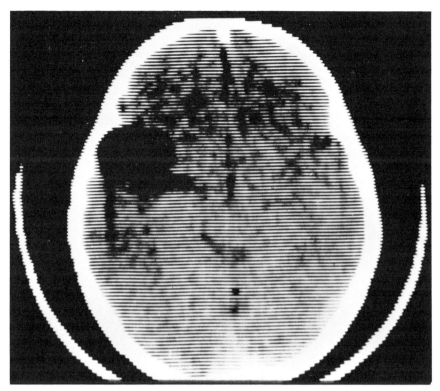

Fig. 3-5. CT scan showing agenesis of the anterior portion of the left temporal lobe. [From Pirozzolo, FJ, & Horner, FA. *Auditory-memory and linguistic deficits in left temporal lobe agenesis: Evidence for linguistic specialization of the left hemisphere* (in press). With permission.]

he had an asymmetric head, which was enlarged in the left temporal region. The results of a computed tomography (CT) scan, angiography, and isotope brain scan suggested agenesis, which was confirmed on surgery. A cystic formation with a thin capsule of water was removed, and his postoperative course was without event (Figure 3-5).

Neuropsychological assessment was conducted and included measures of intelligence, memory, language, oculomotor, and visual-spatial abilities. Postoperative assessment indicated abilities consistent with his school performance, although significant areas of deficit were evident. Table 3-1 presents a summary of his neuropsychological assessment results. The patient's above average performance on the Wechsler Intelligence Scale For Children-Revised (WISC-R) is surprising, considering the extent of the left temporal lobe agenesis. An inspection of Figure 3-5 reveals that the anterior two-thirds of the left temporal lobe failed to develop. Despite the extent of

Table 3-1
Summary of Psychological Test Results of a
Patient With Left Temporal Lobe Agenesis
            (Chronological Age = 9 years)

Test	Score
WISC-R* Verbal Scale IQ	121
WISC-R Performance Scale IQ	134
WISC-R Full-Scale IQ	129
Northwestern Syntax Test—Receptive	1st percentile
Northwestern Syntax—Expressive	50th percentile
Auditory Attention Span for Unrelated Words (Detroit)	Mental age = 5.9

Reprinted from Pirozzolo, FJ, & Horner, FA. *Auditory-memory and linguistic deficits in left temporal lobe agenesis: Evidence for linguistic specialization of the left hemisphere* (in press). With permission.
*Wechsler Intelligence Scale for Children—Revised

the agenesis, he still achieved a verbal IQ of 121, which was more than adequate to project success in most academic endeavors. While his verbal-expressive abilities seemed reasonably well preserved, he did demonstrate significant difficulty in receptive syntactical skills. Specifically, he experienced trouble in comprehending permuted sentences, in replacing missing pronouns, and in recognizing correct sentences that were semantically and grammatically anomalous (e.g., "my favorite desert is radios and cream" or "the best cars in Canada are Fords and Datsuns").

Unfortunately, Pirozzolo and Horner (in press) were unable to report the results of Wada testing or some other direct measure of functional cerebral lateralization. Consequently, it is unknown whether language abilities had actually shifted to the right cerebral hemisphere. Whether they had is a moot point perhaps because, as the authors note, the results are consistent with those observed in young children who have undergone left hemispherectomy. The point is that even in this rather remarkable case in which above average expressive ability was present (an ability not subserved by the temporal lobe), the agenesis of the temporal lobe resulted in auditory comprehension deficits of a rather severe nature. Frankly, this result would be expected, based on our knowledge of functional neuropsychology.

What then is the bottom line insofar as the agenesis literature is concerned with regard to plasticity and brain function? It should seem evident that in the vast majority of cases either gross or, at least, subtle neurologic and/or psychologic deficits accompany the agenesis. Whether the functions affected by the agenesis are subserved by homologous regions in the opposite cerebral cortex, in adjacent cortical areas, or by other commissural or subcortical tracts, neurologic deficits are more the rule than the exception. In some respects it might be difficult to see how this relates to a volume on dyslexia. It does, however, when one considers that some still argue that the mechansim of plasticity is absolute, and therefore the equipotential nature of the brain will allow for recovery of lost or delayed function (Sandoval & Haapanen, 1981). The fact that almost any anomaly in the development of higher cortical structure will result in predictable or, at least, understandable functional deficits should have obvious implications to any remedial-reading teacher or psychologist. When one considers the number of brain structures related to the functional system of reading, it seems reasonable to expect that there exists a high probability that any area that fails to develop normally could very well affect the reading process.

The agenesis literature suggests that other areas of brain not "targeted" to subserve some specified function do so in a less-efficient manner, even when allowed to take over such function from birth. The research on brain-damaged children may provide a different perspective on the recovery of lost functions. While it would be expected that cases of trauma result in more severe deficit, the fact that the trauma is induced allows us to examine the age of trauma and its relationship to the recovery of lost function.

Brain Damage in Children

It is important to study the effects of brain trauma in children for a variety of reasons. First and foremost, it should be obvious that if we can identify the causes of brain damage we can perhaps, in some fashion, control or reduce the factors associated with its occurrence. It has been estimated that in any one year at least one million children incur some type of head injury (Young, 1969). To reduce this number by even 10 percent would certainly be a significant achievement and our study of its etiology may someday achieve this goal.

From a theoretical standpoint, it is important to examine the effects of brain trauma in children. As has been proposed, some agree that deficits arising from acquired brain damage mimic those found in developmental dyslexia (Aaron et al., 1980). Rudel (1978) has so aptly stated that

> It is apparent, however, that the concomitants of dyslexia are virtually the same whether they appear as the result of an acquired lesion or as a developmental deficit of unknown origin. The functional requirements for reading are, after all, identical in the child or the adult and correlative deficits are therefore similar in the developmental or acquired condition. (p. 298)

It is important to develop an understanding of the effects of acquired disorders and the mechanisms for possible recovery of function if we are to comprehend the effects of developmental disorders such as dyslexia. Another reason it is important to study the effects of head injury in children is that many believe that the course of recovery and residual effects are different than in adults. As an example, it is usually accepted that children have a higher likelihood of survival from severe head trauma (Carlsson, Von Essen, & Löfgren, 1968; Schurr, 1979). It is also widely held that the effects of head injuries are less severe in young children than in adults (Heiskanen & Sipponen, 1970; Schurr, 1979). These facts alone argue for important neurodevelopmental considerations in constructing theoretical paradigms for brain-behavior relationships in children. Finally, we can justify the study of brain injury in children on the grounds that such a study will enable us to differentiate those factors that predict recovery-rate curves. Only in this way can we as professionals make intelligent decisions regarding the necessary course of rehabilitation and learn to predict, with at least minimal accuracy, long-term prognosis.

The Nature of Head Injury in Children

In many respects, trauma to the head in children will result in different patterns of injury than in the adult. One of the most important variables in determining the extent of head injury in children is the extent of plasticity of the young child's skull. In very young children in whom the sutures have not yet fused together, the skull has the capacity to expand as the result of intracranial pressure. For this reason alone, fractures are usually rare in the youngest of children (Schurr, 1979).

One study examined 3000 hospital admissions in the greater Boston area and found a significant percentage (34 percent) of children were suffering a concussion and other minor cerebral contusions. Simple skull fractures accounted for 26 percent of the head-injured group. Subdural hematomas were found in 18.3 percent of the children, while depressed fractures were found in only approximately 10 percent. Although the effects of mild head trauma may be minimal and not manifest itself until later developmental plateaus are expected to be achieved, severe head trauma often results in predictable patterns of both behavioral and cognitive deficit. The degree or significance of the deficit varies according to the age at admission and other important predictive factors, such as length of unconsciousness and obvious neurologic aftereffects (Schurr, 1979).

It is widely believed, for example, that at birth both cerebral hemispheres have the capacity to subserve most cognitive-behavioral functions. If severe damage occurs to the left cerebral hemisphere, which has been predisposed for language, then the less efficient but none-the-less-able right cerebral hemisphere will assume the language function. As proof in point that both hemispheres have the capacity to subserve language, Alajouanine and Lhermitte (1965) argue that right- or left-hemisphere damage at an early age will produce speech and language deficits. As the left hemisphere exerts its ever increasing suppressive effect over right-hemisphere language functions, however, this phenomena disappears. From approximately five to seven years of age, left-hemisphere damage will result in aphasia while right-sided damage will usually not (Lenneberg, 1967).

This finding with brain-damaged children is consistent with what we know about feral children or about children who have been raised in severely deprived environments. If these children are identified prior to their eighth or ninth year, there exists a reasonable chance of at least some language development. After age ten or so, however, any hope of reversing the effects of the deprivation is almost nonexistent (Fromkin, Krashens, Rigler, & Rigler, 1974).

Based on this limited presentation, it would seem reasonable to hope that early damage or deprivation of one kind or another would leave a child with sufficient alternate pathways or compensatory cortical structures to accommodate any loss. There are, however, several problems with this notion because brain damage is not always as neat and as clear as one might conceptualize from reading the literature. While any young child may have the capacity to shift language dominance from one hemisphere to another, optimal levels of functioning via the right cerebral hemisphere assumes that no significant damage occurred in this region as a result of the injury. We know that it is often the case in children (or adults) with cerebral concussions that they suffer what are termed *contrecoup* concussions. When the head receives a blow, damage often occurs to the immediate cerebral cortex. Because the brain receives the force of the blow, however, it may well sustain damage to the opposite side as it bounces against the inside of the skull. The child consequently might evidence deficits associated with the neural substrata affected immediately by the blow as well as by the brain being forced onto the skull on the opposite side of the head (Hartlage & Reynolds, 1981).

It is also possible that the effects of head acceleration and abrupt deceleration can cause a torquing of the brain, thus breaking dendritic connections and resulting in subtle learning disorders. In fact, the effects of the subtle brain deficits may be more of an inhibitor to optimal cognitive recovery than a severe head trauma, which totally destroys part of the brain (Dreifuss, 1975; Kinsbourne, 1974; Rudel, 1978). When a functional system such as the one involved in reading is impaired because of several minor areas of dysfunction, the total system is affected. There is ample evidence, however, that if a young child has a left hemispherectomy, language abilities may well be subserved by other remaining cortical areas (Milner, 1974). This phenomena depends, of course, on the age of the child and one's definition of plasticity. Prior to discussing the more specific effects of brain injury on cognitive functioning and its relationship to age of insult, a brief primer on brain mechanisms associated with recovery of function is in order.

   The mechanism of neural plasticity. After any cerebral trauma, a number of physiological events take place and many have a direct bearing on the degree and rate of recovery. Conceptually, Kolb and Whishaw (1980) suggest that three phases follow brain injury: diaschisis, a period of initial recovery, and the phase of chronic disability. For our purposes in this section, we will consider the first two phases.

   In 1881 Munk proposed that when brain tissue was damaged, neural tissue not committed to a given function could assume the responsibility for the lost ability. Any damage which may have occurred could thus be recovered, much the same as a person on an assembly line could easily be replaced should something critical happen to his ability to carry out some important task.

   In 1911 Von Monakow proposed that when one area of the brain's tissue is damaged, not only is that area and its corresponding function disturbed but also are those areas that are connected or related to it. The performance of neural tissue related to that function is depressed temporarily. When recovery of function thus occurs it may actually represent a reemergence of the function of these heretofore depressed areas of the cortex. This process is termed diaschisis and probably occurs after injury because of shock triggered by edema (swelling). There are a number of excellent case studies available (Luria, 1972; Milner, 1975; Rosner, 1974) that serve to demonstrate the possible recovery of function due to diaschisis. Milner (1975), for instance, tested patients who experienced epilepsy prior to surgery. Over time, their IQs were stable, indicating that epilepsy did not affect their IQs. After surgery their IQs declined 10 to 15 points. However, one year postoperatively it returned to normal and in some cases actually increased 5 to 10 points. Did the epilepsy actually serve to depress cognitive ability? As Kolb and Whishaw (1980) suggest, it may be better to have no tissue than to have tissue which is malfunctioning. The main point, however, is that by one year postsurgery any swelling should have disappeared and the adjacent tissue is allowed to return to normal functioning.

   It is possible that the process of diaschisis occurs because of other factors. Kolb and Whishaw (1980) proposed that diaschisis could easily occur because of depressed neurotransmitter production, receptor changes, and variation in axon membrane potentials, to name only a few possibilities. Whatever the reason for diaschisis, it does occur and plays a major role in any discussion regarding recovery of function due to brain damage. Two identifiable periods of recovery of function exist. First, there is the recovery from diaschisis. This period of recovery is characterized by slow change in levels of cognitive ability. Overall, the order of recovery seems to be from lower-level functions toward the recovery of higher-order functions. Teitelbaum and Epstein (1962) suggested that the pattern of recovery parallels the original developmental sequence of the emergence of that function in infants or young children. Both clinical (Barbizet, 1970; Twitchell, 1965; Whitty & Zangwill, 1966) and experimental animal studies (Anand & Brobeck, 1951; Nathan & Smith, 1973; Teitelbaum & Stellar, 1954) support this notion.

A second period of recovery is thought to occur through the reorganization of surviving tissue as first proposed by Lashley (1929). Kolb and Whishaw (1980) suggest several mechanisms. First, regeneration is believed to occur where some connections may very well regrow. We know for a fact that this process can occur in the peripheral nervous system. It seems that the neurilemma develops, thus providing a tube for the axon to develop. There are many questions, however, regarding neural regeneration, especially since it appears not to occur in the central nervous system of adult mammals. It may be that the glial scar at the site of the lesion blocks regeneration. Lund (1978) notes that scar tissue is less impressive in young mammals and that growth may sometimes occur across a glial scar. It is also possible that regeneration can only occur if appropriate feedback from the terminal area exists to promote growth. Finally, it seems that damaged axons may sprout proximal to the lesion and its occupation of abnormal tissue prevents any future stimulus for regeneration (Lund, 1978). Despite these reasons for the failure of regeneration, exciting new developments are occurring and it may actually be possible someday to determine exactly the mechanism of neural regeneration (Björklund, Segal, & Stenevi, 1979; Kolata, 1982; Kromer, Björklund, & Stenevi, 1978; Marx, 1982).

A second mechanism observed during this period of recovery is neural sprouting in which other neurons send in branches to fill the void left by the tissue damaged. Although sprouting in the adjacent neural tissue appears to take place in the first seven to ten days after trauma, there is a question as to whether this sprouting of tissue is functionally useful (Kolb & Whishaw, 1980). Degeneration and disinhibition of compensatory cortical areas are also thought to occur during this second stage of functional recovery. There seems to be an interesting phenomenon that accompanies the mechanism of compensation. Woods and Teuber (1973) studied prenatal or early postnatal cases of brain damage to the left and right hemispheres. They found that language usually survived in cases of left-hemisphere damage, but it seemed to result in a "de-repression" of language areas in the right hemisphere. Many of the children, however, experienced a visual-spatial deficit. It seems that language has a priority and when it crowds right hemispheric visual-spatial functions, deficits in this latter area result. Conversely, when right-hemisphere lesions occur at an early age, visual-spatial functions are impaired as no shift of function to the left cerebral hemisphere occurs. These conclusions have received support from Rasmussen and Milner (1975). Furthermore, if this shift of language function does not occur prior to age five or so, any recovery of function is probably related to reorganization within the impaired left cerebral cortex (Smith, 1981). It is interesting to note that there may be slight variations in this pattern according to the sex of the child (Inglis & Lawson, 1981). What possible implications exist because of possible sex differences are however, unclear.

Now that we have some basic understanding as to the neural mechanics believed to serve as the foundation in recovery of lost function due to brain injury, we can turn our attention to other, more relevant matters. The following three sections will examine the literature as it pertains to general cognitive deficits associated with brain injury in children, recovery from aphasia, and, finally, recovery from acquired alexia. In considering the following evidence, it may be helpful to bear in mind the following quote from Kolb and Whishaw (1980).

> The use of such words as plasticity and the emphasis placed on recovery of function in a great deal of basic research gives the impression that the brain has an unlimited potential for recovery and reorganization after injury. Although there is a paucity of information available on long-term recovery, the available evidence indicates that there are always residual and permanent deficits, and that extensive recovery is the exception, not the rule. (p. 422)

General Cognitive Deficits Associated with Brain Injury

Considering all of the neural mechanisms involved in recovery from brain trauma, it is no wonder that such significant variation occurs on a case-to-case basis in recovery rates from seemingly similar brain lesions. The literature related to the study of age effects on recovery from brain insult is a varied one, indeed. Some investigators have examined age effects on lateralized lesions in children (McFie, 1961, 1975), the effects of age and EEG abnormalities (Fedio & Mirsky, 1969), and age effects in the abilities of hemispherectomy patients (Gott, 1973).

A recently published study by Chadwick, Rutter, Thompson, and Shaffer (1981) deserves special attention due to its sound and complete research design. These investigators sought to examine cognitive deficits and age effects in 97 children with open-head injuries. They argued that by employing children with open-head injuries, it was possible to more clearly specify the exact site of the trauma. Closed-head injuries, on the other hand, presented many problems for study since the locus and lateralization of the lesion (because of the contrecoup effect previously mentioned) is difficult to determine, the skull may act as a buffer displacing the force of the blow, and there is usually widespread cerebrovascular congestion. All of these factors work to confound any firm conclusions that may be drawn from investigations using children with closed-head injuries.

As is typical for head-injury populations, Chadwick, Rutter, Thompson, et al. (1981) found a disproportionate number of boys. The mean age of the entire population was five years, five months, at the time of head trauma. All of these children were evaluated after approximately five years had passed, and the resulting mean age at follow-up was 11 years, 10 months. Due to the long follow-up period, it would be expected that if recovery of function was to occur, it would have become well established at the time of the final evaluation.

In support of other studies, it was found that the likelihood and severity of cognitive deficit was positively associated with the degree of the resulting coma and posttraumatic amnesia. Also consistent with the notion that the immature brain can accommodate lost function more easily than the older brain, Chadwick, Rutter, Thompson, et al. (1981) found that there were "no significant differences in scores on any of the intelligence tests between those with left-sided and those with right-sided lesions" (p. 131). There was, however, a consistent if slight trend for academic dysfunction to be associated with left-hemisphere lesions. In fact, 8 of the 12 children (67.7 percent) who were under 5-years-old at the time of their injury experienced difficulty in learning to read. None of the children aged five and over at the time of insult, however, suffered reading difficulties. This important finding suggests that brain insult results in deficits in learning new material and may affect the more well-established abilities less severely. This finding was the only significant age effect and the authors concluded that, as a whole, cognitive deficits typically associated with lateralized function seem to be less specific in children than in adults. The major effect, consequently, in predicting later deficits appeared to be manifested in factors associated with the severity of head trauma (i.e., coma, amnesia, etc.) rather than the age of the child or the lateralized nature of the trauma.

The case against specific cognitive deficits associated with brain damage may rest on the nature of the trauma. For example, Chadwick, Rutter, Thompson, et al. (1981) utilized children with very discretely defined hemispheric lesions and found no relationship to cognitive deficits. The failure to find the expected pattern of deficit, as found in adults, may relate to the nature of the defined population.

In a study published the same year, Chadwick, Rutter, Shaffer, and Shrout (1981) examined cognitive deficits in children with generalized brain trauma. Twenty-eight such children, who suffered a posttraumatic amensia (PTA) of more than one week but less than three months, were followed up at four months after injury; at one year; and at two years, three months. A closely-matched normal control group was also examined. After one year of recovery, the 10.3 point deficit in VSIQ noted at the initial assessment had all but disappeared. The 30.2 point PSIQ deficit only returned to an 11.5 point deficit. At the one year, three months assessment, the deficits in

PSIQ remained as did also difficulties on a manual dexterity and copying task.

What conclusions can be drawn from these studies that support those reported by other authors using both children and adults (Black, Jeffries, Blumer, Wellner, & Walker, 1969; Boll, 1974; Bond, 1975; Brink, Garrett, Hale, Woo-Sam, & Nickel, 1970; Klonoff & Low, 1974; Klonoff, Low, & Clark, 1977)? First, brain trauma of any nature, whether highly localized or diffuse, will probably result in cognitive deficit of some kind. Effects of highly localized brain injury seem to be less severe than generalized brain trauma. Finally, some deficits may only manifest themselves on tasks requiring new learning ability not tapped previously but nonetheless dysfunctional due to the cerebral insult. In summation, one would have to agree with Rudel's (1978) conclusion that the effects of damage may appear early and disappear, will be seen at all age levels regardless of the age at which the lesion was acquired, and will manifest itself only when developmentally prominent abilities (i.e., reading) are called on.

Recovery From Aphasia and Alexia

Now that we have a reasonable understanding as to the effects of brain damage on cognitive performance, it may be appropriate to examine a bit more closely what the literature suggests about recovery from aphasia and alexia. In addition to Broca's and Wernicke's aphasia, other types of aphasic conditions include conduction, global, transcortical motor, transcortical sensory, and anomic aphasia. All of the aphasias have characteristic language deficits and a thorough evaluation of fluency, repetition comprehension, and naming will suffice in making a clinical diagnosis (Ross, 1980). A discussion of the six other types of aphasia other than Broca's and Wernicke's is beyond the scope of this chapter; if the reader is interested he should consult Benson (1979) or Ross (1980) for excellent discussions on this topic.

Alexia is often seen as an accompanying symptom of aphasia or aphasia-like disorders. It does, however, appear as an isolated symptom of brain damage. Two types of alexia due to brain damage can usually be identified. Alexia with agraphia can usually be traced to a lesion in the left cerebral hemisphere in the region of the angular gyrus (Fig. 3-6, No. 1). As the angular gyrus borders on the speech areas, it is common to find a mild anomia and an accompanying Gertsmann syndrome. Spelling and arithmetic will probably be severely affected. While verbal comprehension is still intact, this patient cannot read nor write. Alexia without agraphia usually is related to a lesion involving the splenium (the posterior portion of the corpus callosum) and the left medial aspect of the occipital lobe, as depicted in the lesion in Figure 3-6, Number 2.

Alexia without agraphia produces a right hemianopsia due to the in-

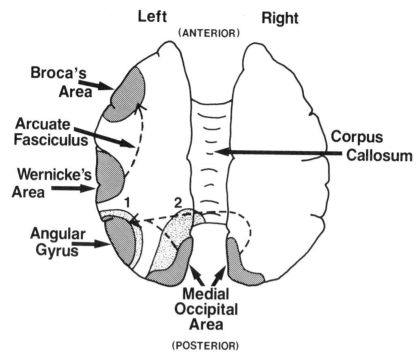

Fig. 3-6. The brain as viewed in horizontal section. The lesions thought to cause alexia with agraphia (1) and alexia without agraphia (2) are shaded and numbered.

volvement of the primary visual cortex. The lesion actually serves to disconnect the visual cortex from the angular gyrus. Since no damage is done to the motor areas or the speech and language centers, the patient can copy well or even write spontaneously but cannot read the material.

It is important to understand that the disorders discussed in this section are acquired disorders but are, nonetheless, mimicked by the syndrome of developmental dyslexia. We shall see in a later section that developmental dyslexics share many of the features of the aphasic or the alexic but also have many unique or more generalized deficits. This factor alone suggests that developmental dyslexics suffer from more than specific lesions and demonstrate a pattern consistent with either multiple lesion sites or generalized impairment. Before addressing this research, we need to have some understanding of the aphasia and alexia recovery literature.

Much of our data base for the recovery literature regarding aphasia comes from soldiers who suffered penetrating head wounds and were followed after World War II (Goldstein, 1948; Newcombe, 1969; Wepman, 1951). As in the literature dealing with generalized brain injury, it seems as though there is agreement that the younger the subject, the less the actual impairment, and the more rapid the recovery. This is a conclusion usually agreed on, although some evidence exists to the contrary (Culton, 1969; Mahut & Zola, 1977; Sarno, Sarno, & Levita, 1971; Schneider, 1979).

Most of the improvement in language abilities seems to occur (perhaps up to 90 percent) within the first nine months after brain injury. The most significant period within this nine months seems to be the first 30 days. Whatever the eventual rate or level of recovery is to be very likely can be predicted from the degree of recovery evidenced in the first 30 days (Culton, 1969). There is some controversy as to whether expressive (Broca's) or receptive (Wernicke's) language abilities recover more rapidly, and evidence seems to exist to support either position (Butfield & Zangwill, 1945; Cummings, Benson, Walsh, & Levine, 1979; Mohr, 1973; Vignolo, 1964; Weisenburg & McBride, 1935). Cummings et al. (1979) make an interesting point that whatever recovery does take place may be more a result of a releasing of right cerebral hemisphere language abilities than due to any other factor. It can also be said with some certainty that traumatic aphasics will fare better in recovery than those who suffer aphasia due to cerebrovascular accidents (Kertesz & McCabe, 1977; Luria, 1970).

In 1964 Vignolo published the first study that compared a group of subjects who received language therapy with those who did not. No significant differences between groups were found. Sarno et al. (1971) found similar results. As in many areas of neuropsychology, however, evidence seems to exist to the contrary that shows that treatment is effective, especially when it is individualized (Basso, Capitani, & Vignolo, 1979; Woertz, Collins, Brookshire, Friden, Kurtzke, Pierce, & Weiss, 1978). Writing abilities seem to emerge from the literature as that ability most amenable to treatment effects. From all of this, however, it is clear that no case of aphasia has ever returned to pretrauma levels of functioning.

Many early cases exist describing cases of alexia (Bastian, 1898; Charcot, 1877, 1889; Franz, 1918; Goldstein, 1942; Paterson & Bramwell, 1905). In some respects, alexia presents a more complex problem for study since the process of reading is the result of a variety of brain functions, any one of which could produce the disorder (Gardner, Denes & Zurif, 1975; Pirozzolo & Kerr, 1981). Despite this fact, and possibly because of it, the alexia literature is equally as confusing as the aphasia literature, although in both, recovery never seems to return to premorbid levels (Gardner & Zurif, 1975; Kapur & Perl, 1978; Kurachi, Yamaguchi, Inasaka, & Torii, 1979; Newcombe, 1969; Newcombe & Marshall, 1973; Wechsler, 1972; Wechsler, Weinstein, & Antin, 1972). To gain a better understanding of the literature regarding recovery from alexia, it might be helpful to examine a couple of studies: one with adults and one with a child.

Newcombe, Marshall, Carrivick, & Hiorns (1974) qualitatively examined the improvement in reading in three patients with acquired alexia. The patients all originally suffered aphasia due to trauma but the reading difficulties persisted long after the speech abilities returned to their optimal level of recovery. These investigators make note that very few studies have ever addressed the pattern of recovery in acquired alexia. Although several such studies do exist (Ajax, 1967; Denckla & Bowen, 1973), it is indeed surprising how few exist, especially when one considers the considerable literature on acquired aphasia.

Based on studies that have indicated that the greatest percentage of recovery of function will occur between two to three months after trauma (Butfield & Zangwill, 1945; Head, 1926), Newcombe, et al. (1974) proposed that recovery from acquired alexia would also follow this pattern of recovery with some significant improvement being noted over a long course posttrauma. They studied three patients. The first patient was operated on for a large cranial abscess in the left occipital lobe at the age of 41 years. Three months after the operation she was discharged with a persistent right homonymous hemianopsia. A slight right hemiparesis cleared over the course of recovery. A month after the operation she could not read or name letters. Three months later, however, she could call all of the letters of the alphabet but still could not read. The second and third patients studied included two 17-year-old men who had suffered closed-head injuries due to traffic accidents.

To examine the effects of recovery on the acquired alexia, Newcombe, et al., (1974) constructed two lists: one consisted of 40 CVC (consonant-vowel-consonant) words, including 20 nouns and 20 verbs; the second list consisted of 60 words of four to seven letters comprising 20 nouns, verbs, and adjectives. No training was given and the subjects were simply told the lists that they were to read were designed to measure progress. The first patient was followed for 166 weeks (41.5 months) and the other two for 14 and 17 months, respectively. The plotted rates of repeated performance by the patients on these two lists indicated a dramatic reduction in the number of errors over the period of time assessed. In the first patient, the most dramatic recovery rate was observed in that, on the second list of words, her number of word-calling errors at 20 weeks postoperatively fell from approximately 60 percent to approximately 10 percent.

Any study such as this would be sure to make an experimental psychologist or remedial-reading teacher question the results. Although the results are interesting, the effects of practice alone confound any possible conclusions. The greatest problem, however, is that presumably the subjects were fluent readers before their brain insult and have now recovered some limited word-recognition abilities over a one- to three-year period. As these authors (Newcombe, et al., 1974) modestly suggest, "this preliminary approach to the study of recovery is limited to performance in experimental tasks. It does not consider the relationships between test performance and functional efficiency in everyday life" (p. 132). This is a considerable understatement. All that can be reasonably concluded from this all-too-typical study is that on repeated tasks using the same-word stimuli word recognition, errors do show a decline over time; with maximum recovery, as minimally measured here, occurring within approximately the first 20 weeks.

Levine, Hier, and Calvanio (1981) offer us a much better case study of recovery from learning and reading deficits due to brain injury in a young child followed for several decades. Levine et al. (1981) proposed that in the general population of disabled readers only a relatively few have had a history of brain injury (Ingram, Mason, & Blackburn, 1970; Rutter & Yule, 1975). They suggestd that children who have identifiable brain injury with resulting impairment in reading may offer important clues as to the neuropsychological basis for reading disabilities. These investigators presented a case study that met four criteria: the typography of the cerebral lesion was known, the age at which the lesion occurred was known, it was possible to determine correlated deficits in perception, language, and memory, and the extent to which reorganization in neuronal activity contributed to later functional recovery could be estimated.

Their subject appeared normal until five years, eight months of age, at which time he developed nighttime spells of screaming, stiffening of the arms and pallor. Bifrontal headaches were also reported. Admitted to the hospital five months later with his first clonic seizure, he was examined both medically and psychologically. The medical examination was essentially normal except for bilateral retinal hemorrhages. Psychological evaluation suggested impoverished comprehension and a Stanford-Binet IQ of 88. Electroencephalographic (EEG) testing revealed slowing in the left anterior temporal region, and a ventriculogram indicated a left temporal lobe mass. A craniotomy was performed in the frontotemporal region and 26 ml of blood was withdrawn from the anterior region of the left temporal lobe. At age seven years, eight months, the left anterior portion of the temporal lobe was removed to aid in controlling seizures.

As would be expected, postoperatively the child was experiencing word-finding difficulties and his verbal IQ on the WISC had dropped to 60. Three months later he was again given the WISC and his verbal IQ had risen to 75. After the lobectomy, his performance IQ was 79, and after three months it had risen to 90. School proved to be a problem, and he left the public schools at age 13 years, but continued to receive remedial assistance in reading until age 24 years. Those remedial courses were usually not of benefit. Seizures continued to be controlled through the use of primidone and phenytoin. Further evaluation at 17 years of age using the Wada technique revealed essentially no language abilities of the intact right cerebral hemisphere; and evaluation at age 31 years, using a CT scan confirmed that the site of the lesion was restricted to the left temporal region.

The uniqueness of this study, and for its detailed report here, is that at age 33 years, the patient was administered a complete neuropsychological evaluation. This degree of long-term follow-up is very unique in the literature. It well represents an attempt to study the mechanism of neural plasticity and the associated long-term rate of recovery. Although it is impossible to determine premorbid levels of functioning, the fact that he spoke at 9 months of age and walked at 12 months suggests at least normal development of linguistic and psychomotor abilities. His scaled score on the Block Design subtest of the WISC/WAIS, furthermore, did not vary significantly over the 24-year period in which he was evaluated. This score was always measured to be in the normal range. This is an important finding because it suggests that had he not experienced the circumscribed lesion due to his operation, the likelihood of normal reading achievement would have been good. Any differences or changes in verbal-linguistic abilities as measured by the WISC/WAIS verbal scale subtests, or changes in IQ, should consequently reflect the recovery of function after his craniotomy.

Over the 24-year follow-up his vocabulary subtest score (it correlates highest with verbal scale IQ) rose from zero to five (10 = average), with his verbal scale IQ ranging from a high of 75 down to 70. This level of performance places his verbal-linguistic skills in the borderline range. As would be hypothesized, he experienced a complete inability to learn to read or write, despite consistently intense assistance over a long period of time. Apparently his best achievement over the follow-up period consisted of naming only a few printed words. Typically, he could not name with any degree of accuracy all of the letters of the alphabet.

The most important point to be made here is that in a strict sense his deficit in verbal-linguistic learning cannot be considered dyslexia since he had never learned to read or write preoperatively with any degree of skill. As Levine et al. (1981) note, abilities that are mastered before deficit usually reemerge after the initial trauma of the operation. However, emerging skills or abilities such as the patient's early reading abilities seem most severely affected. Also, the results of the Wada testing and application of dichotic listening and visual half-field procedures showed that no shifting of speech or language mechanisms ever occurred. This result is consistent with Rasmussen and Milner (1977) and others cited previously who suggest that the transfer of linguistic function to the opposite (in this case, right) hemisphere rarely occurs after the preschool years. Finally the obvious parallel between the neuropsychological performance of this subject and that of dyslexic children suffering verbal-linguistic dyslexia cannot be ignored. The authors note that similar auditory-verbal and visual-verbal processing may also be present in this subgroup of dyslexic children. As will be seen in Chapter 6, such speculation has an excellent foundation and merits more in-depth consideration later in this volume. Levine et al., (1981) summarize their conclusions in this important case study by stating:

> The occurence of this pattern of deficits after left temporal lobe damage should draw attention to this region as a possible site of dysfunction in children with

developmental dyslexia. Although gross temporal lobe damage is unlikely in most children with developmental dyslexia, there may be more subtle lesions, or there may be anomalies of development that result in adverse left-right anatomic asymmetries of the brain. Therefore, developmental dyslexia of this type may result from malfunction of a hemisphere with well-developed language dominance—not from delayed or weak hemispheric lateralization of language. Such dyslexic patients should show the normal pattern of ear and visual field asymmetries in auditory and visual span tasks. The magnitude of the asymmetries may be even greater than normal, and Wada tests should show well-lateralized speech. (p. 263. With permission.)

This rather lengthy quote has been cited because it stands out as exceptionally important both in terms of serving as a conclusion for this well-done study and as a guidepost for the remainder of this chapter. Three possible statements may be generated from this quote that are supported by research in other related areas.

The easiest statement to address is the notion that children with learning or reading deficits are normal in their lateralization of cerebral function. Although Chapter 5 addresses this important topic in considerable detail, it can be stated at this point that a variety of studies have examined the hypothesis of Levine et al. (1981). Contrary to the ideas of Orton (1937) and those who supported his model of delayed lateralization, the more current literature indicates that reading- and learning-disabled children are, in fact, similarly lateralized as their normal counterparts. Studies consistently show that the left hemisphere is prepotent for language abilities (Hynd & Obrzut, 1981), and in some cases the disabled children even outperformed the matched normals (Hynd, Obrzut, & Obrzut, 1981) as suggested by Levine et al. (1981).

Two other statements seem to arise from the conclusions of Levine et al. (1981): some dyslexic children may show reversed left-right anatomic asymmetries, and some dyslexic children may suffer subtle lesions in neurological development that result in the psycholinguistic deficits associated with this disorder. So that these ideas can be more fully explored, the following sections will be devoted to expanding on these important ideas about neurological development and functioning in dyslexic children.

NEURODEVELOPMENTAL ASYMMETRIES IN DYSLEXIC BRAINS

Based on the seminal work of Geschwind and Levitsky (1968), who found that the area roughly equivalent to Wernicke's area was larger on the left than on the right cerebral hemisphere, Hier, LeMay, Rosenberger, and Perlo (1978) suggested that such an obvious asymmetry may have functional

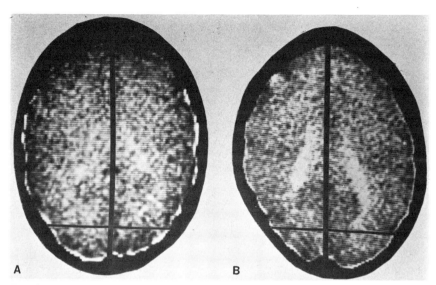

Fig. 3-7. Computerized brain tomograms of two dyslexic patients. Both transaxial sections are at the level of the bodies of the lateral ventricles. The heavy black stripe lies vertically along the interhemispheric fissure; the thin black stripe lies horizontally across the posterior parietooccipital region. (A) Brain at left (Table 3-2, case 18) shows the common pattern of cerebral asymmetry with the wider left parietooccipital region. (B)   Brain at right (case 4) shows a marked reversal of usual cerebral asymmetry with a wider right parietooccipital region. [From Hier, DB, LeMay, M, Rosenberger, PB, & Perlo, VP. Developmental dyslexia: Evidence for a subgroup with a reversal of cerebral asymmetry. *Archives of Neurology*, 1978, *35*, 90–92. Copyright 1978, American Medical Association, reprinted with permission.]

correlates. By being so enlarged, the left planum temporale may serve as a logical anatomical substrata for linguistic competence. The fact that such asymmetries are observed both in prenatal and newborn brains (Chi, Dooling, & Gilles, 1977; Wada, Clarke, & Hamm, 1975; Witelson & Pallie, 1973) suggests that language functions are indeed preordained to be lateralized to the left temporal region. Hier et al. (1978) hypothesized that some forms of dyslexia may be related to a reversal of this normal pattern of anatomical development.

Incorporating 24 developmental dyslexics ranging in age from 14 through 47 (mean age was 25), CT scans were obtained so that this hypothesis could be evaluated. The relative widths of the two cerebral hemispheres were evaluated by drawing a midline down the interhemispheric fissure and by measuring the symmetry of the left and right parietooccipital regions (Fig. 3-7).

The results of this assessment first confirmed that all patients had not

Table 3-2
Clinical and Radiological Data From 24 Dyslexic Patients

Patient	Sex	Age	Handed-ness	Reading Level*	IQ Verbal	IQ Performance	Widths of Parieto-Occipital Regions	Delayed Speech ‡
1	M	21	R	HX†	113	116	R>L	Yes
2	F	33	R	1.6	74	94	R>L	Yes
3	M	30	R	1.9	97	99	R>L	No
4	M	17	R	2.8	71	83	R>L	Yes
5	M	40	R	4.2	91	100	R>L	No
6	M	18	R	HX	74	97	R>L	No
7	M	16	R	3.2	88	95	R>L	No
8	M	14	L	HX	95	104	R>L	Yes
9	M	17	L	HX	94	86	R>L	No
10	M	31	L	0.0	76	82	R>L	No
11	M	22	R	2.8	94	107	R=L	No
12	M	30	R	HX	110	118	R=L	No
13	F	35	R	HX	84	98	R=L	No
14	M	45	R	0.0	93	99	R=L	No
15	M	20	R	HX	124	106	R=L	No
16	M	35	R	HX	88	93	R=L	No
17	M	47	R	HX	105	109	R<L	No
18	M	22	R	1.9	93	109	R<L	No
19	M	22	R	0.0	92	98	R<L	Yes
20	M	24	R	4.4	99	97	R<L	No
21	M	17	R	HX	114	102	R<L	No
22	M	28	L	HX	105	118	R<L	No
23	M	17	L	HX	103	120	R<L	No
24	M	43	L	0.0	91	75	R<L	No

Reprinted from Hier, DB, LeMay, M, Rosenberger, PB, & Perlo, VP. Developmental dyslexia: Evidence for a subgroup with a reversal of cerebral asymmetry. *Archives of Neurology,* 1978, *35,* 90–92. Copyright 1978, American Medical Association, reprinted with permission.
* Grade level equivalent as determined by the Gray Oral Reading Test. † HX indicates patients who scored above 5.0 but who read at least two grades below grade level while in school. A score of 0.0 indicates a nonreader. ‡ Onset of speech in phases after age three years.

suffered any neurological insult to the brain, and thus the subjects could truly be considered as developmental dyslexic. As can be seen in Table 3-2, ten patients demonstrated that the right parietooccipital area was wider than the same area on the left. Fourteen patients had the more normal pattern of the left parietooccipital region being significantly larger than the homologous area on the right (see Table 3-3). Interestingly, and supportive of what we know about the application of psychometric assessment proce-

Table 3-3
Intelligence Test Scores According to Pattern
of Cerebral Asymmetry

Asymmetry	No. of Patients	Mean IQ (± SD)	
		Verbal	Performance
Right parietoccipital region wider than left	10	87 ± 13*	96 ± 10
Left parietoccipital region wider than or equal to right	14	99 ± 11*	103 ± 12

Reprinted from Hier, DB, LeMay, M, Rosenberger, PB, & Perlo, VP. Developmental dyslexia: Evidence for a subgroup with a reversal of cerebral asymmetry. *Archives of Neurology,* 1978, *35,* 90–92. Copyright 1978, American Medical Association, reprinted with permission.
*Difference is significant ($p < .01$).

dures to neurological fuctioning, the verbal IQ of patients with the atypical pattern of hemispheric asymmetry was significantly less ($p<.01$) than that group with the normal asymmetry. The performance IQ did not vary significantly ($p<.05$) between these groups. Of the patients with reversed asymmetry, 40 percent reported delays in speech acquisition while only 7 percent did in the group with normal asymmetry.

As Hier et al. (1978) noted, only approximately 9 percent of most normal right-handed people and 27 percent of left-handed people have this pattern of reversed asymmetry found in this sample of dyslexics. The authors suggest that the lower verbal-scale IQ found in the group with atypical asymmetry may result in a disruption between the normal correlates of structural and functional asymmetry. Most right-handed people have a correspondingly enlarged left parietoccipital region, whereas this reversed asymmetry group did not. It is suggested by Hier et al. (1978) that this pattern of reversed asymmetry reflects a "mismatch between hemispheric specialization for language and structural asymmetry of the hemispheres" (p. 92). They also conclude that the pattern of reversed asymmetry by itself does not result in dyslexia but rather (like gender and other risk factors) acts as a potential contributor to the condition should other factors (e.g., family history) predispose the child to dyslexia. This is a strong statement since, according to their results, children with this reversed cerebral asymmetry would have approximately five times the potential to be dyslexic when compared with a child with the normal pattern of cerebral hemispheric asymmetry.

This study is important in that it provides anatomical evidence in a group of developmental dyslexics that a deviant pattern of neurological organization may be related to at least one subtype of dyslexia. It may well be that in those dyslexics who suffer significantly depressed verbal skills relative to even the normal population of dyslexic children, an atypical neurodevelopmental organization of the brain may exist. This is in keeping with the conclusions of Levine et al. (1981) and may help explain why those children with mild verbal-performance discrepancies have correlated mild reading deficits while a smaller subgroup has severe discrepancies in verbal and performance skills. Although it would have been desirable, as in the Pirozzolo and Horner (in press) case, if Hier et al. (1978) had conclusively determined language dominance using either the Wada, the dichotic listening, or the visual half-field procedures, as well as competence in a subset of reading abilities, their study nonetheless is vital in demonstrating a correlation between a functional disability (i.e., reading) and neurodevelopmental organization.

In a follow-up study, Rosenberger and Hier (1980) examined verbal abilities in a population of 53 learning-disabled children and reported a 42 percent incidence rate for reversed cerebral asymmetries. While the evidence seems convincing that cerebral asymmetries may be related to functional problems in reading and learning, some limited evidence exists that suggests caution in interpreting these results (Haslam et al., 1981).

It will be recalled that Levine et al. (1981) also suggested that subtle lesions may be at the foundation of developmental dyslexia. Throughout this chapter it has been suggested that this may indeed be the case and it is now time to evaluate the related literature. Two sets of evidence will be presented in support of this notion. First, the focus of the discussion will be on the electrophysiological evidence. Second, the only two autopsy cases available on the brains of dyslexics will be presented.

EEG CORRELATES IN DYSLEXIA (BEAM)

Although EEG abnormalities are not in and of themselves pathological since they seem to occur in "normal" children with no learning or reading disabilities (Bryant & Friedlander, 1965; Cohn, 1961), they do seem to occur more frequently in children with reading problems (Ayers & Torres, 1967; Hughes, 1968; Hughes, Leander & Ketchum, 1949; Muehl, Knott, & Benton, 1965). As Pirozzolo and Hansch (1982) note, it is disappointing that despite general slowing usually being noted in the posterior region, no correlation exists between EEG abnormalities and the degree of reading retardation.

The confusing state of affairs in the area of electroencephalographic research with dyslexia may be undergoing a change as investigators have begun to utilize EEG power-spectrum analysis in varying frequency domains (Ahn, Prichep, John, Baird, Trepetin, & Kaye, 1980). The brain electrical activity mapping (BEAM) procedure developed by Duffy and his co-investigators offers new insights into the regional differences in brain electrical activity in dyslexic children.

In a series of studies these investigators evaluated the utility of an analysis of between electrode values from brain electrical activity (Duffy, 1981; Duffy, Burchfiel, & Lombroso, 1979; Duffy, Denckla, Bartels, & Sandini, 1980a; Duffy, Denckla, Bartels, Sandini, & Kiessling, 1980b). Operating on the assumption that EEG and evoked potential (EP) analysis present too much data to be easily understood, they sought to display values on a computer-driven color video screen, thus providing maps of regional differences in electrical activity in dyslexic children.

In an early study, Duffy et al. (1979) examined the BEAM spectral plot for three dyslexics who had no history of neurological difficulties. In addition to the EEG analysis, EP studies were also conducted with the adolescent dyslexics. A standard analysis of the EEG and EP data showed no atypical patterns at rest. When the dyslexic subjects were required to attend to speech, which should activate the left cerebral hemisphere, alpha dysyncronasion was not noted. This is important because when a given area of the brain is activated, the percentage of alpha (band of electrical activity indicating an alert but passive cognitive state) should decrease rather dramatically. The failure to find a suppression of alpha activity over the left parietal lobe during a linguistic task would add support to the notion that the region of the angular gyrus is important in reading disability.

The results of this preliminary study were intriguing and suggested that the BEAM procedure had clinical utility not only with dyslexics but also with tumor patients and those suffering psychopathic personality disturbances. In their conclusions the authors recommend the BEAM procedure for both clinical and experimental purposes, noting that the computation time by computer to generate a topographic map was only four seconds. The entire assessment procedure took less than 15 minutes per patient. The investment in terms of equipment and technical time seemed to be minimal and the procedure did seem viable for further study.

It was the follow-up investigation of Duffy et al. (1980a) that is of major importance to the present volume. Proposing that EEG data using the BEAM technique can be valuable in the study of dyslexia because it can localize brain activity that characterizes these children, and can provide for a culturally less-biased criteria for clinical diagnosis, Duffy et al. (1980a) studied eight dyslexics using this procedure. They chose to differentiate between "dyslexia-pure" and "dyslexia-plus" as proposed by Hughes and Denckla (1978). Consequently, subjects were omitted who evidenced the dyslexia plus other common behavioral manifestations (e.g., hyperactivity, math difficulties, motor deficits, etc.). In addition to receiving a negative neurological examination, none of the subjects had a history of psychopathology. Oral reading scores were at least 1.5 years below their expectancy level and all were males with IQs ranging from 94 to 114. A closely matched population of normal control children were selected, representing a socioeconomic level similar to that of the dyslexic children.

EEG data was collected using standard electrodes in the international 10–20 format. Ten different conditions of approximately three minutes each were used. The conditions were designed such that several were expected to activate the left hemisphere, as they were linguistic in nature; others were designed to activate the right cerebral hemisphere using music or spatial stimuli; while still other stimuli were designed to involve both cerebral hemispheres (e.g., paired visual-verbal associations). Three additional EP conditions were also included in the experimental procedures. Mean image matrices from each EEG and EP conditions were developed for the dyslexics and their matched controls, and significant differences were then computed using a t statistic. A percentage index was then computed and a color topographic map was constructed with each color representing a specific percentage index value.

The maps revealed that the dyslexics evidenced less state-alpha–dependent activity distributions than the normals who showed more variation in state-alpha distributions. Predictably, differences between the controls and the dyslexics were evidenced on every state-dependent condition. Most importantly, the areas of greatest difference were observed in the supplementary motor area (bilateral medial frontal zone), Broca's area, the left temporal region, and an area roughly equivalent to Wernicke's area, the parietal and visual association areas. This latter area would incorporate the cortex of the angular gyrus (Color Plate 3-1).

Based on our understanding of the brain, as outlined in Chapter 2, and of the neuropsychological aspects of language as discussed previously in this chapter, it seems a safe conclusion to state that at least three of the four areas noted above are critical to the language and, presumably, the reading process in dyslexic children. As Duffy et al. (1980a) state:

> So the regions that we have shown to differ electrophysiologically between the brains of dyslexic and normal boys appear to be among the regions normally involved in speech and reading. Thus, dyslexia-pure may represent dysfunction within a complex and widely distributed system, not a discrete brain lesion. (p. 417)

One of the especially interesting findings to come from this study is that between-group differences were noted in the region of the medial frontal lobe (supplementary motor area). As Duffy et al. (1980a) note, this region has been associated with some speech deficits (Hanley & Sklar, 1976). It may well be that frontal lobe dysfunction plays an important role in the production of speech in dyslexics. Also, it has been suggested elsewhere

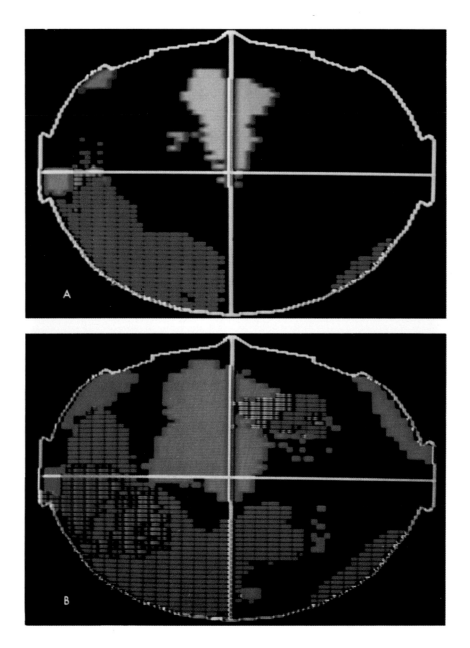

Color Plate 3-1. Summary maps of between-group differences of normal and dyslexic subjects. Colored areas represent regions of between-group differences reaching a PI (percent index) of at least 2 (A) or 5 (B) at least once during all EEG and EP states. Solid red represents the contribution from the ten EEG states (alpha plus theta); the dashed red represents the contribution from the three EP states. The blue region represents overlapping contributions from both EEG and EP states. Note four prominent between-group regions of differences at PI = 2: bilateral frontal, left anterolateral frontal, left midtemporal, and left posterolateral quadrant. It is suggested that dyslexia represents dysfunction of much of the cortex normally involved in speech and reading. Note the bilaterality of the between-group difference. Note also that differences shown by EEG lie anterior to the interaural line, whereas EP differences lie posterior to that line. [From Duffy, FH, Denckla, MD, Bartels, PA, Sandini, G, & Kiessling, LS. Dyslexia: Automated diagnosis by computerized classification of brain electrical activity. *Annals of Neurology*, 1980, 7, 421–428 (b). With permission.]

that frontal lobe dysfunction in adolescents may be the cause for behavioral anomalies such as hyperactivity (Golden, 1981). Duffy et al. (1980a) suggest that this area could play, "a previously underemphasized role in aphasia and in concepts of dyslexia and dysgraphia" (p. 419). Clearly, the result of this study indicate that in a carefully defined population of dyslexics, brain electrical abnormalities exist in areas of the brain that we know to be critical in normal language and reading ability.

In an attempt to validate and extend the utility of their automated classification of brain electrical activity in dyslexics, Duffy et al. (1980b) developed a system of classification rules derived from linear discriminant analysis of their data. A total of 24 subjects (13 normal, 11 dyslexic) were used, all having participated in the ten EEG states and three EP conditions. Stepwise linear-discriminant function analysis incorporating the ten best measurements resulted in a maximum separation between groups (Wilks' lambda = 29.35, $p<.00001$), correctly classifying 96 percent of the subjects. All of the dyslexic children were correctly classified according to the ten best measurements, while 12 of the 13 normals were correctly classified. When the classification rules were applied to a population not used in the initial study, 80 to 90 percent success rates in classification were achieved.

The investigations by Duffy and his colleagues well represent a major advance not only in the application of EEG and EP procedures, but also they are important because they provide direct evidence that abnormal brain electrical activity is correlated with dyslexia. It may well be, as they claim, that the failure to consistently find this result in the past, using EEG techniques, was the result of having too much data at hand, thus confounding diagnosis. By using the BEAM technique, meaning is drawn to the vast and complex information generated through electrophysiological procedures.

While the findings reported in this series of investigations are complementary to the aphasia literature and correspond well with what we know about the functional system involved in reading (Fig. 3-2), there are some problematic issues unresolved at present. It should seem evident that, for instance, the fact that differences exist between normal and dyslexics does not strictly imply neurological deficit. It could well be as some have suggested (Snyder, 1980), that the results merely reflect developmental delay and that the dyslexics would have eventually caught up. As Snyder (1980) suggested, it would perhaps be more meaningful to have compared the brain electrical activity of the dyslexics with a younger population of normal boys rather than with their chronological-age peers. The research using other experimental procedures would tend to suggest that this is not a factor. Duffy (1980) has indicated, however, that such an investigation is underway and this point will be addressed in the near future.

A second concern relates to the notion that dyslexia may actually represent several distinct subtypes. It could be that a further investigation would

reveal variable patterns of brain electrical activity among subgroups of dyslexics according to the area of deficit functioning. Despite these ideas for
further research, Duffy's investigations have been exceptional in pointing
to areas of the brain long thought to be deficit in dyslexic children and has
provided concrete evidence to this suspicion.

CYTOARCHITECTONIC STUDIES OF
DYSLEXICS' BRAINS

Scant evidence existed prior to the research of Hier et al. (1978) and
Duffy et al. (1980a, 1980b) that clearly affirmed a neurological base to severe reading problems in children. The recent advances in computerized
tomography and brain electrical mapping using computerized-assisted top-
ographical analysis has provided more direct evidence as to some of the
neurological factors associated with reading failure. This evidence stands in
stark opposition to those who propose that, "studies aimed at the brain
functions of learning disabled children have failed to find evidence for brain
damage" (Ross, 1976, p. 83).

The evidence provided by Hier et al. (1978) demonstrates a correlation
between deviant brain asymmetry and functional abilities known to be important in reading. The work by Duffy et al. (1980a, 1980b) indicates EEG
correlates associated with dyslexia. What would be most desirable is direct,
observable pathological deficits in the brains of dyslexics, which would help
convince these skeptics as to the neurological basis of dyslexia. Some have
even suggested that should autopsies be conducted on dyslexics, no identifiable abnormalities would be apparent (Critchley, 1964).

The argument that dyslexia is the result of neuropathology would be
strengthened significantly if autopsy reports were, in general, available on
dyslexics. Since dyslexia is not a life-threatening disorder, it will never be
presented to the pathologist as the manifest disorder. Consequently, directly observable neuropathological correlates of dyslexia are usually not
available. The clinical and pathological studies that are available (Drake,
1968; Galaburda & Kemper, 1979) provide very strong evidence in favor of
the neurological conceptualization of dyslexia as presented in this volume.
Since these two landmark studies are so critical to our understanding of the
neuropsychological processes involved in dyslexia, they will be reviewed in
some detail.

Pathological Findings in a Child with
Developmental Dyslexia

The first autopsy report correlating clinical with neuropathological
findings in a dyslexic child was published by Drake in 1968. His report

detailed the course of a 12-year-old boy who experienced marked difficulty in reading comprehension. He also had difficulty in arithmetic and was exceptionally slow in completing his homework. Written work was marked by poor writing and spelling. He was originally referred to school personnel because of his academic and associated behavioral problems. This boy experienced violent outbursts, was unusually active, had staring spells, enuresis, recurring unilateral headaches, and was considered manipulative by his parents. Interestingly, and consistent with the characteristics of some dyslexic children, he had a family history of reading problems associated with mixed dominance (hand-eye). This family history seemed to be transmitted through the male members of his family and affected both the child and his younger brother.

School performance was always average to below average, showing a marked decline from first grade, where he earned average marks, to fifth grade, where he consistently earned Ds. Intellectual abilities as measured on two separate occasions fell within the average range. Word-recognition abilities were assessed to be in the above-average range (measured at the seventh grade, fourth month level) when tested last in the sixth grade at age 12 years, 2 months. Importantly, however, his performance on word-meaning and paragraph-meaning measures resulted in abilities at the 8th percentile and 14th percentile, respectively. In some respects, his profile of abilities and disabilities resembles that of a hyperlexic (superior word-calling ability with little or no comprehension). Behaviors observed during reading included a monotone voice, omission of words, substitutions, frequent repetitions, whispering during silent reading, and inaccurate return sweep-eye movements when moving from line to line.

Although the child's history and classroom behavior suggested emotional problems that may have compounded his reading difficulties, those behaviors associated with reading coupled with the family history would indeed suggest a neurological base to the reading comprehension difficulty. Based on our prior discussion of functional neuroanatomy one might even speculate that the area of neurologic deficit, if it exists in this case, could be found in the region of the parietal lobe where the angular gyrus is found. It has already been proposed that this cortical area is critical in intersensory integration and, consequently, in reading comprehension in which meaning and associations must be paired with the visual stimuli (i.e., words).

On the day that the patient died, he experienced a temper outburst, complained of a mild headache, and felt lethargic. He died in his sleep that same night. The cause of his death was a massive hemorrhage in the inferior portion of the cerebellum. The hemorrhage extended into the subarachnoid and ventricular regions. On gross inspection of the brain, an abnormal convolutional pattern was noted in the parietal region bilaterally. Deep gyri that appeared unconnected were obvious. Also, the associated region of the corpus callosum seemed thin. Other microscopic anomalies included nerve cells that were spindle shaped and many ectopic neurons in the white matter. It should be stressed, however, that the cerebellar hemorrhage was due to an angioma and in no way could have produced the abnormal neuropathological findings that may have been associated with the dyslexia.

The pattern of educational disability manifested as a severe difficulty in comprehending written material is consistent with the findings of the autopsy case. Acquired alexia and learning disabilities have a long history in clinical neurology as being associated with neuropathological findings in the region of the angular gyrus (Bastian, 1898; Broadbent, 1872; Charcot, 1877, 1889; Dejerine, 1892). The autopsy findings in this case of developmental dyslexia are consistent with other earlier reports of acquired alexia.

It is, of course, impossible to directly correlate observed behavior and the neuropathological findings in this case. It is interesting to hypothesize whether the application of Duffy's BEAM technique would have recorded conclusive electrophysiological anomalies in the region of the angular gyrus during reading. The correlation between the studies of Duffy et al. (1980a) and Drake (1968) is certainly striking and one would suspect a direct relationship between observed pathology and associated EEG readings during reading.

A More Recent Cytoarchitectonic Case Study

In addition to the report by Drake (1968), only one other autopsy study is available for consideration. The investigation provided by Galaburda and Kemper (1979) is especially important because it examines the neuroanatomical structure in serial sections that can potentially provide more meaningful information than the procedures used in the brief report by Drake (1968).

The patient described by Galaburda and Kemper (1979) evidenced no prenatal or postnatal complications and seemed to achieve important developmental milestones at the expected chronological ages. Only clumsiness seems to be a general observation of any clinical significance. Speech, however, apparently presented somewhat of a problem. He reportedly did not speak in full sentences until after three years of age. Once in school, the patient had considerable difficulties in reading and spelling and had to repeat first grade because of his failure. He was diagnosed at that time as developmental dyslexic. A Stanford-Binet IQ of 105 was reported. His reading problems persisted despite intensive tutoring, and at age 13 years, his grade equivalents in paragraph meaning, word meaning, and spelling were 2.4, 3.0, and 3.0, respectively. Oral reading was equal to a normal child in the first grade, sixth month.

Although he continued to receive intensive assistance, by age 19 years little significant improvement was noted. At 13 years of age he was administered a second psychological test battery that resulted in a full-scale IQ score of 88. Despite this low average estimate of ability, he should still have had the capacity to learn to read, as his verbal-scale IQ was 95 while his performance areas seemed to be slightly more depressed (IQ = 83). Unlike Drake (1968), who used a measure of hand and eye dominance to assess laterality, the patient reported by Galaburda and Kemper (1979) received a dichotic listening test (discussed in Chapter 5). His performance on this measure of central language processing indicated that he was strongly lateralized to the left cerebral hemisphere for language representation. Despite this normal pattern of brain organization, he was left-handed, as were a number of other immediate family members. Similar to the case reported by Drake (1968), both brothers and the father were reading-retarded. Seizures were manifested at age 16 and were easily controlled. There was no evidence of other neurological deficits other than those associated with the dyslexia.

Death was caused by a fall at his first job as a sheet metal worker at age 20. Multiple internal injuries were the cause of death. At autopsy the brain showed no evidence of trauma or gross abnormalities associated with the fall.

Unlike the case described by Drake (1968), gross inspection of the brain revealed no obvious neuroanatomical abnormalities. Serial sections of the brain were made and comparison with the brains of normal age-matched subjects revealed no abnormalities of the subcortical white matter of other subcortical structures. All serial sections demonstrated the normal pattern of hemispheric asymmetry with the left cerebral hemisphere being larger than the right. Relative to the theories by Hier et al. (1978) about reversed cerebral asymmetry, this particular brain would appear to represent the larger subgroup of dyslexics with normal asymmetry. Interestingly, however, the planum temporale was approximately equal on both sides of the brain, which is in contrast to the more normal pattern of the left being larger than the right, as reported by Geschwind and Levitsky (1968).

The abnormalities that were found on microscopic examination were restricted to the left cerebral hemisphere. The most important area of abnormality was confined to the region posterior to the planum temporale in which polymicrogyria were observed. This malformation may be due to genetic or environmental factors and is usually correlated with impairment of function normally associated with the brain region (Jacobson, 1972). As might be expected, Galaburda and Kemper (1979) found fused molecular layers, dysplasia, and no cell-free layer; and, normal cytoarchitectonic landmarks could not be identified on close inspection. The region of deficit was determined to be directly posterior to the auditory cortex (Fig. 3-8).

As the authors of this study note, their patient exhibited many of the

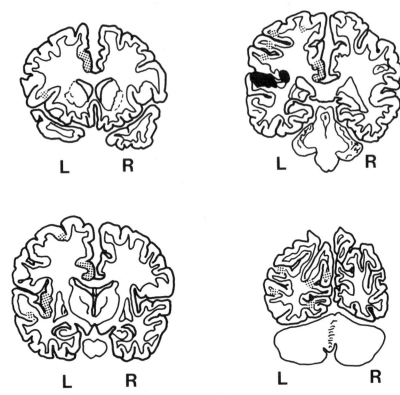

Fig. 3-8. The brain at several coronal levels. Cross-hatching represents areas of mild cortical dysplasia in the left cingulate gyrus, rostral insula, and focally throughout the left hemisphere. Note the increased frequency of focal lesions posteriorly. Area in black represents the polymicrogyria. [From Galaburda, AM, & Kemper, TL. Cytoarchitectonic abnormalities in developmental dyslexia: A case study. *Annals of Neurology*, 1979, *6*, 94–100. With permission.]

classical symptoms of developmental dyslexia. These symptoms included an inability to learn to read despite apparent intellectual ability, a family history of reading failure, increased tendency toward left handedness and delayed speech. The dysplasia observed in the left temporal region was confined to an area thought to be important in forming auditory associations with perceived auditory stimuli. While it is impossible to know for sure if it was the abnormal cortical tissue that was responsible for the dyslexia, the fact that the pathological condition existed in an area known to be critical in reading comprehension is good evidence that, in this case, there existed an excellent correlation between structural and behavioral deficit. This is an especially important conclusion in this case since we know, based on the dichotic listening task, that it was indeed the left temporal region that was responsbile for language perception. It should also be noted that in a follow-up study of this same patient, Galaburda and Eidelberg (1982) found bilateral disruption of normal pathways in the thalamus. Both cortical and subcortical abnormalities may hence contribute to neuropsychological deficits in dyslexia.

Although only two autopsy reports on dyslexics exist, it does seem highly significant that in both cases neuropathological anomalies existed in regions of the brain that we would expect to be related to reading failure. Based on these reports, it seems highly probable that other dyslexics may likewise suffer from inadequate neural structures subserving the functional system involved in reading. The fact that a functional system is involved in reading, as outlined earlier in this chapter, is supported by the fact that the same symptom (i.e., reading failure) was the result of abnormal neural structures localized in different, but equally important, regions of the cortex and the thalamus that are critical to successful reading. It seems reasonable to project that additional autopsy reports will reveal similar neuropathological correlation in patients suffering from developmental dyslexia.

CONCLUSIONS

The purpose of this chapter was to present an overview of what is believed to represent the functional system involved in reading. The neuropsychological correlates of reading behavior were reviewed with specific emphasis on the region of the angular gyrus. In an attempt to provide the reader with some understanding of the brain mechanisms involved in the recovery from brain trauma, physiologic correlates and factors associated with the recovery of function were reviewed. Finally, evidence was presented that suggested strongly that developmental dyslexia has its genesis in neuropathology. Based on the material presented in this chapter, it seems that the following conclusions are warranted.

The cortical region known as the angular gyrus seems to lie at the junction of the parietal, occipital, and temporal lobe association cortex, as suggested by Geschwind (1974a). By its strategic location it serves the vital purpose of facilitating cross-modal integration, a task necessary for fluent reading.

Since the functional system involved in reading includes many cortical regions primarily localized to the left cerebral hemisphere, any deficit within the system may manifest itself behaviorally in reading failure. The reported autopsy cases would support this conclusion, as different neuropathology consistent with our model of the neurological basis of reading were associated with dyslexia.

The agenesis literature and the research on recovery from brain damage both support the conclusion that complete recovery from any neurological anomaly, whether developmental in nature or induced, will result in some impairment in cognitive functioning. While age may play some vital role, it is only in exceptionally rare cases in which no neuropsychological deficits are found.

When brain trauma or insult does occur, such factors as length of post-traumatic amnesia predict with some certainty the rate and extent of recovery. Furthermore, the greatest extent of recovery seems to occur within the first 30 days, and up to 90 percent of the eventual recovery occurs within the first year post-trauma. The mechanism of plasticity probably relies more on intrahemispheric adjustments, than on other cortical areas in the opposite hemisphere assuming brain function once it is damaged. It is only in extremely young or rare cases in which functions actually switch to the undamaged hemisphere.

It seems that two factors may serve as the foundation for developmental dyslexia. First, it seems possible that variations in neurodevelopmental asymmetries may be related to at least one subtype of dyslexia in which language functions are served by a hemisphere which is ill equipped to do so. A second group of dyslexics who may also suffer from the above anomaly evidence diffuse EEG differences in brain electrical activity. The regions of greatest electrical difference, when compared with normals, were in regions of the brain known to be vital in the reading process.

Autopsy reports on the brains of dyslexics demonstrate neuropathology in regions of the brain consistent with reading failure. For this reason, it seems appropriate to conclude that there exists a positive correlation between deviations in cortical structure and function. The neurological basis to developmental dyslexia seems well established when sample populations are carefully defined, and established procedures for educational, neuropsychological, and medical evaluations are utilized. With these conclusions in mind, it is now appropriate to critically examine the research on dyslexia.

———Chapter 4———

Single Factor Research with Dyslexics: The Perceptual-Deficit Hypothesis and Cross-Modal Integration Research

The single-factor approach to the study of developmental dyslexia comprises the largest collection of hypothesized explanations for this disorder. They include theories that propose deficits or delays in areas such as visual perception, cross-modal integration, and cerebral dominance, just to name a few. While all of these theoretical approaches differ as to the proposed underlying cause of developmental dyslexia, they all have certain methodological and theoretical similarities. First and foremost, all of these studies make the underlying assumption that the population of dyslexic children is a homogeneous etiological and clinical entity exhibiting a random distribution of characteristic errors in reading. A second commonality within this approach involves the methodology employed to study this group of children. Almost all of the studies reviewed in this chapter have been designed to compare the levels of performance of normal and dyslexic children on a particular task thought to be related to reading achievement. Not until recently have researchers begun to explore developmental trends within the dyslexic population. Finally, all of these studies assume that there is some form of neurological dysfunction (deficit or delay) as the underlying basis for the reading disability. It is important to keep these points in mind as we explore the literature focusing our attention on the perceptual-deficit hypothesis and dysfunction in cross-modal integration. An important variation of the single-factor approach to the study of dyslexia is that of dealing with notions of incomplete cerebral dominance. This important concept will be dealt with in the following chapter.

DYSFUNCTION IN VISUAL PERCEPTION: THE
PERCEPTUAL-DEFICIT HYPOTHESIS

One of the most popular theories for developmental dyslexia is that these children have difficulty in the perception of visual symbols. As mentioned in Chapter 1, Orton (1928, 1937) was the first to propose that the characteristic letter and word reversals, commonly observed in these children, were the result of a perceptual dysfunction that stemmed from a delay in the development of lateral dominance for language. Orton hypothesized that words were stored correctly in the dominant hemisphere and that the mirror images were stored in the minor hemisphere. The retrieval of words from the minor hemisphere resulted in confusion in reading characterized by letter reversals (*b* for *d*) and word reversals (*was* for *saw*) as well as the orientation errors observed in the writing of dyslexic children. This "mixed" dominance theory was viewed by Orton as a developmental delay and not as a cognitive deficit, thus spawning a major controversy in the developmental dyslexia literature that still remains unresolved.

Orton's work gave rise to several other theories stressing this basic dysfunction in visual processing. For example, Bender (1956, 1957) proposed that reading disability was likely associated with poorly established lateral dominance, but unlike Orton, she felt this delay resulted in faulty figure-ground organization. Hermann (1959), while being in agreement with the notion of faulty visual-spatial processing as the cause of reading disability, felt that this deficit was the result of a genetic disposition toward directional confusion. Finally, another group of authors (Frostig, 1964; Kephart, 1971) have proposed that reading disability may be the result of deficient perceptual-motor integration.

Support for the Perceptual Deficit Hypothesis

Support for the visual perception theory can be drawn from a series of studies by Lyle and Goyen (Lyle, 1969; Lyle & Goyen, 1968, 1975). In a factor analytic study of 54 reading-retarded and 54 normal readers aged 6 to 12, Lyle (1969) found that based on the results of a comprehensive test battery, two distinct factors were associated with reading retardation. One factor was related to tasks in which there was a strong perceptual component, while the second factor was related to tasks requiring verbal skills. Looking at the variable of age, Lyle found that the reading-disabled readers below 8 years of age were more likely to demonstrate difficulties on perceptual tasks, while the older disabled readers were more likely deficient on the verbal-factor tasks.

Lyle and Goyen (1968) compared 20 good and 20 deficient second- and third-grade readers on tasks of visual recognition. Children deemed reading deficient were at least nine months below grade level. Through tachistoscopic presentation, the children were shown letters of the alphabet that are commonly confused by poor readers and asked to indicate which letter they had seen from multiple-choice response cards. Three conditions were employed: that of immediate recall, that of testing after a short delay, and that of three consecutively presented stimuli requiring order of presentation to be given; the children had to clasp their hands and recite multiplication tables while waiting for the response card in order to avoid verbal or kinesthetic rehearsal. The results indicated that the retarded readers performed significantly below the good readers on all tasks, with the younger retarded readers erring most. The authors interpreted these results to indicate that young retarded readers do, in fact, have a perceptual deficit.

Finally, Lyle and Goyen (1975) compared the performance of 21 retarded readers and 21 nonretarded readers, aged six and seven, on speed of processing information, perceptual discrimination, and short-term memory. Reading retardation was defined as at least nine months below age level for the six-year-old children, and at least one year below age level for the seven-year-old children. The children were asked to view rectangular shapes through a tachistoscope and asked if they were the same or different. Some children viewed both items in a pair simultaneously, while others viewed each item separately between a two-second delay or a seven-second delay. Results indicated that when stimuli were presented rapidly, the retarded readers had more difficulty than adequate readers in recognizing these stimuli. It must be noted that these differences only occurred when the stimuli presented were different and not when they were the same. Difficulty in perceptual discrimination ability was thus posited.

Further support for a perceptual-deficit hypothesis has come from investigators who report significant correlations between performance on figure-drawing tests and measures of reading achievement (deHirsch, Jansky, & Langford, 1966; Jansky & deHirsch, 1972; Silver & Hagen, 1971). In addition, the results of two longitudinal studies (Rourke, 1976; Satz, Friel, & Rudegeair, 1974) appear to concur with Lyle and Goyen by concluding that visual-perceptual and visual-spatial abilities are somewhat less important at advanced stages of the learning-to-read process than they are during the initial stages of reading acquisition.

Controversy Over the Perceptual Deficit Hypothesis

While this body of research appears to support the notion of perceptual deficit as an underlying cause of developmental dyslexia, there is a considerable amount of research evidence that does not support this contention. For example, Vellutino and his colleagues (Vellutino, Smith, Steger, & Kaman, 1975; Vellutino, Steger, & Kandel, 1972) administered visual presentations of three-, four-, and five-item words; scrambled letters and numbers;

as well as geometric designs, to poor and normal readers aged 7 to 14. In these studies, Vellutino classified poor readers as those children with normal intelligence who were scoring two or more years below their grade placement on a test of oral reading. Difficulty in single-word recognition and component-sound analysis were also present. The children were asked to copy the stimuli from memory, pronounce and spell the verbal stimuli in correct order, or spell out the scrambled letters and numbers in correct order. Results indicated that poor readers performed considerably better in the copying of verbal stimuli than they did in the naming of those same stimuli. Furthermore, the performance of poor readers was comparable to that of the good readers on the copying of the geometric designs until item number (four- and five-letter words) began to tax visual short-term memory. An interesting observation was also made in the poor reader group. The children were often found to copy the stimulus (*was* or *calm*) correctly but misread them as *saw* or *clam*. When Vellutino and his colleagues looked at the group-by-age interaction, they found that only the second graders faltered in copying and naming (in correct order) the letters in four- and five-letter words, with the poor reader making more errors than the normal readers. In the sixth-grade group, copying and naming errors were negligible. The authors concluded that the visual perception of a given word is not necessarily reflected in the pronunciation or verbal labeling of that word, casting serious doubts about the validity of perceptual deficits in reading disability.

Additional support for the above conclusions is derived from Vellutino and his colleagues (Vellutino, Steger, & Pruzek, 1973; Vellutino, Steger, Kan in, & DeSetto, 1975). In these studies, good and poor readers (similarly defined), aged 7 to 12, were presented with three-, four-, and five-letter words printed in Hebrew in order to control for previous experience with letters and words. Subjects were asked to reproduce each stimulus from memory. Results indicated that poor readers performed as well as good readers. In contrast, neither group performed as well as children learning to speak Hebrew. In addition, both good and poor readers exhibited left-right scanning tendencies while the reverse effect was observed in those children learning Hebrew. While these results again cast considerable doubt on the perceptual-deficit hypothesis in general, they also appear to discredit the left-right scanning deficit theory of Hermann (1959) in particular.

In order to summarize the work of Vellutino and his associates in this area, a quote from Vellutino (1978) is most pertinent:

> It is suggested that the positional and directional errors commonly observed in the reading and writing of poor readers (i.e., b/d, was/saw) and long thought to be compelling evidence in favor of a perceptual deficit explanation of reading disability, are in fact linguistic intrusion errors caused by imprecision in

verbal mediation, rather than visual distortion caused by dysfunction at the level of the central nervous system. (p. 73)

and, Vellutino (1978) also stated that:

> In simpler terms, it is our contention that children who call "b" "d" or "was" "saw" do not literally "see" these configurations differently than normal readers, but, because of one or more deficiencies in verbal processing, cannot remember which verbal label is associated with which printed word. (p. 73, both quotations with permission of Oxford University Press.)

Further evidence against the perceptual-deficit theory comes from a study by Nielson and Binge (1969) who compared normal and reading-disabled 9 and 10 year olds on the Frostig Test of Visual Perception, the Bender-Gestalt Test, and the Goodenough Draw-A-Person Test. Unlike the previously mentioned studies (deHirsch et al., 1966; Jansky & deHirsch, 1972; Silver & Hagen, 1971), the samples under study were carefully screened to exclude extraneous variables such as IQ, emotional factors, and cultural disadvantage. On analysis, Nielson and Binge (1969) reported more similarities than differences in performance between the two groups, and they concluded that impaired visual perception and visual-motor dysfunction do not seem to be important correlates to reading disability.

Before concluding this section of the research literature, it is necessary to examine two studies done by Libeman and her colleagues that serve to emphasize some of the major research difficulties in this area. In their initial study, Libeman, Shankweiler, Orlando, Harris, and Bertt (1971) explored the kinds of reading errors normal children make at various stages of learning to read. Specifically, the authors explored the occurrence of reversal errors in an entire school population of second graders. It was found that letter confusions and reversals of sequence occurred with appreciable frequency on a standard test of reading achievement only among the children in the lowest third of the class. Even among this bottom group, reversals of order and sequence accounted for only 10 and 15 percent of the reading errors. Furthermore, within this group of "poor readers," only a few reversed to an appreciable extent, and no sinistral directional bias was present (right-left scanning tendency). The authors concluded that these results did not support Orton's (1937) contention that reversals are symptomatic of a tendency to scan words in a right-to-left manner. Instead, they proposed that these errors were the result of linguistic intrusion (mislabeling) rather than perceptual distortion.

In a more recent article (Fischer, Libeman, & Shankweiler, 1978) these authors went on to compare the pattern of reading errors (in context and isolation) of the original "school group" with those of an "institute group" consisting of children eight to ten years of age who had previously been diagnosed dyslexic according to medical and psychoeducational criteria.

The results the study of Fischer et al. (1978) indicated that although there was only a small difference between mean-reading levels on the Gray Oral Reading Tests, (1.4 versus 1.7), the institute group was significantly less proficient in decoding isolated words out of context. Also, the institute group did not differ significantly from the school group in incidence of either word or letter reversals, and errors of reversal only accounted for a small proportion of the total errors in reading. Consonant and vowel errors were far more frequent in both groups. Lastly, the authors noted that the two groups were found to differ with respect to the directional characteristics of their reversals; the institute group made significantly more reversals in the horizontal plane with a 2:1 bias toward a right-to-left transformation. This trend was consistent across letter, as well as word, reversals. The school-age group, while also tending toward horizontal reversals, showed no consistencies toward sinistrad directional bias as mentioned in the previous study.

Based on this result, the authors concluded that the institute children consistently demonstrate a failure to establish stable left-to-right habits of scan, thus giving support to the sinistral directional scanning hypothesis by Orton (1937). The authors went on to state that while directional problems were found in some of the dyslexic children, the majority of reading errors made by both groups reflect common difficulties in phonemic segmentation of words, phonetic recoding, and mastery of orthography. Fischer et al. (1978) thus concluded that the reading difficulties of both groups are more reflective of the linguistic characteristics of words rather than with their visual properties.

Major Problems in Research Design

While the results of these two studies appear to lend more fuel to the argument against the perceptual-deficit hypothesis of developmental dyslexia, they also serve to emphasize some major problems with the research in this area.

Many of the studies mentioned in this review as being in support of the perceptual-deficit hypothesis appear to have failed in adequately differentiating the population of dyslexic children from the population of backward readers according to the guidelines set down by the World Federation of Neurology (as discussed in Chapter 1). Since most studies used children who were defined according to different criteria as being dyslexic, the results of these studies cannot be compared nor can any conclusions be drawn. This is a crucial error that can drastically affect the validity of the studies in question as they pertain to the dyslexic population.

Another problem that is common to all of the studies in this area is that they treat the dyslexic population as a homogeneous entity. It is very possible (and, as we will see later, quite probable) that the population of dyslexic children is not homogeneous but heterogeneous. This contention may account for the two factor findings of Lyle (1969) and the finding in the Fischer et al. (1978) study that noted that some of their dyslexic population did exhibit perceptual distortion and scanning difficulties, while the majority did not.

A final problem with the research in this area pertains to the age across reader-group variable. While it appears that there is a fair amount of evidence supporting the contention that visual-perceptual abilities are more important in the early stages of the learning-to-read process (Lyle & Goyen, 1968; Rourke, 1976; Satz, Friel, Rudegeair, 1974), future work will be needed in order to delineate the role that perceptual difficulties have in young readers. In conclusion, the authors must agree with Benton (1975) when he states, "The importance of visuoperceptive and visuomotor difficulties as determinates of reading failure has been overrated by some authors" (p. 8).

DYSFUNCTION IN CROSS-MODAL INTEGRATION

A second popular explanation for developmental dyslexia comes from the work of Birch and Belmont (1964, 1965). Playing on a similar theme as Luria (1980), these authors proposed that one of the factors that contributes to dyslexia is a deficiency in the ability to integrate auditory and visual stimuli. They feel that there may be a group of poor readers who have not developed cortical connections among the sensory areas of the brain that are necessary for the development of adequate reading and related skills. In accordance with this theory, several cardinal assumptions are made by Birch (1962): development within sensory systems takes place prior to the establishment of relationships between systems; the distal senses (external) become dominant over the proximal (internal) senses; poor readers would be differentiated from normal readers on tasks requiring the ability to establish equivalent sensory representations; and such a difficulty should not be unique to any specific modality.

Birch and Belmont provided support for their theory in two studies. In the initial study (Birch & Belmont, 1964), the authors compared a sample of good and poor readers, aged nine to ten, on their ability to match (establish equivalence) between simple rhythmic patterns tapped out with a pencil and their visually equivalent dot pattern presented in a multiple choice fashion. Results indicated that, as a whole, the good readers performed significantly better on this task than poor readers. It must also be stated that some poor readers performed as well as the good readers and vice versa;

based on these results, the authors concluded that deficiencies in cross-modal integration are characteristic of some poor readers and not others.

In a follow-up study (Birch & Belmont, 1965), the authors administered the same task to samples of good and poor readers from kindergarten to sixth grade. Results indicated that audiovisual integration was correlated with reading ability only in the first and second graders, while intelligence was more highly correlated with reading ability in the higher grade levels. Birch and Belmont concluded that cross-modal integration ability was an influential factor in the early stages of the learning-to-read process and improved with age.

Criticism of Studies by Birch and Belmont

After careful analysis of these results, Sterritt and Rudnick (1966) criticized the methodology employed by Birch and Belmont on the following grounds. First, the task which Birch and Belmont employed required them to tap out a rhythm with a pencil. Birch and Belmont did not mention the use of a screening device to shield the pencil from view of the subject, thus the subject received both visual and auditory cues. Sterritt and Rudnick concluded that Birch and Belmont may have been measuring the ability to transpose from visual-temporal to visual-spatial (intramodal integration) rather than the ability to transpose from auditory to visual stimuli. Second, Birch and Belmont did not control for the effects of intelligence. As a result of these criticisms. Sterritt and Rudnick sought to replicate Birch and Belmont's findings by employing three conditions. Condition One was identical to that used by Birch and Belmont. Condition Two involved the presentation of auditory tone patterns through a tape recorder and required matching to visual patterns as in Condition One. Condition Three involved visual-temporal patterns flashed with a red light and required matching as in Condition One. The subjects were 36 boys in the fourth grade of a middle class school. Each child was administered a group intelligence test and the Iowa Test of Basic Skills. Results indicated that after IQ was controlled for (50 percent of the variance of reading scores), the auditory-to-visual task was the only one of the three that was a significant predictor of reading scores (23 percent of the variance). The authors concluded that the above finding can be interpreted in two ways: the ability to transpose from auditory-temporal to visual-spatial formats may be the critical function involved in reading, or the auditory-pattern perception ability by itself is the primary function related to reading.

In a follow-up study, the same authors (Rudnick, Sterritt, & Flax, 1967) sought to replicate their procedure in a group of third graders in order to validate the finding of Birch and Belmont (1965), which reflected developmental trends in the ability to integrate information cross-modally. As in the initial study, the variable of intelligence was controlled for. The children in both groups came from the same school. Results indicated that in this sample of third graders, both the auditory-temporal to visual-spatial, and the visual-temporal to visual-spatial tasks were significant predictors of reading ability (11 and 14 percent of the variance, respectively). The Birch and Belmont task was not significant. As in the initial study, intelligence was also found to be a significant predictor (30 percent of the variance). The authors concluded that the results of the two studies appear to indicate that with age, visual-perceptual abilities, visual-temporal–visual-spatial (VT-VS), decline in importance, while auditory and/or cross-modal perceptual abilities become more important as predictors of individual reading ability, thus opposing the developmental process predicted by Birch and Belmont.

Another group of researchers who found fault with the conclusions of Birch and Belmont were Blank and her associates (Blank & Bridger, 1966; Blank, Weider, & Bridger, 1968). They questioned the findings of Birch and Belmont on two grounds, one of which was that depending on the task requirements, cross-modal or intersensory integration can have different levels of difficulty. For example, recognition of the same stimulus through different modalities is much easier than recognizing analogous stimuli presented in different modalities. A further contention was that the second task, which is similar to that used by Birch and Belmont, involved complex conceptualization. Blank and her colleagues concluded that what Birch and Belmont were measuring may have been the ability to establish equivalence within a modality (VT-VS), rather than intramodal transfer.

In order to test these hypotheses, Blank and Bridger (1966) evaluated 13 retarded and 13 normal readers aged 9 years, 4 months to 9 years, 11 months (fourth graders). The subjects were matched for IQ and all came from a public school in New York City. The average reading level for the retarded readers was 3.4 while that of the good readers was 6.4 as measured by the Metropolitan Reading Achievement Test. The children were administered three separate tasks that measured their ability to convert temporal stimuli (light flashes) into spatial stimuli (dot arrays) within the same modality; their ability to perceive the dot patterns; and, their ability to report the exact sequence in which the light was flashed.

The results indicated that the retarded readers did significantly less well than the normal readers on intramodal transfer, as measured by task one. The retarded readers were thus unable to convert temporally distributed stimuli into spatially distributed stimuli, even within the same modality. On task two, the retarded readers did equally as well as the normal readers, indicating that there was no significant difference between the groups on the ability to match successively presented spatial material from memory. Finally, in task three the retarded readers performed significantly below the level of normals on their ability to report the exact sequence in which the lights were flashed. While all children employed some sort of number coding device to achieve this task, the retarded readers had difficulty in reporting both the number of lights and the placement of the pauses. Blank and Bridger concluded that retarded readers had difficulty in intra-modal transfer of visual stimuli (temporal to spatial) and that this difficulty appears to be the result of an underlying deficit in the ability to apply the correct verbal labels to temporally presented stimuli (abstract verbal conceptualization). What appeared to be a cross-modal deficiency thus seems to be instead a failure to verbally code the temporally presented components of an intra-modal task.

In order to test the developmental aspects of their hypothesis, Blank et al. (1968) presented the same tasks, with slight modification, to both normal and poor-reading first grade students matched for IQ. These children ranged in age from 6 years, 4 months to 7 years, 3 months, with good readers scoring on a 2.3 level or above and poor readers scoring below 2.0 on the Gates Primary Reading Test. As mentioned above, the tasks were essentially the same as in the initial study with the following exceptions: the task measuring equivalence between visual-temporal and visual-spatial stimuli had to be shaped over three progressively harder tasks due to the age of the subjects employed; and, a rhythm perception test was added to explore the perception of temporal stimuli in a manner that did not require coding strategies. Imitation of a rhythm by the subject was thus all that was required.

The results indicated that, as in the initial study, the retarded readers again experienced significantly more difficulty on the task requiring them to establish equivalences between temporal and spatial stimuli. As in the initial study, the groups did not differ on their ability to perceive and remember the visual-spatial dot patterns (task two), or in their ability to imitate the rhythm pattern on the additional task (task four). The two groups of subjects, however, were also found to differ on their ability to verbalize the pattern of the temporally presented lights (task three). As in the initial study, the retarded readers were found to be significantly deficient in this ability. Based on these results, and those found in the initial study, the authors concluded that regardless of whether a task is intramodal or cross-modal, retarded readers will have difficulty in coding those aspects of the task (in this case temporal-to-spatial) that demand a high level of abstraction. Thus, "a deficiency in symbolic mediation rather than perception is present at the onset of reading retardation and this deficiency may be responsible for the poorer performance of young reading retardates on tasks which seemingly are perceptually based" (Blank et al., 1968, p. 833).

Bisensory Memory Investigations

A different methodological approach to the evaluation of the intersensory integration theory has been conducted by Senf and his associates. In a series of three studies (Senf, 1969; Senf & Feshback, 1970; Senf & Freundl, 1971) the authors employed an audiovisual adaptation of Broadbent's (1956) Dichotic Listening Technique called the Bisensory Memory Task. In this procedure, an auditory and a different visual stimulus were presented simultaneously (or staggered), with three such pairs comprising each trial. The subject's task was to recall all six stimuli, under two general types of recall: free and directed. In all three studies, the "learning disabled" sample, which closely fit a diagnosis of dyslexia, met the following criteria: normal or above normal IQ, 1.5 years or more below grade level in reading, not diagnosed as severely neurologically impaired or emotionally disabled, and not severely perceptually impaired. Controls were matched for age and IQ.

In the initial study (Senf, 1969) the author compared three different age groups (mean ages 9 years, 5 months, 12 years, 2 months, and 14 years, 6 months) of "learning-disabled" children with matched controls, ranging in age from 7 to 15 across three separate experimental conditions. In the first condition, half of the children were directed to recall the items under free-recall conditions, the other half were directed to recall the items in pair order. In the second condition, half the children were directed to recall the items in pair order, the other half in modality order. The third condition attempted to assess the generality of the findings of the second condition by using very different stimuli: pictures and colors instead of digits.

Results indicated that the learning-disabled children were less sensitive than normals to an instructional set designed to induce them to order the six bisensory stimuli in three audiovisual pairs. Instead, they preferred to recall the stimuli in two modality sets. This finding was coupled with a marked inferiority in their ability to recall the stimuli in pair-ordered sets when they were required to do so. A second finding was that the failures of the learning-disabled children were usually specific to the ordering of stimuli, not to their accuracy of recall. Finally, an age by reader-group by condition interaction was found. At the early ages, the learning-disabled group was deficient in modality recall (favoring auditory stimuli) but the two groups did not differ on their ability to recall the stimuli in pair-order form. While the normal readers showed a marked improvement in the pair-ordered skill with age, however, the learning-disabled children did not. Senf concluded from these results that the deficiency found in the learning-disabled group indicated that perhaps some integrating mechanism or at least some process more complex than short-term memory is deficient.

In a second study (Senf & Feshback, 1970), the authors sought to replicate the findings of the initial study, while at the same time extending these results to a culturally deprived group of children also deficient in reading skills. The learning-disabled group was defined as in the initial study and matched for IQ with the control and culturally deprived group. Results indicated that replication with the learning-disabled population was successful. These children again showed a failure in developing the ability to organize the bisensory stimuli into audiovisual pairs, thus supporting the original contention by Senf (1969) that this deficiency was related to some cross-modal integrating mechanism. Two other findings characteristic of the learning-disabled group that were found to be consistent with the initial study was their inability to remember the order of the stimuli rather than the actual stimuli themselves and the deficient modality recall (favoring auditory stimuli), found only in the younger learning-disabled group.

In addition to replicating the results of the initial study, the authors found that while the culturally deprived group also had severe reading problems, they showed no substantial deficit or pairing behavior on the bisensory memory task. Their performance was thus not found to be significantly different from the normal group. The authors concluded that the reading problem of the culturally deprived children is functionally different from that of the learning-disabled group.

The final study in this series of three articles (Senf & Freundl, 1971) was undertaken in order to replicate the finding that showed young learning-disabled children to be inferior to normal readers in modality recall but to be as capable in audiovisual pairing. The second purpose of the study was to test whether the deficiency was related to sensory factors or higher-order processes. Subject selection and methodology was again similar to the initial study. As shown in the previous studies, the younger learning-disabled group (mean age 8 years, 9 months) was found deficient in modality recall. Altering of the stimulus presentation allowed the authors to rule out sensory masking as a cause of this deficiency. The authors thus concluded that some higher-order processes were involved and postulated three different explanations. First, based on the previous finding that learning-disabled children are heavily auditory preferent in free-recall conditions (Senf, 1969), the authors proposed that this group may be stimulus bound in that their attention is captured by auditory stimulation. They may thus be unable to deploy sufficient attention to visual material when auditory stimulation is present. Second, the learning-disabled child may be disproportionally inferior at discriminating, encoding, or recalling visual material independent of auditory material. This could also account for both gross and order errors in both modalities. Lastly, the learning-disabled child may be deficient in the organizational aspects of the task as related to the dimension of time. What is evidenced as a bisensory modality-recall deficit may thus result from higher-order memory organization disabilities that are not specific to the two-modality situation.

It is important to note here that, by making these hypothesized explanations, Senf and his associates are suggesting that their initial conclusion, which stated that reader-group differences on the bisensory memory task were the result of cross-modal transfer, was incorrect. In fact, two later

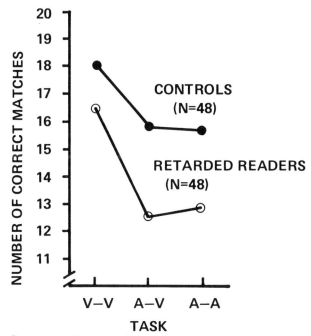

Fig. 4-1. Correct matches as a function of sample and task. Each point is the mean of the 48 Ss; maximum score = 20. [From Van de Voort, L, Senf, GM, & Benton, AL. Development of audiovisual integration in normal and retarded readers. *Child Development*, 1972, *43*, 1260–1272. With permission.]

studies by this group (Vande Voort & Senf, 1973; Vande Voort, Senf, & Benton, 1972) appear to support this shift in conceptualization. In both studies retarded readers and controls, matched for age (8–12 years) and IQ, were compared on a matching-to-standard task (same-different) over the following modalities: visual-visual, auditory-auditory, and auditory-visual.

The following findings were reported. With age, improvement in controls is seen on all three tasks with improvement being similar for within-modal tasks as on the cross-modal task. Controls were found to be superior to the reading-retarded group on all three tasks, with the most discrepancy found on the auditory-auditory task (Fig. 4-1). Lastly, with age, the retarded readers failed to show improvement in all three tasks, not just the intersensory task as Birch and Belmont hypothesized (1965) (Fig. 4-2). Taken together, these results suggest that when within-modality controls for encoding and memory processes are accomplished, it appears that retarded readers fail to develop skill required by within-modal as well as by cross-modal tasks. These results thus fail to support the hypothesis that intersensory integration deficits are the sole or primary developmental ability accounting for the reading disability in dyslexic children. The authors go on

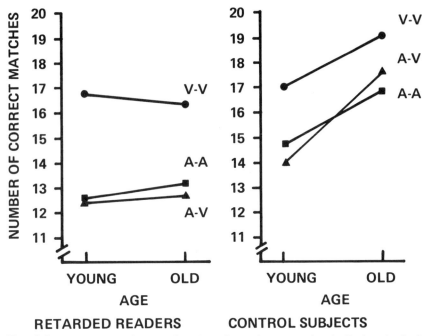

Fig. 4-2. Correct matches as a function of sample, age, and task. Each point is the mean of the 24 Ss; maximum score = 20. [From Van de Voort, L, Senf, GM, & Benton, AL. Development of audiovisual integration in normal and retarded readers. *Child Development*, 1972, *43*, 1260–1272. With permission.]

to conclude that faulty attentional and/or stimulus encoding problems, possibly associated with "central perceptual deficit" of deficiencies in "memory" could more likely explain the results in these studies as well as the results of their initial studies.

Investigations of Temporal-Order Recall

Bakker, referencing the work done in the cross-modal studies by Blank (Blank & Bridger, 1966; Blank et al., 1968) and Senf (Senf, 1969; Senf & Feshback, 1970; Senf & Freunal, 1971), as well as the results of his own studies (Bakker, 1967, 1972; Groenendaal & Bakker, 1971), has proposed a theory of developmental dyslexia, which has as its underlying deficiency a dysfunction in temporal-order recall. Underlying this theory are two major contentions. First, Bakker (1972) conceived of temporal-order and gross (item) memory as separate entities and suggested that the dyslexic child is especially deficient in temporal-order memory. In fact, there is support for this contention from Luria (1973), who proposed that the simultaneous and sequential processing of information are primarily subserved by different systems within the brain. Second, Bakker (1972) suggested that the left hemisphere (assuming the left hemisphere is dominant for language) is responsible for the sequencing of verbal stimuli, while the right hemisphere is responsible for the sequencing of nonverbal stimuli, and Bakker cites the work of Milner (1962, 1967) in support of this contention.

In his initial study (Bakker, 1967), the author attempted to explore the retention of temporally presented material as a function of the type of material presented. Fifty-four boys from a school for children with learning and behavior problems, aged 9–15, were divided into two groups: "better readers," who were on the average two years behind in reading on a standard achievement test, and "worse readers," who were four years behind in reading. The groups were matched for age and IQ as well. Each child was presented 30, four-item series, in tachistoscopic fashion. After each presentation the child was shown the same items scrambled on a card and was asked to order the items as in the visual presentation. The series was composed of either nonsense figures, meaningful figures, letters, or digits.

Results indicated that, in general, "worse readers" made more errors than "better readers." With regard to the type of material presented, the "worse readers" made significantly more errors than "better readers" on both the letters and meaningful figures. The group differences for the digits did not approach significance, and no difference was found with the meaningless figures. Bakker concluded that the results of this study supported the contention of Blank and Bridger (1966) and suggested that poor readers have difficulty using the verbal labels inherent in the meaningful figures to aid in the temporal-order recall. Children who are able to mediate verbally thus achieve better results in perceiving and retaining meaningful sequences than children who cannot employ good verbal mediation.

In a second study (Groenendaal & Bakker, 1971) the authors sought to replicate their initial finding, to explore possible differences in children who are mediators and those who are nonmediators, and to look at age relationships. Subjects were below-average and average readers (reading equivalents not given), matched for IQ, and further divided into seven-year-old and ten-year-old age groupings. Each subject was administered a test of nonverbal mediation in addition to the temporal sequencing task, which was made up of meaningful and nonmeaningful series.

Results indicated that, as in the initial study, children who are good readers are better able than poor readers to perceive and retain the temporal-order sequences of meaningful figures, while performing equally as well on the same task with meaningless figures. Second, children who mediate, according to the mediation task given, also achieve better results on the retention of temporally ordered meaningful figures than non-mediators. Finally, it could not be shown that more good than poor readers were able to mediate verbally. It is important to note here, as Bakker himself points out, that it may be false to assume that verbal mediation was used by all subjects on the mediation task, which also was nonverbal.

Bakker thus concluded that poor readers are deficient only in perceiving the temporal order of verbal stimuli (letters and meaningful stimuli) and do not differ from normal readers in the temporal perception of nonverbal (meaningless) stimuli. Bakker draws further support for his contention from the work of Senf (1969), who found that failures made by the learning-disabled group on their task were usually specific to the ordering of the stimuli and not to their accuracy of recall. Bakker also finds support in his own work (Bakker, 1972), which demonstrated differences between good and poor readers on measures of serial memory for letters presented visually, auditorally, and haptically.

On the surface, this theory would appear promising. Vellutino (1978), however, in his review of this area, finds fault with this theory on two major grounds. First, Vellutino cites several studies that failed to support Bakker's underlying contention that item and order information are processed by two separate memories. The final word is thus not in on this subject. Second, since Bakker has found good and poor readers to differ only on measures involving the temporal ordering of verbal stimuli, the explanation given by Blank and her associates (1966, 1968) that poor readers may be more deficient than normal readers in their ability to employ verbal mnemonics to facilitate the recall of temporally ordered stimuli would seem more plausible. Finally, the work by Blank and Senf that Bakker cited in support of his theory employed digits, dots, and light flashes, which, according to Bakker, are nonverbal meaningless stimuli.

CONCLUSIONS

While the research evidence cited in this chapter does not appear to support the belief that the underlying deficit in developmental dyslexia is one of cross-modal integration, the studies do appear to support the following conclusions.

Some higher-order function common to both cross-modal integration and within-modal integration of information is deficient in many dyslexic children. Whether the deficit is in verbal mediation, temporal-order memory, or faulty attention and/or stimulus encoding skills remains to be seen. Based on the cytoarchitectonic evidence provided by Drake (1968) and Galaburda and Kemper (1979), as well as that from the brain electrical activity mapping research (Duffy, 1981; Duffy et al., 1979; Duffy et al., 1980a, 1980b), it might be reasonable to speculate the deficits in cross-modal and within-modal performance merely reflects subtle neurological deficits. Any neurological deficit, whether in a primary sensory area such as vision or audition or in an association zone, will be manifested in the experimental procedures employed by the investigators cited in this section. All that can be safely concluded is that such processing deficits exist and they may be manifested on some or all integrative tasks.

The relative importance of the age differences reported in these studies cannot be adequately assessed due to the inconsistencies in the ages attributed to the categories of young and old readers. It would thus seem that the disparity of the results obtained in this area again points to the need for studies that look at longitudinal factors associated with different dyslexic-reader subgroups. The investigations discussed in the next chapter are an important step in this direction.

─────Chapter 5─────
Cerebral Dominance and Dyslexia

In Chapter 1, Orton's hypothesis (1928, 1937) that a negative relationship existed between the development of cerebral dominance for language (typically the left cerebral hemisphere) and strephosymbolia, as he termed it, was presented. According to this theory, the left cerebral hemisphere had to establish dominance for all linguistic functions if language abilities were to develop to their ultimate potential. This theory has generated not only a large professional following but also an enormous volume of literature, most of it seemingly contradictory.

There appear to be two reasons why Orton's hypothesis of delayed lateralization has been so widely embraced not only by the psychological community but also by the educational community. First, the idea that cerebral dominance "develops" offered encouragement to those who proposed to help children with learning problems "catch up." It is a most appealing idea that if someone is "delayed" in the normal achievement of some task or developmental milestone, we can simply provide appropriate enrichment experiences in order to foster the person's development. Based on the encouraging work of Sequin and his physiological method (Hynd, Cannon, & Haussmann, 1983; Kaufman & Kaufman, 1983), many educators in the United States developed programs of educational intervention aimed at facilitating the development of functional cerebral lateralization. The Orton-Gillingham method that attempts to train the development of directionality is a good example of this approach. The interested reader may want to refer to Hynd and Obrzut (1981) for an alternate explanation as to why such an approach may prove beneficial to children experiencing learning problems.

A second reason why the incomplete cerebral dominance hypothesis has gained so much widespread popularity is its great degree of face validity. As Obrzut and Hynd (1979) note, one needs little experience with reading-disabled children to validate the idea that these children suffer mixed or incomplete cerebral dominance. Dyslexic children often evidence weak or inconsistent laterality ("eyedness," "footedness," or "handedness") and commonly make reversal errors in reading or in letter recognition. There is hence ready subjective support for Orton's ideas. The problem is that word and letter reversals and mixed cerebral dominance for preferences in laterality may be due to either a delay in development or to a neurological deficit. As will be seen in the chapter dealing with remediation, this distinction between a developmental delay and a neurological deficit is an important one and has critical theoretical as well as practical implications.

Investigations related to articulating the relationship between cerebral dominance and dyslexia can be conceptualized into those that use measures of lateral preference and those that are thought to include measures of central processes, such as audition and vision. For the purposes of the discussion, the research concerning lateral preferences will be dealt with first. As will be seen, this area of research is fraught with many problems and has little to contribute to our present understanding of brain-behavior relationships in dyslexic children. The more direct noninvasive measures of central language and spatial processes have much more to offer in increasing our understanding of the dyslexic child, so proportionally more space will be devoted to these investigations. As such, the final two sections of this chapter will focus on the dichotic listening and the tachistoscopic visual half-field research, respectively.

ASYMMETRIES IN LATERAL PREFERENCE

Early investigations of preferences in lateral asymmetries were fairly comprehensive in that studies related deficits in academic achievement to poorly established eyedness, footedness, and, handedness. The aspects of handedness have without doubt, received by far the greatest attention, and it is often concluded that dyslexics show weak handedness preferences. A closer inspection of the voluminous literature, however, (Corballis & Beale, 1976; Diamond & Blizard, 1977; Harnad, Doty, Goldstein, Jaynes & Krauthamer, 1977; Herron, 1980; Kinsbourne & Hiscock, 1981; Neville, 1976) reveals that most, if not all, studies in this area are fraught with either conceptual or methodological problems.

It is assumed that the deficits observed in dyslexic children on measures of handedness (when compared with controls), for example, is reflective of reversed or of poorly established functional laterality. In other words, if a child is dyslexic and left-handed it is typically thought that the left handedness reflects the fact that language abilities have been lateralized to the right (nondominant) cerebral hemisphere. The dyslexia is but a symptom of this reversed cerebral asymmetry in which language abilities are lateralized to a hemisphere clearly not suited to subserve language skills. In the vast majority of cases this notion is absurd, especially when it is based on measures of handedness since manual preferences are so well known to be amenable to the effects of training and socialization. It is especially an absurd notion because we know from the aphasic literature as well as from the use of the Wada testing that nearly two thirds of all left-handers are lateralized to the left cerebral hemisphere for speech much the same as approximately 95 percent of all right-handers (Annett, 1975; Goodglass & Quadfasel, 1954; Hécaen & Piercy, 1956; Humphrey & Zangwill, 1952; Luria 1970; Penfield & Roberts, 1959; Rasmussen & Milner, 1975, Rossi & Rosadini, 1967). Despite such knowledge, left-handers and children with sinistral tendencies have always, it seems, received "bad press" as the now infamous Cyril Burt (1937) best exemplified:

> They squint, they stammer, they shuffle and shamble, they flounder about like seals out of water. Awkward in the house, and clumsy in their games, they are fumblers and bunglers at whatever they do. (as quoted by Corballis, 1980, p. 287)

Certainly, an argument can be made that deficient right-handed performance or lateralization to the left hand may reveal underlying damage to the cerebral cortex. Such a conclusion, however, cannot be made on the basis of handedness-observation data or performance on a handedness questionnaire, as some would advocate (Coren, Porac, & Duncan, 1979; Dean, Schwartz, & Smith, 1981). The only way in which such a clinical conclusion can be reached is with supporting evidence regarding central language processing, as can be derived from dichotic listening or visual half-field studies. This fact is further supported by those well-controlled studies that have investigated the lateral-preference patterns evidenced by children and the relationship of the patterns to performance on measures of cognitive performance (Hardyck, Petrinovitch, & Goldman, 1976; Kaufman, Zalma, & Kaufman, 1978; Ullman, 1977). As would be expected, no relationship existed between poor achievers and their laterality quotient.

In sum, the authors are tempted to agree with Money (1966), who concluded, "a great deal of material about mixed cerebral dominance adds up to make sheer anatomical nonsense" (p. 91). Our clinical experience and recognition that deficits in lateral performance may have diagnostic value when complemented with other more relevant data, however, has allowed us to offer the preceding brief discussion. The literature that focuses attention on central processing offers more meaningful theoretical as well as practical information and will be discussed in considerably more depth.

DICHOTIC LISTENING RESEARCH

The first nonobtrusive procedure to be discussed here is dichotic listening. This technique requires the subject to recall two different auditory messages that are presented simultaneously, one to each ear. This area was pioneered by the study of Kimura (1961). Working with normal subjects, she demonstrated that the majority of subjects would correctly identify more stimuli presented to the right ear if the message was verbal, and more stimuli presented to the left ear if the message is nonverbal (Fig. 5–1). She then

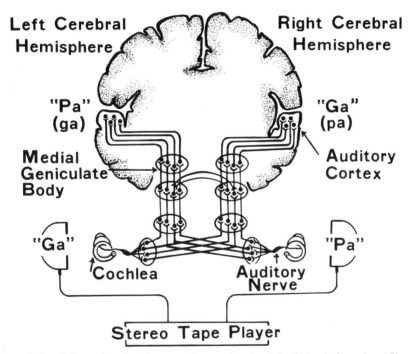

Fig. 5-1. Schematic of auditory pathways involved in dichotic listening. Since crossed auditory pathways are more numerous/prepotent, a dichotic stimuli presented to the right ear ("Pa") is perceived in the left auditory cortex. The dichotic ear effect occurs because the right perceptual field (right ear) is favored in linguistic stimuli recognition by the left auditory cortex. The crossed auditory pathways are more numerous and seem prepotent in auditory stimulus recognition, since pathways cross at both the level of the pons at the trapezoid body and at the level of the midbrain at the inferior colliculus.

compared the performance of neurological patients in whom cerebral dominance had been established by the sodium amytal test. Those with known left-hemisphere representation of language function showed the normal right-ear superiority on verbal material, and those with known right-hemisphere representation for language function showed a left-ear superiority. This suggests that the superiority of each ear on a particular class of material reflects the functional specialization of the contralateral hemisphere (Kimura, 1967).

When a verbal dichotic listening task, similar to the one described above, was presented to 14 nine-year-old dyslexic boys and 14 matched controls, Zurif and Carson (1970) reported that the normal-reader group demonstrated a right-ear (left hemisphere) advantage that bordered on statistical significance. The dyslexic group, in contrast, exhibited a slight tendency to identify information to the left ear more accurately than to the right ear. The authors interpreted this result as supporting a dyslexia theory of incomplete cerebral dominance.

Witelson and Rabinovitch (1972) similarily administered the dichotic listening task to a homogeneous group of reading-disabled children (mean lag, two years), all of whom were demonstrating auditory-linguistic deficits such as poor auditory discrimination and sound-blending skills, as well as to a group of normal children with no history of academic difficulty. The learning-disabled group consisted of 24 children (21 boys, 3 girls) ranging in age from 8 to 13 years (mean age 10.1 years) with normal IQ, who were free from psychiatric disturbance, known brain damage, sensory handicaps, or inadequate school experiences. The control children, 17 boys and 7 girls, ranged in age from 9 to 11 years (mean age 9.7 years) and also had normal intelligence. The results indicated that the reading-disabled children tended toward a left-ear (right hemisphere) advantage for verbal information, whereas significantly more of the normal children (71 percent) demonstrated a right-ear (left hemisphere) advantage.

This result would appear to support the interpretation of Zurif and Carson (1970) of incomplete cerebral dominance in dyslexic children. After closer investigation of their data, however, Witelson and Rabinovitch found that the reading-disabled children were not showing a lack of preference for either ear, as would be expected if the hypothesis of Zurif and Carson (1970) were correct. The reading-disabled children, in fact, showed a greater difference in accuracy between ears than did the normal children. Witelson and Rabinovitch (1972) suggest that the reading-disabled children do have definite lateralization of speech functions, and further suggest that the slight tendency toward a left-ear preference, by this group, is an indication of a higher-than-normal incidence of right-hemisphere superiority for speech functions. What thus appears to be a lack of preference for either ear is merely the result of statistical averaging of those reading-disabled children

Table 5-1
Mean Total Accuracy* for Each Ear for
Normal and Clinic Subgroups

Measure	Subgroups With Greater Right Ear Accuracy		
	Normal	Clinic	t
Number of subjects	17	14	
Left ear accuracy	125.4	103.6	3.67†
Right ear accuracy	135.9	119.9	3.58‡
R−L accuracy	+ 10.5	+ 16.3	1.69
	Subjects With Greater Left Ear Accuracy		
	Normal	Clinic	t
Number of subjects	7	10	
Left ear accuracy	128.0	124.2	0.61
Right ear accuracy	113.7	76.5	3.08‡
R−L accuracy	− 14.3	− 47.7	2.42§

Data from Witelson, SF, & Rabinovitch, MS. Hemispheric speech lateralization in children with auditory-linguistic deficits. *Cortex*, 1972, 8, 412–426.
Note: These children were language disordered and may not represent the general population of dyslexic children.
*Maximum accuracy score for each is 150.
†$p < .001$; ‡$p < .01$; §$p < .05$.

having a right-ear superiority (14 children) with those having a left-ear superiority (10 children). The authors proceeded to compare these two clinical subgroups, with the corresponding subgroup of normal children demonstrating the same-ear superiority (Table 5–1).

On analysis, the two reading-disabled subgroups were found to differ in their pattern of accuracy scores relative to the matched control groups. The right-ear–superior reading-disabled group was significantly impaired in accuracy on both ears relative to its control group. Witelson and Rabinovitch (1972) found this pattern to be strikingly similar to the test performance of adult patients with dysfunction in the left, speech dominant, temporal lobe (Kimura, 1961). They went on to speculate that this subgroup of disabled readers may have speech functions represented in the left hemisphere, but that they may also have a dysfunction present in the region of their brain that, in a child, is functionally comparable to the left-temporal areas of the adult brain. The left-ear–superior reading-disabled group was found to be significantly impaired in only right-ear accuracy, as compared with its control group. The authors found this pattern to be similar to adult patients with a dysfunction present in the right temporal lobe, which is nondominant for speech, who have been found to be impaired only on the contralateral (left) ear on verbal dichotic tasks (Kimura, 1961). The authors speculated that this subgroup of disabled children are right-hemisphere dominant for speech, with a dysfunction in the contralateral (left) hemisphere. Drawing from the work of Benton (1964), Witelson and Rabinovitch go on to propose that the children comprising the left-ear–superior reading-disabled group may have suffered early left-hemisphere damage that resulted in a impetus for right-hemispheric speech lateralization. Left-hemispheric dysfunction thus is proposed as a key factor in all the reading-disabled children in this study; but, the time of onset, the extent, and/or the localization of the dysfunction may differ, so that while speech function remained in the dysfunctioning (left) hemisphere in the right-ear–superior subgroup, it shifted to the right and possibly more intact hemisphere in the left-ear–superior subgroup.

While the overall (main effect) of the two studies just cited appeared to demonstrate that the dyslexic children under study tended to show a nonsignificant left-ear (right hemisphere) superiority for verbal material, other investigators have demonstrated a significant right-ear advantage for both normal and dyslexic readers. Employing a similar experimental design, McKeever and Van Deventer (1975) compared nine dyslexic and nine normal male adolescents (mean age 13.7 years) on the dichotic listening task. The dyslexic children were defined according to the following criterion: All were two or more years behind grade level in reading; all were of normal intelligence; all were free from visual or auditory deficits, sociocultural deprivation, known neurological impairment, and emotional or behavioral problems; and none were from a bilingual background. The only difference in the dyslexic children in this study and the studies discussed previously was their more advanced chronological age. The results indicated that while these older dyslexic children made considerably more errors in both auditory channels than did control children, they, like the control children, demonstrated a significant right-ear (left hemisphere) lateralization for language.

In another study, Yeni-Komshian, Isenberg, and Goldstein (1975) also compared a somewhat older (age range 10.6–13.4 years, mean age 11.8 years) group of 19 poor readers with a group of 19 normal readers. It must be stated that while the poor-reader group was of normal intelligence and on the average was found to be reading three grade-levels below the normal readers, the authors failed to mention if the poor readers also met the other criterion needed for a diagnosis of dyslexia that were employed in the studies mentioned above. Comparison of each group's performance on the dichotic listening task indicated that there was a significant main effect for ears, indicating an overall right-ear (left hemisphere) advantage for both the poor- and normal-reader groups, with the difference in ears being somewhat larger for the poor-reader group, although not statistically significant. It is interesting to note that this main effect held across both the attended (material reported first) and the unattended (material reported last) ear conditions. The authors concluded that these results seem to contradict the hypothesis that disabled readers are not as well-lateralized for language functioning as are normal readers.

Finally, Leong (1976) has also administered the dichotic listening task to a group of 58 dyslexic boys (age nine) and to a group of above-average readers matched for age, sex, and IQ. The dyslexic children were found to be reading at least 2.5 grade levels below expectancy; were of normal intelligence; and were free from gross emotional, visual, and auditory disabilities. The results indicated that both the dyslexic and normal-reader groups demonstrated a significant right-ear (left hemisphere) advantage on the dichotic listening task, with the normal-reader group obtaining higher scores for both ears than did the dyslexic group. Leong concluded that this result was evidence for the notion of a lag in functional cerebral development in dyslexic readers.

The Concept of Maturational Lag

Looking at age effects as an independent variable in developmental dyslexia, Satz, Rardin, and Ross (1971) performed a cross-sectional study of dyslexic and normal readers in order to test a theory (Satz & Sparrow, 1970) that postulated that the pattern of deficits found in developmental dyslexia could be best explained as a lag in the maturation of the central nervous system. More specifically, this theory involves the concept of a maturational lag in the lateralization and differentiation of motor, somatosensory, and language functions subserved by the dominant left hemisphere. The theory predicts that skills that develop ontogenetically earlier (visual-motor and auditory-visual integration) would be more delayed in younger dyslexic children, while skills that develop later (language and formal operations) would be more delayed in older dyslexic children. The dichotic listening task comprised just one of several developmental-cognitive measures administered to a younger (aged 7–8 years) and an older (aged 11–12 years) group of dyslexic boys. Both groups were individually matched for age, sex, race, and IQ, with normal-reader control groups. The dyslexic subjects were, in addition, free from gross physical, sensory, or neurological handicaps. The results indicated a significant right-ear (left hemisphere) advantage in both the younger and in the older dyslexic and normal-reader groups. The tendency toward left-hemisphere dominance for speech, in other words, was evident in both the dyslexic and the normal readers at both ages. Second, and most important to the authors' hypothesis, was the finding that the magnitude of the right-ear advantage was significantly greater in the older normal group as compared with the older dyslexic group, with no statistically significant differences being found between younger normals and dyslexics. The authors concluded that this finding supported their theory that the brain evidences increasing maturation and functional lateralization with age, but does so at a slower rate than normal in dyslexic readers.

Taking an identical theoretical position, Bakker and his associates (Bakker, 1973; Bakker, Smink, & Reitsma, 1973) performed a series of studies (employing a cross-sectional design), the aim of which was to test the hypothesis that efficient reading performance is associated with low ear-dominance at younger ages and with high ear-dominance at older ages. The authors extended their theorizing somewhat from that of Satz and Sparrow (1970) by postulating that a relatively advanced degree of language lateralization (left hemisphere) may also interfere with the acquisition of the perceptual reading skills necessary at younger ages.

In their initial study, Bakker et al. (1973) looked at the performance of various age groups of normal readers on a monaural listening test of ear dominance and related the ear-dominance effects obtained with the reading ability of the children. The results indicated the following conclusions. At younger school ages (7 years to 7.5 years of age) the best readers showed the lowest absolute between-ear differences. As children get older (ages 8.5 years to 11 years of age), those showing a difference between ears with respect to accuracy of recall read better than those children who do not. While efficient reading appears to be associated with a lack of ear dominance at early ages and the development of moderate ear dominance at older ages, a too-advanced lateralization seemed to hamper reading efficiency. It must be stated that this latter result did not show a distinct age-based dichotomy, and so did not reach statistical significance. The authors went on to conclude that these results support the hypothesis of Satz and Sparrow (1970) and confirm the results of the Satz, Rardin, and Ross (1971) study, thus, the process of learning to read appears to be coupled with the gradual progress of increased lateralization.

In a second study, Bakker (1973) employed a similar experimental design with dyslexic children. The results indicated that the relationship between dominance and reading for dyslexic children aged 9–10 and 11–13 years were very similar to the relationships found for the normal readers aged 7–8 and 9–11 years in the Bakker et al. (1973) study. The pattern of the dominance-reading relation as well as the reading-performance level of dyslexic children were thus found to be two years behind those of normal children. Bakker concluded that this result gave further support to a developmental delay in lateralization in dyslexic children.

Witelson (1976) has also employed a cross-sectional design to explore hemispheric specialization in developmental dyslexia. In this study, Witelson administered a series of different tests (dichotomous tactual stimulation, lateral tachistoscopic stimulation, and dichotic listening) to a group of 85 dyslexic boys ranging in age from 6 to 14 years and to a group of 156 normal boys, comprising a similar age range, in order to assess both left- and right-hemispheric functioning in the dyslexic children. The dyslexic children were at least 1.5 grade levels behind in reading, as measured by the Wide Range Achievement Test (mean lag 2.6 grade levels); of normal intelligence (mean IQ = 102); and free from emotional disturbance, detectable brain damage, or sensory difficulties. In order to assess left-hemispheric specialization for language, each child was administered the verbal dichotic listening test. The results indicated a significant right-ear (left hemisphere) advantage for both the dyslexic and the normal readers at all age groupings (6–7, 8–9, 10–11, and 12–14 years of age), except for that of the youngest dyslexic group. The overall accuracy, in addition, for the normal group was significantly greater at all age levels than that of the dyslexic group. Based on these results, Witelson concluded in part, that like normal male readers, dyslexic boys employ the left hemisphere for linguistic processing. The level of ability to process the linguistic information in this task, however, is markedly lower in the dyslexic children and may be suggestive of a disorder in left-hemispheric functioning in dyslexic children.

In his review of the literature on cerebral dominance and reading disability, Satz (1976) reports the results of a study (Darby, 1974) that employed a longitudinal design in order to examine the developmental parameters of the ear asymmetry in dyslexia. Darby selected a group of severely reading-retarded male children who were identified as such at the end of first grade (age 7), and who were originally tested two years earlier at the beginning of kindergarten (age 5.5), as part of a longitudinal-predictive study of dyslexia (Satz, Friel, & Rudegeair, 1976). Each child included in the dyslexic category had to be predicted as severe high risk, based on the initial testing done at the kindergarten and the first-grade levels; as well as demonstrating reading below preprimer level at the end of first grade. In addition, children were excluded from the dyslexic category if they had a low socioeconomic rating, showed emotional immaturity, had one or more sensory handicaps, or had a Peabody IQ score below 90. Controls were selected from the population who evidenced no predicted or assessed reading problems during the first two years of the longitudinal-predictive study cited above. In order to assess the full range of age comparisons, a third group of older dyslexic children (aged 11–12 years) were selected and matched for socioeconomic status (SES), sex, and IQ with the dyslexics in the longitudinal study. These children had to show evidence of severe reading disability of greater than two years in duration, in the absence of sensory handicaps and brain damage. Controls for this group were selected under similar matching conditions as those employed for the younger dyslexic subjects. The results indicated that, for the normal-reader control children (Fig. 5–2), the magnitude of the ear asymmetry increased with age

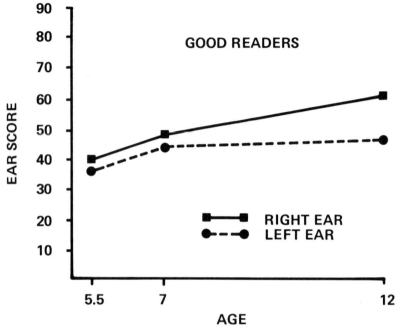

Fig. 5-2.   Mean dichotic listening scores by ear and by age for good readers. [From Satz, P. Cerebral dominance and reading disability. In Knights, RM, & Bakker, DJ (Eds), Neuropsychology of learning disorders: Theoretical approach. Baltimore, University Park Press, 1976. With permission.]

with a significant right-ear (left hemisphere) advantage evident only in the older group (aged 11–12 years). The trend in favor of a right-ear advantage, however, was evident as early as age 5.

The dyslexic children, in contrast, failed to develop a significant right-ear (left hemisphere) advantage at any age level, although the trend toward a right-ear advantage also increased with age (Fig. 5–3). The author concluded that these results supported the maturational lag theory of Satz and Sparrow (1970), which predicts an age relationship between reading ability and lateralization, especially at older ages when the lateralization of speech is thought to be complete.

Finally, in a recent study, Sadick and Ginsburg (1978) grouped good and poor readers, as measured by either the Gates-McGinite or the Metropolitan Reading Readiness Test, into three age categories (5 and 6, 7, and 8 to 11 years). A dichotic listening assessment resulted in the following indications. Good readers showed a consistent decrease in ambilaterality from 61 percent of the population in the 5- and 6-year-old children, to a 25 percent decrease in the 8- to 11-year-old children. This was accompanied by a steady development of right-ear superiority from 31.7 percent in the 5- and 6-year-old children, to 68.8 percent in the 8- to 11-year-old children. On the other hand, poor readers showed almost no shift in ambilaterality

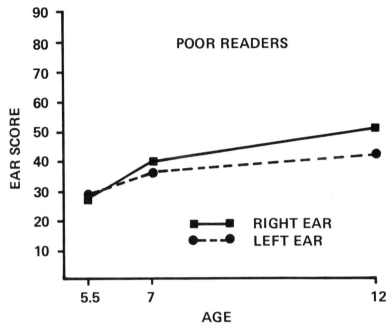

Fig. 5-3. Mean dichotic listening scores by ear and by age for poor readers. [From Satz, P. Cerebral dominance and reading disability. In Knights, RM, & Bakker, DJ (Eds), Neuropsychology of learning disorders: Theoretical approach. Baltimore, University Park Press, 1976. With permission.]

with age. They instead exhibited an increase in right-ear advantage from 37.5 percent to 60 percent over age, with a corresponding decrease in left-ear advantage of 12.4 percent to 0 percent with age. The authors thus conclude that there appears to be a developmental trend in good readers from ambilaterality at the very early stages of the learning-to-read process to increasing laterality in the later stages of reading development.

Sex and age differences in normal readers have been explored by Bakker, Teunissen and Bosch (1976). The authors compared three age groups of boys and girls (mean ages 7.6, 9 and 11 years) on the dichotic listening task and on a word-naming task, in which the child had to read as many words as possible within a minute. Results indicated that in the youngest group, boys read well if there was an advantage for either ear, but girls read well only when there was a right-ear advantage. In the older group, both sexes read well only when a right-ear advantage was demonstrated. On the basis of these findings, Bakker and his associates proposed that the learning-to-read process develops in stages that are passed through first by girls and then by boys. Both cerebral hemispheres initially possess the capacity to mediate written language, but later on only the left hemisphere has this capacity. The authors go on to state that the reading proficiency in right-hemisphere–dominant subjects appears to be achieved differently than in left-hemisphere–dominant subjects. Young left-dominant children read rapidly, at the risk of making many errors. Young right-dominant children read slowly but accurately. This slow but accurate strategy, while appropriate at the early stages of the learning-to-read process, may be disavantageous at later stages.

In conclusion, the results of the studies presented in this section, which have explored the relationship between language lateralization of the brain (as believed to be measured by the dichotic listening task) and reading ability, suggest that different degrees of hemispheric asymmetry for language appear to be advantageous as different phases of the learning-to-read process are approached. It would seem that at the earliest stages of this process during the ages of five- and six-years-old, a maximum interplay between linguistic and visual-perceptual skills is required. It would appear likely, as a result, that ambilaterality would be a characteristic of good readers at this age. It would also seem likely as reading becomes more automatic, that the emphasis on visual-perceptual skills would diminish. With increasing age (approximately seven years of age and up) it is thus not surprising that good readers continue to show an increasing trend toward greater lateralization (presumably in the left hemisphere). This, in fact, is what the cross-sectional and longitudinal studies with normal control readers done by the Satz (1976), Bakker et al. (1976), and Sadick and Ginsburg (1978) research groups appear to be telling us. In addition, the Bakker et al. (1976) study seems to have gone one step further by showing that girls proceed through this developmental process at a faster rate than do boys.

After analysis of the data accumulated on the dyslexic population, it appears safe to say that the results are not as clear cut. Looking at those studies that simply compare dyslexic and normal readers without control for developmental effects we find some studies (Witelson & Rabinovitch, 1972; Zurif & Carson, 1970) reporting dyslexic children as possessing a slight left-ear (right hemisphere) advantage which led these researchers to postulate "incomplete cerebral dominance" or a "left hemisphere dysfunction for speech" as a possible cause in the etiology of dyslexia. Still other researchers (Leong, 1976; McKeever & Van Deventer, 1975; Yeni-Komshian et al., 1975), employing a similar research design with older subjects, reported that their dyslexic children, like the normal reader controls, demonstrated a significant right-ear, (left hemisphere) advantage. This result, taken together with the finding that the dyslexic children showed a lower overall right-ear superiority than normal readers, let Leong (1976) to conclude that his results supported the notion of a lag in functional cerebral development in dyslexic readers. Further support for a developmental-delay model of dyslexia can be obtained from the longitudinal studies done by Satz and his colleagues (Darby, 1974; Satz, Rardin, & Ross, 1971), as well as the cross-sectional studies done by Bakker and his colleagues (Bakker, et al., 1976). Witelson (1976), however, interprets her cross-sectional data as being suggestive of a disorder in left-hemispheric functioning in dyslexic children.

The differences reported in these studies can be explained in several ways. Many of the studies appear to be suffering from methodological errors. Satz (1976), for example, in his review of the literature in this area, has pointed out that the failure of some studies to show normal or atypical between-ear differences in dyslexic children may be the result of "ceiling and floor effects" in the tests used. Second, many of the studies did not control for sex differences or seek to explore the significance of this factor. Third, the studies employing a cross-sectional design to assess age-difference trends will encounter difficulties in interpretation when spurts and plateaus in development are overlooked. Finally, all of the studies mentioned here viewed the dyslexic population as a homogeneous entity. As mentioned previously, it would seem very possible and, in fact, probable that the disparity in the results is in part the result of multiple etiology within a single diagnostic category.

While it thus appears safe to conclude that the dyslexic children under study do differ from normal readers in their performance on the dichotic listening task, it would seem unwarranted to interpret this difference as evidence for either a neurological deficit or a developmental delay in cerebral functioning when, in fact, the neural-deficit hypothesis does not preclude the observation of a lag in the development of cognitive skills.

TACHISTOSCOPIC VISUAL HALF-FIELD RESEARCH

A second noninvasive procedure used in studying the relationship between cerebral dominance and developmental dyslexia involves the tachistoscopic presentation of verbal or spatial stimuli to either the right or the left visual field. Comparisons are then made between response latency and/or percentage of correct responses within the two visual fields. It should be reiterated here that the anatomical pathways for vision are such that stimuli perceived in the left visual half-field are received in the right cerebral hemisphere, while stimuli perceived in the right visual half-field are received in the left cerebral hemisphere (Fig. 5–4). Keeping this in mind, it has been reliably found that in normal readers, verbal stimuli are more accurately perceived in the right visual half-field (left hemisphere) than in the left visual half-field (right hemisphere) (Kimura, 1966). Similarly, nonverbal or spatial material is more accurately perceived in the left visual half-field (right hemisphere) (Kimura & Durnford, 1974).

Relatively few researchers have employed this technique in the comparison of dyslexic and normal readers, and those who have employed this technique report mixed results. In one of the early studies, McKeever and

VISUAL FIELDS

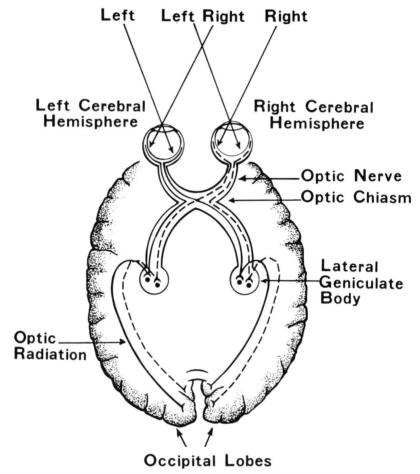

Fig. 5-4. Schematic of the visual pathways involved in tachistoscopic visual half-field paradigms. Stimuli of a linguistic nature presented in the right visual field will be perceived with greater accuracy in the left occipital cortex.

Huling (1970) compared the performance of two groups of seventh grade children on the unilateral tachistoscopic presentation of four-letter nouns. The normal-reader group consisted of ten children whose mean reading level and mean IQ according to the Peabody Picture Vocabulary Test (PPVT) were 8.1 and 117.2, respectively. The poor-reader group also consisted of ten children with a mean reading level of 3.8 and a mean IQ (PPVT) of 86.6. While the poor-reader children were found to be delayed in their reading ability by over four full grade levels, it must be stated that the authors made no mention of controlling for such confounding variables as psychiatric disturbance, neurological impairment, sensory handicaps, and inadequate school experience. A diagnosis of dyslexia thus must remain questionable. The results indicated that both groups demonstrated a superior recognition for words presented to the right visual half-field (left hemisphere) under both monocular and binocular conditions. The magnitude of the asymmetries for both groups, in addition, appeared similar. Although these results provide no support for the theory of incomplete or delayed cerebral dominance for speech, they must be viewed with caution due to the limitations cited above.

In a second study, Marcel, Katz, and Smith (1974) assessed the performance of two groups of boys and girls (mean age 7.6–8.7 years) on the unilateral tachistoscopic presentation of five-letter verbs and concrete nouns. The good- and poor-reader groups were each comprised of ten boys and ten girls, all but two of whom were right-handed. Reader ability was measured by the National Foundation for Educational Research Reading Test. As in the McKeever and Huling (1970) study, the authors made no mention of any effort to control for IQ, neurological impairment, sensory handicaps, psychiatric disturbance, or inadequate school experience. The children were instructed to report the word if they saw it or, if not, to report as many letters as possible. Analyses were thus made on correct word and letter responses. The results indicated a significant right visual half-field asymmetry (left hemisphere) for word and letter reports in both the good and poor readers. Marcel and his colleagues, however, also found that this right visual half-field supcriority was greater in the good readers. After carefully ruling out eye movements or attentional artifacts in their data, Marcel et al. (1974) concluded that good readers store linguistic data more asymmetrically than do poor readers, and also that the differential nature of the extent of functional lateralization is most likely to be the causative factor of their results.

In a later study (Marcel & Rajan, 1975), Marcel and his colleagues sought to replicate the findings of the Marcel et al. (1974) study with a group of good and poor readers (ten boys and ten girls in each group), ranging in age from 7.0 to 9.1 years. Assessment of reading ability and tachistoscopic procedure were similar to the initial study. The results indicated a consistent right visual half-field (left hemisphere) superiority for both reader groups with the good readers, demonstrating a greater asymmetry than the poor readers. As in their initial study, they attributed these results to the difference in the extent of linguistic specialization in the function of the left hemisphere between readers.

Yeni-Komshian et al. (1975), in a study cited previously in the dichotic listening research, also administered a digit numeral and word tachistoscopic task to a group of 19 poor readers (age range 10.6–13.4 years, mean age 11.8 years) and to a group of 19 normal readers of similar age. The material presented was linguistic, and the response was in the verbal mode.

It must again be stated that while the poor-reader group was of normal intelligence and on the average was found to be reading three grade levels below the normal readers, the authors failed to mention if the poor readers also met the other criterion needed for a diagnosis of dyslexia. The results indicated a significant right visual half-field (left hemisphere) asymmetry for both numerals and words only in the poor readers. This result led the authors to conclude that the poor readers demonstrated more lateralization than did the good readers. This assumption is highly questionable due to the fact that the authors failed to show a reliable right visual half-field (left hemisphere) asymmetry in their normal-reader group. The authors went on to note that the major difference between the two reading groups was the significantly lower left visual half-field (right hemisphere) performance of the poor-reader group. This result led Yeni-Komshian et al. (1975) to further speculate on a right-hemispheric deficit in their poor-reader group. Because of the nature of the material presented and the verbal response mode, the authors concluded that either there is some form of processing deficit in the right hemisphere of poor readers, or, their right-to-left hemisphere transmission has somehow broken down.

McKeever and Van Deventer (1975), in a study that was previously discussed in the dichotic listening research, were the first researchers to administer the tachistoscopic task (unilateral and bilateral presentation) to a group of nine dyslexic and nine normal control readers. The dyslexic group ranged in age from 11 to 18 years (mean age 12.9 years) and were all found to be reading at least two years below their expected grade level. In addition, the dyslexic children were of normal intelligence and were free from visual or audition deficits, sociocultural deprivation, neurological impairment, emotional or behavioral problems, and bilingual backgrounds. The normal-reader group were all reading on or above grade level and possessed normal intelligence, hearing, and vision, with no history of emotional or neurological involvement. The results indicated that the mean word-recognition levels for both visual half-fields was considerably lower for the dyslexic group on the unilateral as well as on the bilateral modes of tachistoscopic presentation; the normal reader group demonstrated a significant right visual half-field (left hemisphere) superiority on both the bilateral and unilateral word-recognition tasks; the dyslexic group demonstrated a strong trend toward a significant right visual half-field advantage on the bilateral presentation but failed to show a similar trend on the unilateral presentation; and, although the bilateral presentation resulted in a reduction in overall recognition relative to unilateral presentation for both groups, the visual half-field pattern was very different for the two groups. Under unilateral presentation, the dyslexic group was markedly inferior to the normal readers in the recognition of right visual half-field words but on left visual half-field recognition the performance of the two groups appeared similar. With bilateral presentation the dyslexic group showed a greater drop in left visual half-field recognition efficiency relative to right, whereas in the normal readers the reduction occurred exclusively in right visual half-field recall. The bilateral word-recognition task thus suggested left-hemisphere dominance for the dyslexic readers, but the unilateral word-recognition task failed to show left-hemispheric dominance.

Due to the brief exposure time employed in the bilateral task, the interpretation of visual half-field differences for this mode of presentation remains questionable. The authors, as a result, decided to replicate their study with the same subjects one year later. The word-recognition tasks were readministered exactly as before, except the exposure durations were increased for all subjects. As in the initial study, the results indicated that the mean word-recognition levels for both visual half fields was considerably lower for the dyslexic group both on the unilateral and on the bilateral modes of tachistoscopic presentation; the normal-reader group demonstrated a significant right visual half-field (left hemisphere) advantage both on the unilateral and on the bilateral word-recognition tasks; the dyslexic group demonstrated a significant right visual half-field asymmetry on the bilateral presentation, but again they failed to show a similar trend on the unilateral presentation; and, as in the first study, the dyslexic group showed greater impairment of right visual half-field recognition than left visual half-field recognition when compared with normal readers on the unilateral condition. With bilateral presentation, the dyslexic group showed a greater reduction of left visual half-field recognition than right visual half-field recognition as compared with the normal readers. No significant differences between unilateral and bilateral recognition existed for either visual half-field for the normal readers.

Based on the results of these two tachistoscopic studies and the dichotic listening study discussed earlier, McKeever and Van Deventer (1975) concluded that their older "chronic" dyslexics possess clear left-hemispheric language lateralization even though the unilateral tachistoscopic word-recognition task, if considered in isolation, would seem to support an incomplete cerebral-dominance hypothesis. According to the authors (McKeever & Van Deventer, 1975), the absence of a right visual half-field asymmetry on the unilateral task seems more parsimoniously explained as the result of a dysfunction of the left hemisphere. The authors go on to hypothesize that two deficits may exist in chronic dyslexics: the left hemisphere may have a dysfunction in the visual-association cortex, and their auditory memory may have high-rate and/or sequential language input deficits. These may cause even simple reading to be slow and error-prone.

Kershner (1977) was the second researcher to administer a bilateral tachistoscopic word-recognition task to a group of ten-year-old dyslexic readers and ten-year-old good readers. A gifted-reader group was also assessed in order to help control for intelligence. The dyslexic-reader group was comprised of three boys and seven girls of average intelligence, all of whom were right-handed, at least two years behind in reading level, and free from emotional problems, gross neurological disorder, and sensory handicaps. The good-reader group was comprised of three boys and eight girls matched for age, IQ, and handedness with the dyslexic group. The gifted-reader group was comprised of five boys and seven girls who had been advanced from sixth grade to seventh grade. In addition, they were also matched for age and handedness. The results indicated the following findings. All three reader groups were able to recognize more words presented to the right visual half-field (left hemisphere) than to the left visual half-field. While all three groups demonstrated a right visual half-field advantage, the gifted and good readers demonstrated a significantly higher right visual half-field score as compared with the dyslexic group. The left visual half-field comparison revealed that although the dyslexic group scored higher than both the gifted and good readers, a significant difference was only reached with the gifted-reader group. Lastly, controlling statistically for differences in IQ had no impact on the visual half-field differences found between the gifted and dyslexic reader groups, while controlling for reading ability eliminated the cerebral dominance effect.

These findings, taken together, led Kershner (1977) to conclude that although IQ and proficient reading are known to be interacting variables, it appears that reading disability is associated with nonintellectual, lateralized word-processing functions.

> The results suggest that reading impairment is related to hemispheric differences in processing reading material. We are not dealing with cerebral dominance for language when measuring visual half field asymmetries but with a specific linguistic ability-decoding print, which appears to be a function that the left hemisphere can learn to perform more efficiently than the right. (p. 65)

Kershner (1977) goes on to state that,

> It can be hypothesized that reading disability may be the result of a perceptual coding strategy (right hemisphere as opposed to left) that is inappropriate to the processing demands made by comprehending text and inefficient for the achievement of academic success via orthodox reading instruction. (p. 66)

Witelson (1976), in an article previously discussed in the dichotic listening research, also employed the unilateral tachistoscopic presentation of unfamiliar figures of people as well as the dichotomous tactual-stimulation test with nonsense shapes as a means of studying right-hemisphere specialization for spatial processing in dyslexic and in normal subjects. As prevously noted, the children under study were a group of 85 right-handed dyslexic boys and a group of 156 right-handed boys who were normal readers. Both groups ranged in age from 6 to 14 years. The dyslexic children were at least 1.5 grade levels behind in reading as measured by the Wide Range Achievement Test (mean lag 2.5 grade levels); of normal intelligence (mean IQ = 102); and free from emotional disturbance, gross brain damage, or sensory difficulties.

The tachistoscopic presentation of pictures of people in a unilateral fashion required each child to view two pictures of people in either the left or right visual field and indicate whether the two stimuli were the same or different. It was reasoned that since the right hemisphere is specialized for spatial processing, one might predict that stimuli that require the perception of spatial relationships (faces, figures) would be better perceived when presented to the left visual half-field. Witelson cited the work with adults of Kimura and Durnford (1974) as support for this prediction in children. The results indicated that normal-reader group demonstrated a significant left visual half-field (right hemisphere) advantage while the dyslexic-reader group showed a similar but nonsignificant trend in the same direction. In addition, the left visual half-field score of the normal reader group was significantly greater than the score of the dyslexic group, while both groups obtained right visual half-field scores that were compatible. These results, when taken together, appear to indicate that while the normal-reader group, like adults, possesses right-hemispheric specialization for visual-spatial processing, the dyslexic group appears to lack right-hemispheric specialization or possesses bilateral spatial representation.

The dichotomous tactual-stimulation test required each child to palpate, out of their view, two different nonsense shapes simultaneously for ten seconds, one with each hand. The child then had to choose those two stimuli from a visual-recognition display of six shapes. The use of nonsense shapes and having the child point to a visual match ensured that verbal processing was not required in the cognitivie process. It must also be stated here that tactual-shape discrimination has been shown to depend on the contralateral somethetic pathways (Sperry, Gazzaniga, & Bogen, 1969). The consequence of this relationship would be the production of a competing situation between the right and left inputs. If the right hemisphere is more effective in processing spatial information, then this task would be expected to result in some advantage to stimuli presented to the contralateral (left) hand. The results indicated that while the accuracy scores for both groups were similar and that both groups demonstrated greater left-hand (right hemisphere) scores, the normal-reader group obtained a significantly greater left-hand score than right-hand score, while the dyslexic group did not. In addition, while the left-hand scores for the two groups were compatible, the right-hand score for the dyslexic group was significantly greater than the right-hand score for the normal-reader group. These results again appear to indicate that the dyslexic group, unlike their normal-reader counterparts, seems to be lacking right-hemispheric specialization for special processing or that they possess a bilateral spatial representation.

The results of the above-mentioned studies combined with the results of the dichotic listening study previously dicussed led Witelson (1976) to conclude the following. First, on the basis of the dichotic listening data it is hypothesized that the dyslexic boys have left-hemisphere specialization for linguistic processing, as do normal boys. The level of processing linguistic information in this task, however, is markedly lower in the dyslexic child and may be suggestive of a disorder in left-hemisphere functioning. Second, on the basis of the tachistoscopic and dichotomous tactual-stimulation tests, it is suggested that dyslexics have a bilateral representation of spatial functions that may interfere with the processing of linguistic functions by the left hemisphere. Witelson thus (1976) suggested that the absence of specialization in the right hemisphere regarding spatial processing as well as abnormal linguistic processing in the left hemisphere's functions are two neural dysfunctions that may be associated with the developmental dyslexia syndrome.

CONCLUSIONS

The sparsity of research studies that employ tachistoscopic visual half-field procedures that have adequately differentiated the dyslexic population from the general reading-retarded population, the use of unilateral presentation in some studies versus the use of bilateral stimulus presentation in others, and the apparent conflict over possible scanning bias in the procedure, as well as the paucity of developmental and subgroup research, make generalization difficult. With these considerations in mind, if we consider the studies that have adequately defined the dyslexic population (using the definition by the World Federation of Neurology [Critchley, 1970] or some similar criteria) and who have made an effort to control for scanning bias (Kershner, 1977; McKeever & Van Deventer, 1975; Witelson, 1976), some tentative conclusions may be offered.

The results of those studies that have employed a bilateral tachistoscopic presentation of verbal material (Kershner, 1977; McKeever & Van Deventer 1975) in order to assess left-hemisphere specialization for language seem to support the findings of the dichotic listening research discussed in a prior section. That is, dyslexic children, like their normal-reader counterparts, appear to have left-hemispheric specialization for linguistic processing, but not at the same level that is demonstrated by normal readers. This conclusion is also consistent with the research conducted with learning-disabled children (Hynd, Obrzut, Weed, & Hynd, 1979). The question of whether this difference in the degree of lateralization found in the dyslexic children is the result of developmental delay or is the result of neurological deficits cannot be answered conclusively from the data at hand.

Since the dyslexic children demonstrated deficit performance on tasks assessing all modalities, it could be speculated that a more general, nonspecific deficit underlies the dyslexic syndrome. As mentioned in Chapter 2, Dykman et al. (1970, 1971) implicated the RAS (reticular activating system) as being deficient in its arousal function in children with learning problems. The arousal function of the RAS as discussed by Luria (1980, 1969) and the relationship to frontal-lobe functions may possibly be correlated with the generalized deficits in performance as reported in this chapter. It should be pointed out that this is speculation awaiting further research.

The study conducted by Witelson (1976) appears to have gone one step further in that it characterized right-hemispheric involvement as well as left-hemispheric involvement in the etiology of the dyslexic syndrome. Based on her findings, Witelson proposed that dyslexia may be the manifestation of bilateral representation of spatial processing (normally thought of as a right-hemispheric function) that interferes with the processing of linguistic functions by the left hemisphere, or may be the result of a dysfunction in the left hemisphere, as speculated by other researchers.

By proposing this model of dual causation in the dyslexic syndrome, Witelson (1976) has opened the door to a reevaluation of the dyslexic syndrome. More precisely, dyslexia may not be the result of a specific deficit or characteristic developmental delay. It may instead be more productive from a conceptual and practical viewpoint to view dyslexia as having multiple etiologies. Multiple etiologies as well as expected variation in the manifestation of dyslexia would result in different subgroups of dyslexic readers, each with their own pattern of cognitive deficits. As will be seen in Chapter 6, important new developments are taking place along this line of inquiry.

────Chapter 6────
Subgroups of Dyslexia

It has been assumed until recently that children comprising the diagnostic population entitled "developmental dyslexia" constituted a homogeneous group. As mentioned previously, one of the most basic assumptions underlying all of the single-factor theories of developmental dyslexia is the notion of a single etiological entity that exhibits a random distribution of reading errors. Research evidence will be presented in this chapter that supports the view that the dyslexic population is not a homogeneous entity, but is rather a heterogeneous entity comprised of different subgroups of dyslexic children who manifest different subtypes of reading deficiency. The underlying notion is that if the development of reading requires the complex integration of several higher-order processes, then a deficit in any one of these critical processes can be the sufficient cause of developmental dyslexia.

The first research evidence to be cited in support of this conception does not come from any one theorist or researcher, but comes instead from the entire body of single-factor research. As suggested in Chapter 5, the major finding of this research approach has been that there is, in fact, more than one underlying cause for this disorder. As we have seen, dyslexic children have been found to differ from normal readers in the areas of visual perception, intersensory integration, temporal-order sequencing, language development, and cerebral dominance; in short, they differ in almost every perceptual-cognitive function necessary for the development of reading. It is also of interest that many of these deficits would be manifested in the association and tertiary areas (e.g., angular gyrus) of the cerebral cortex whether the lesion or deficit actually occurred there. This finding, taken together with the fact that no single child diagnosed as developmental dyslexic exhibits all of these deficits, is strong evidence in and of itself for the conception of developmental dyslexia as a heterogeneous diagnostic entity.

INITIAL CONCEPTUALIZATION

Perhaps the first individual research study undertaken to explore the possibility of distinct subgroups of dyslexic children was accomplished by Kinsbourne and Warrington (1963) at the National Hospital in London. They divided children referred because of reading backwardness into two groups on the basis of Wechsler Intelligence Scale for Children (WISC) or Wechsler Adult Intelligence Scale (WAIS) Verbal-Performance IQ discrepancies. Group 1 was composed of six children who had at least a 20-point verbal-performance discrepancy in favor of the Performance Scale IQ (PSIQ). These children were termed the language-retarded group. Group 2 was comprised of seven children who had at least a 20-point verbal-performance discrepancy in the opposite direction, favoring the Verbal Scale IQ (VSIQ). These children were termed the Gerstmann Group. The children in both groups ranged in age from 8 to 14 years.

Based on tests commonly used in a neurological evaluation, the following results were reported. Group 1 children (VSIQ < PSIQ), in addition to their verbal-performance pattern noted on the WISC, exhibited delays in speech acquisition, verbal comprehension, and verbal expression. In short, the language-retarded group presented a picture analogous to that of aphasia in the adult. In the Group 2, or Gerstmann Group, children (PSIQ < VSIQ), finger agnosia, as characterized by poor performance on tests of finger order and differentiation, was always present. In addition, significant retardation in right-left orientation and in arithmetic, as well as constructional difficulty, was found.

While drawing the analogy between the language-retarded group and acquired aphasia (due to lesion) in the adult, and between the developmental Gerstmann syndrome group and the adult with acquired Gerstmann syndrome, the authors were quick to caution that the analogy between these syndromes of acquired cerebral deficit in adults and developmental cerebral deficit in children was solely on a functional level. No anatomical correspondence was thus to be assumed. The fact that a lesion in a certain part of the brain may cause a particular syndrome in the adult in no way implies that a child with a similar developmental syndrome had a localized cerebral lesion. Kinsbourne and Warrington (1963) noted that the full syndrome need not be present in every Gerstmann or language case. The symptomatology presented would depend on not only the level of severity of the deficit but also on the degree of compensation to it. Finally, the authors pointed out that there could be other conceivable disorders of perception and movement that could lead to difficulties in reading and writing. The authors speculated, for example, on the possibility of cases in which both the Gerstmann and language syndromes were present in the same child. Kinsbourne and Warrington (1963) concluded by stating the following:

> Rather than regarding specific dyslexia as a single condition, it would seem preferable to accept the occurrence among the population of backward readers and writers of cases based upon developmental cerebral deficit. Insofar as the acquisition of reading and writing skill is a complex procedure, involving a variety of cerebral functions, it is not surprising to find that retarded development of one or other of the functions subserved by the cerebral hemispheres may delay this acquisition, and do so in different ways, depending upon the exact nature of the function which is insufficiently developed (p. 153, with permission.)

Evidence in Support of Kinsbourne and Warrington

Another notable contribution to the idea that developmental dyslexia is comprised of heterogeneous subgroups was the delineation of auditory and visual dyslexia by Johnson and Myklebust (1967). The auditory dyslexic child, according to these authors, experiences difficulty in remembering auditory symbols and in stringing them into sequences. The visual dyslexic child, on the other hand, appears to experience deficits in visual perception and in memory. These children, as a result, have visual discrimination problems that result in confusion of letters and words that look the same. These children can make discriminations, but they will be made very slowly.

Bannatyne (1966a) has also identified two main subgroups of dyslexic children. The first subgroup, the genetic dyslexic group, is viewed as representing the lower end of a normal continuum in verbal ability within the general population. Bannatyne characterized these children as having difficulty with fine auditory discrimination, with auditory sequencing, and with the association of sound-symbol relationships. The second subgroup, referred to as the minimal neurological dysfunction dyslexia group, is viewed as being neurologically involved. Bannatyne characterized this group as being deficient in a wide variety of skills such as visual-spatial and auditory perception, tactile integration, and conceptualization.

In contrast to her predecessors, Bateman (1968) identified three subgroups of dyslexic children based on test profile analysis of the Illinois Test of Psycholinguistic Abilities (ITPA). The three groups were characterized as follows: children with poor auditory memory but with good visual memory; children with poor visual memory but with good auditory memory; and children who have deficits in both of these processes. Bateman stated that the third group was felt to be the most severe and would be far more persistent than the first or second group. She recommended that remediation strategies for the first group incorporate a whole-word approach to reading, while the second group would profit most from a phonetic approach. Bateman felt that the third group would respond best to a tactile-kinesthetic approach to reading.

Support for the delineation of three, as opposed to two, subgroups of dyslexic readers comes from the work of Ingram and his associates (Ingram et al. 1970). These researchers divided their sample, which was preselected to eliminate environmental, mental, educational, and emotional factors, into one specific category in which the disability was limited to reading and spelling and into a general group who also were deficient in arithmetic skills. The two research groups were then assessed as to their pattern of errors on a reading test. Of concern here are the results of the specific research group that most closely fit the definition of developmental dyslexia. This group was found to be comprised of three subtypes of severely reading-retarded persons. One subgroup made only audiophonic errors, another subgroup made only visual-spatial errors, and a third subgroup was identified that made both types of errors. The study showed that the specific and general categories of readers were grossly different in that within the general category there was an absence of children who made audiophonic errors, and there was a high percentage (40 percent) of children who made neither audiophonic nor visual-spatial errors.

THE CONTRIBUTION OF ELENA BODER

A major contribution to the contention that the diagnosis of developmental dyslexia can be broken down into three distinct subgroups of poor readers came from the work of Elena Boder (Boder, 1970, 1971, 1973a, 1973b). Unlike other approaches, her approach sought to analyze the performance of dyslexic readers in both reading and in spelling. The underlying assumption was that reading and spelling are interdependent functions that are strongly related. From this assumption, Boder hypothesized that if developmental dyslexia was due to an underlying cerebral dysfunction, regardless of its etiology, there should be direct evidence of that dysfunction in the reading-spelling performance. Such evidence should not be able to differentiate the dyslexic child from children with nonspecific reading disorders, but also should permit the direct identification of subgroups within the disorder (Boder, 1971).

The purpose of Boder's screening procedure was thus to make a qualitative analysis of the child's reading and spelling pattern rather than to make merely a quantitative assessment of the child's reading or spelling grade level. It was the analysis of the reading and spelling pattern rather than an assessment of a grade level that enabled the clinician to make a diagnosis of developmental dyslexia. Boder was quick to caution that this procedure was an integral part of a more comprehensive neuropediatric evaluation completed with each child. It was the combined results of this evaluation, and not just the screening procedure by itself, from which the diagnosis of developmental dyslexia was made.

Boder's diagnostic screening procedure, as implied above, revealed three distinct patterns of reading and spelling among dyslexic children. Boder stated that one or another of these three patterns was consistently found in all children who conform to the standard operational definitions of developmental dyslexia, and none of the patterns are found among normal readers. In addition, a direct correlation was found between the reading and spelling performance of a dyslexic child, so that how he reads and how he spells are mutually predictive. Of note here is Boder's finding that the spelling achievement was consistently found to be below that of reading. Follow-up observations also indicated that the reading-spelling pattern of a dyslexic child remained stable, even when reading achievement level rose significantly (Boder, 1970, 1971, 1973a, 1973b). The three dyslexic subgroups described by Boder are dysphonetic dyslexia, dyseidetic dyslexia, and alexia.

The dysphonetic dyslexia group reflects a primary deficit in letter-sound integration and in the ability to develop phonetic skills. They read globally, responding to whole words as configurations or gestalts. Lacking phonetic skills, these children are unable to decipher words that are not in their sight vocabulary. Their numerous misspellings are nonphonetic and thus often unintelligible. Their most striking errors are semantic substitutions such as *funny* for *laugh*.

The dyseidetic dyslexia group reflects a primary deficit in the ability to perceive whole words as gestalts. These children read phonetically, sounding out most words, familiar and unfamiliar, as if they were being encountered for the first time. Their misspellings are phonetic and thus intelligible. An example would be *laf* for *laugh*.

The alexia group reflects a primary deficit in both the ability to develop phonetic-word analysis (synthesis skills) as well as in the ability to perceive letters and whole words as visual gestalts. This child can be differentiated from the dysphonetic child by a significantly lower sight vocabulary, and from the dyseidetic child by a lack of word-analysis skills. This group is the most severely handicapped and, without intensive remediation, may remain nonreaders through high school.

In addition to the qualitative differences discussed within the definitions of the subgroups, Boder (1971, 1973a, 1973b) has found consistent quantitative differences. Normal readers have been found to correctly write to dictation from 70 to 100 percent of their sight vocabulary at grade level or below. They can also develop good phonetic equivalents for 80 to 100 percent of the words that are not in their sight vocabulary. In contrast, all three of the dyslexic subgroups are seldom able to correctly spell 50 percent of their sight word vocabulary. The children in the dysphonetic and alexic groups are also unable to develop (0 to 30 percent) good phonetic equivalents for words that are not in their sight vocabulary. Children in the dyseidetic group, on the other hand, are able to give good phonetic equivalents (80 to 100 percent) for words that are not in their sight vocabulary. The dysphonetic and alexic groups can be differentiated from each other on the basis of the degree of reading retardation. The reading level of the alexic group is far below that of the dysphonetic group at all age levels and seldom is found beyond the primer level if there has not been intensive remediation.

In order to determine the distribution of the three subgroups within the general population of children with the diagnosis of developmental dyslexia, Boder (1971, 1973a, 1973b) has reported the results of a study that employed 107 children seen in her clinic. All of the children had normal intelligence as measured by the Stanford-Binet test, were free from gross neurological disorder or psychiatric disturbance, and were at least two years delayed in reading on the Wide Range Achievement Test (WRAT). There were 92 boys and 15 girls in the sample.

The results of her study indicated that of the 107 children in the sample, 100 clearly exhibited one of the three reading-spelling patterns. Of these 100 children, 67 were classified as dysphonetic, 10 were classified dyseidetic, and 23 were found to be alexic. Of note was a difficulty in differentiating young dyseidetic children from the young alexic children. On the basis of a long follow-up period (seven years in some cases), Boder found that the reading-spelling pattern of these two groups often remained indistinguishable until the dyseidetic children have been exposed to remedial phonics, after which their relatively good ability to develop word-analysis skills will become evident. This may account for the higher number of alexic children in Boder's sample. A second difficulty reported by Boder was in the differentiation of some of the dysphonetic and alexic children on the basis of their spelling pattern alone. The alexic child, as stated above, will show a lower reading level in general and may have no sight-vocabulary or letter-recognition skills.

It is also interesting to note that the largest subgroup, according to Boder's analysis, was the dysphonetic group. This finding appears to be consistent with a number of the studies cited in Chapters 4 and 5, which indicated that deficits in auditory perception, auditory discrimination, sequencing, and sound-symbol relationships are far more frequently associated with developmental dyslexia than with visual-perceptual deficits.

Further Differentiation of Dyslexic Subtypes

Mattis and his associates (Mattis, 1978; Matis et al., 1975) have also reported research evidence that has delineated three independent clusters of deficiencies or syndromes that underlie dyslexia in children. In their initial study Mattis et al. (1975) divided 113 children, age range 11 to 12 years, into one of three groups: a brain-damaged reader group, a brain-damaged dyslexic group, and a non–brain-damaged dyslexic group. The use of a brain-damaged reader group was employed to exclude as causal those neurological deficiencies that are not associated with dyslexia. Each child had a verbal or performance IQ of at least 80 and showed no evidence of severe emotional psychopathology. Dyslexia was defined as reading retardation two or more grade levels below the level appropriate for the child's age on the WRAT. Each child was then administered a comprehensive battery of neuropsychological tests.

As stated above, three distinct subgroups of dyslexic children were isolated. Similar to Boder's findings, these groups were able to account for 90 percent of the children under study. The features of the groups were as follows.

The language disorder syndrome group (39 percent) presented with an anomia and one additional impairment of language functioning such as a disorder in comprehension, imitative speech, or speech-sound discrimination.

The articulatory and graphomotor dyscoordination syndrome group (37 percent) presented with speech articulation deficiencies but without a demonstrable language deficit. The majority in this group were maladroit on tasks requiring rapid protrusion of the tongue and demonstrated marked graphomotor dyscoordination.

The visual perceptual disorder syndrome group (16 percent) presented with significant visual-spatial impairments as measured by a verbal IQ more than 10 points above the performance IQ, and scores on the Raven's Coloured Progressive Matrices and on the Benton Test of Visual Retention below the level expected based on the performance IQ (Table 6–1).

Of further interest here is the comparison between the brain-damaged and non-brain-damaged dyslexic groups. It was found that although the two groups differed as to the number presented with each syndrome, there were no differences between the two dyslexic groups within the same syndrome. This suggests that dyslexic children again function as if they were in fact suffering from a pathological condition as found, for instance, by Galaburda and Kemper (1979).

Table 6-1
Quantitative Criteria for Each Dyslexia Syndrome*

Language Disorder
    Anomia: 20 percent or greater proportion of errors on the Naming Test and *one*
      of the following:
    Disorder of Comprehension: Performance on Token Test at least one standard
      deviation below the mean
    Disorder of Imitative Speech: Performance greater than one standard deviation
      below the mean on the Sentence Repetition Test
    Disorder of Speech Sound Discrimination: 10 percent or greater proportion of
      errors on discrimination of *e* rhyming letters

Articulatory and Graphomotor Dyscoordination
    Performance on ITPA Sound Blending subtest greater than one standard
      deviation below the mean
    Performance on Graphomotor Test greater than one standard deviation below
      the mean
    Acousto-sensory and receptive language processes within normal limits

Visual-Spatial Perceptual Disorder
    Verbal IQ more than 10 points above performance IQ
    Raven's Coloured Progressive Matrices percentile less than equivalent
      performance IQ
    Benton Test of Visual Retention (ten-second exposure immediate reproduction)
      score at or below the borderline level

Data from Mattis, S, French, JH, & Rapin, I. Dyslexia in children and young adults: Three independent neuropsychological syndromes. *Developmental Medicine and Child Neurology,* 1975, *17,* 150–163. With permission.
*These criteria have in large part been adopted by the Child Neurology Society in the development of their proposed Nosology on Disorders of Cortical Function in Children (1981).

In a follow-up study reported by Mattis (1978), the same research group attempted to replicate their original work with a slightly larger but younger population (age range eight to ten years) of Black and Hispanic origin. Results indicated that the three dyslexic syndromes previously isolated were again observed. The largest percentage of dyslexic children was found within the language-disorder syndrome as in the initial study. The percentage of children represented by each syndrome differed from the initial study, however, and were: language-disorder syndrome, 63 percent; articulatory and graphomotor dyscoordination syndrome, 10 percent; and visual-perceptual disorder syndrome, 5 percent. Unlike the initial study, 9 percent of the children presented two of the syndrome patterns and 10 percent findings that suggested a sequencing disorder group.

Based on the results of the two studies, Mattis and his associates concluded that the three subgroups of dyslexic children that they have identified appear to be consistent across age; and that while a fourth syndrome appears to have been isolated, Mattis is hesitant to affirm its presence until a more carefully controlled study with a larger brain-damaged reader group is accomplished. Also, Mattis repeatedly emphasized the need for a brain-damaged reader control group in any study seeking to identify causal factors related solely to dyslexia. Lastly, Mattis (1978) states that "regardless of the number of syndromes to be eventually determined, there appears to be sufficient evidence to date to submit that a dyslexia syndromes model which presumes several independent causal defects is a tenable working hypothesis to guide future research" (p. 52).

Finally, Pirozzolo (1979, 1981) has also been able to identify two neuropsychological subtypes of developmental dyslexia based on profile analysis of a comprehensive neuropsychological test battery that included the WISC-R, the Raven Progressive Matrices, and neurolinguistic analyses of reading and writing errors. The children falling into the auditory-linguistic subtype of dyslexia showed symptoms of a language disorder characterized by having a lower Verbal IQ relative to their Performance IQ and their Raven IQ; by developmentally delayed language onset; by articulation disorders; by an anomia; and by reading and writing errors involving faulty grapheme-to-phoneme translation (Table 6–2). The children falling into the visual-spatial subtype of dyslexia showed symptoms of higher-order visual disturbances characterized by having a higher Verbal IQ relative to their Performance IQ and their Raven IQ; and by showing evidence of right-left disorientation, finger agnosia, spatial dysgraphia, and reading and writing errors involving the faulty encoding of visual informantion.

Pirozzolo pointed out that while a strong case can be made for the incorporation of several different subtypes of developmental dyslexia other than the auditory-linguistic and visual-spatial subtypes discussed here, these two neurobehavioral syndromes may represent the two most common forms of the disorder. He also suggested that if this diagnostic strategy was employed in the assessment of dyslexic children, the results of prior research that sought only to compare normal readers and dyslexic readers on a particular cognitive task or psychometric test would have been drastically different. In support of this contention, Pirozzolo cited his own work with dyslexic and normal readers on the ITPA (Pirozzolo and Hess, 1976). In this study, the authors compared the ITPA test profiles of normal and of dyslexic readers and found that the group data showed no significant differences. On re-analysis of the data using this diagnostic strategy described above, Pirozzolo found that the ITPA profiles of the two dyslexic subtypes not only differed from the normal readers but from each other as well. The auditory-linguistic group performed poorly on the auditory-vocal channel subtests but performed well on the visual-motor channel subtests, while the visual-spatial group demonstrated the reverse pattern. The apparent normality thus seen in the dyslexic grouped data was the result of a regression

Table 6-2
**Neuropsychological Criteria for the Differential Diagnosis
of Dyslexia**

Subgroup Type	
Auditory-Linguistic	*Visual-Spatial*
Average to above average Performance IQ	Average to above average Verbal IQ
Low Verbal IQ (relative to Performance IQ)	Low Performance IQ (relative to Verbal IQ)
Developmentally delayed language onset	Right-left disorientation
Expressive speech defects	Early evidence of preference for mirror or inverted writing
Anomia, object-naming, or color-naming defects	Finger agnosia
Agrammatism	Spatial dysgraphia (poor handwriting, poor use of space)
Reading errors mainly involving the phonological aspects of language	Reading errors involving visual aspects
Spelling errors characteristic of poor phoneme-to-grapheme correspondence	Spelling errors characteristic of letter and word reversals, omissions, etc.
Letter-by-letter decoding strategy	Use a phonetic decoding strategy
Normal eye movements	Faulty eye movements during reading
Relatively intact visual-spatial abilities	Oral language abilities relatively normal

Modified from Pirozzolo, FJ. Language and brain: Neuropsychological aspects of developmental reading disability. *School Psychology Review,* 1981, *10,* 350–355. With permission.

to the mean effect, which obscured the significant differences between the two neuropsychologically distinct subgroups of dyslexia.

Based on the studies reviewed in this section, it seems clear that it can be concluded that evidence exists for at least two, and possibly several, subtypes of dyslexic children. The remainder of this chapter will be devoted to a presentation of the limited research in this area, which has incorporated a multifactor model into the research design.

ARTICULATING THE NEUROPSYCHOLOGICAL CHARACTERISTICS OF THE DYSLEXIC SUBTYPES

It should be realized that the literature broadly supports the conceptualization of at least three distinct subgroups of dyslexics. For this reason, the present section focuses on the most usually agreed on subtypes incorporating children with verbal-linguistic deficits; visual-spatial difficulties; and a third, less well-defined subgroup evidencing characteristics common to both the aforementioned subgroups. Our knowledge of individual differences would predict, however, that other, more discrete subgroups must also exist. In general, it would seem reasonable to expect that these more discrete subtypes will emerge from a further differentiation of the above-noted groups.

The case of hyperlexia is probably a good case in point since it may be a variation of the auditory-linguistic dyslexic child. The hyperlexic child may have VSIQ < PSIQ, be a fluent oral reader, be defective in comprehension, have superior visual-perceptual skills, and evidence behavior frequently found in borderline or autistic children (e.g., preoccupation with numbers, unusual calendar skills, echolalia, etc.). Since hyperlexia is not typically included in the subtype literature on dyslexia (despite its recognition as a definable subtype by the Child Neurology Society, 1981), it has not been the focus of our review. The interested reader is referred to reports on this disorder by Healy (1982) and by Richman and Kitchell (1981).

Seeking to clarify the relationship between hemispheric specialization and developmental dyslexia, Keefe and Swinney (1979) suggested that the discrepancies reported in this area (left-hemispheric–deficit versus right-hemispheric–deficit) are due to the fact that previous studies have failed to examine the performance of individual subjects. In accordance with one of the major criticisms of the single factor theories cited in this volume, these authors rejected the contention that the developmental dyslexic population is homogeneous and chose instead to study the possibility that the conflicting results of the cerebral dominance research were, in fact, due to a heterogeneous population.

In order to do so, these investigators administered a dichotic listening test (numbers) and a tachistoscopic task (letters) to separate groups of dyslexic and normal readers in two different experiments. In both experiments, the dyslexic group was defined as being at least two years below their grade level on the Gray Oral Reading Test, of normal intelligence, and free of diagnosed brain trauma. The control groups were matched for age, sex (all male), and intelligence.

In the dichotic listening experiment, a group analysis indicated that both groups showed a right-ear (left hemisphere) superiority for number recall. The individual subject analysis indicated, however, that for the normal-reader group, the scores distributed themselves in a normal distribution with a single mode that coincided with the group mean (-5 to $+15$). In contrast, the distribution of the scores within the dyslexic group was bimodal, with a modal point falling on either side of the group mean (Fig. 6–1). The groups mean scores thus concealed subject distribution differences observed between the two groups.

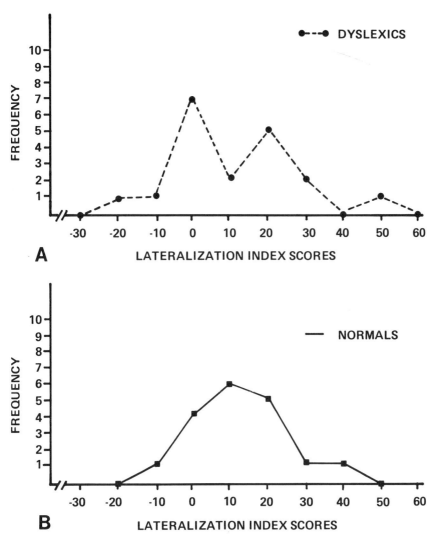

Fig. 6-1. (A) Frequency polygon of distribution of individual lateralization index scores of dyslexic subjects on dichotic listening test. (B) Frequency polygon of distribution of individual lateralization index scores of normal subjects on dichotic listening test. [From Keffe, B, & Swinney, D. On the relationship of hemispheric specialization and developmental dyslexia. *Cortex*, 1979, *15*, 471–481. With permission.]

In the tachistoscopic experiment, group analysis indicated that although the normal readers responded more accurately, both groups showed a right visual half-field (left hemisphere) superiority for letter recall. The individual subject analysis again indicated, however, that although the normal-reader group demonstrated a unimodal distribution, the dyslexic distribution was bimodal.

Keefe and Swinney (1979) concluded that these results appeared to support their contention that the dyslexic population was not homogeneous with regard to cerebral lateralization but was instead heterogeneous. There thus appeared to be at least two categories of dyslexic children with respect to hemispheric lateralization of linguistic material. One type demonstrated a left-hemispheric deficit while the other demonstrated a right-hemispheric deficit, as compared with the normal readers. These results are interesting in view of the single-factor studies reported earlier that supported only one or the other of these etiological explanations. The results in this study, in fact, seem to correlate very nicely with multifactor studies that uncovered at least two subgroups of dyslexic children. The first subtype, which is reported to be deficient in auditory-linguistic skills, corresponds to what one might expect from the left-hemisphere–deficit group, while the second subtype, said to be deficient in visual-spatial skills, would correspond to the right hemisphere deficit group.

Support for the findings of Keefe and Swinney (1979) can be obtained from an excellent study done by Pirozzolo and Rayner (1979), who also proposed a similar theoretical position, that the lack of agreement among the laterality studies may be due to a heterogeneous population of dyslexic children.

In order to explore this possibility, the authors presented faces or five-letter words tachistoscopically to a group of normal and dyslexic readers (mean age 12.5 years, matched for age and IQ). The dyslexic children were reading at least two years below their expected grade level while the normal readers were on grade level or slightly above. The dyslexic group, in addition, was limited to those children thought to represent the auditory-linguistic subgroup; they had a verbal-performance discrepancy of 15 points in favor of the performance area.

Their results indicated that there was no difference between the dyslexic subgroup and normal readers in their ability to recognize faces, with both groups exhibiting a left visual half-field superiority (right hemisphere). The normal readers, in addition, identified words presented to the right visual half field more accurately than to the left visual half field (left-hemispheric superiority), while the children comprising the auditory-linguistic dyslexic subgroup demonstrated no clear asymmetry (Fig. 6–2).

The authors concluded that the dyslexic subgroup did not show the right-hemispheric deficit for spatial functioning proposed by Witelson (1976, 1977), thus providing evidence that processing within the right hemisphere is ostensibly normal in this subgroup. It remains feasible, however, that the subgroup of dyslexic children exhibiting visual-spatial deficits may in fact demonstrate a right-hemispheric dysfunction. The dyslexic children in this

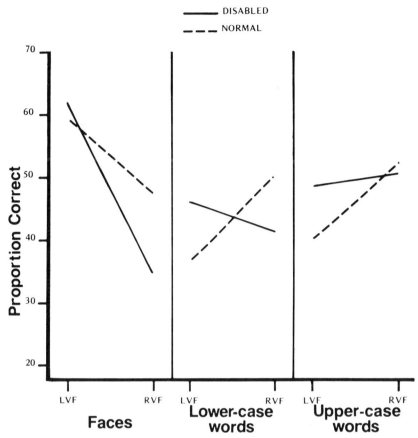

Fig. 6-2.   Proportion correct for face and word recogition for normal and disabled readers. [From Pirozzolo, FJ, & Rayner, K. Cerebral organization and reading disability. *Neuropsychologia*, 1979, *17*, 485–491. With permission.]

study did not, however, show the left-hemispheric superiority for linguistic information found in normal children. These results, taken together, appear to support the contention of Keefe and Swinney (1979) that the auditory-linguistic subgroup of dyslexic children does, in fact, exhibit a left hemisphere dysfunction in the lateralization of linguistic material.

Employing the Boder (1971, 1973a, 1973b) classification system, Obrzut (1979) administered a dichotic listening task and a bisensory memory task to normal, nonspecific, dysphonetic, dyseidetic, and alexic readers in order to assess cerebral dominance, auditory recall ability, and auditory-visual integration ability. The subjects were further divided into two grade levels, second and fourth grades; matched for normal IQ; and were free of physical, emotional, or sensory deficits.

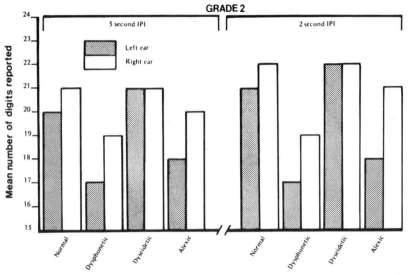

Fig. 6-3. Mean number of digits recalled by reader groups. A total score of 24 was possible for each ear. [From Obrzut, JE. Dichotic listening and bisensory memory skills in qualitatively diverse dyslexic readers. *Journal of Learning Disabilities*, 1979, *12*, 304–314. With permission.]

Results of the dichotic listening task indicated that at both the second and the fourth grade levels, normal and dyseidetic readers recalled significantly more digits from both ears than did the dysphonetic or the alexic groups (Figs. 6–3 and 6–4). It thus appears that normal and dyseidetic readers show better processing and recall of auditory information. The results of ear asymmetry were, however, inconsistent with this finding and with prior expectations. While all groups showed a slight right-ear (left hemisphere) advantage, the only group that consistently demonstrated a significant right-ear advantage was the dysphonetic reader group, who presumably have difficulty with phonetic and linguistic processing. Obrzut explained this discrepancy from expectation on the basis of selective attention of the subjects as a means of relieving boredom. Results of the bisensory memory task indicated that, in general, all groups made more visual than auditory recall errors. With the exception of one experimental condition (fourth grade, fast rate), however, the normal and dyseidetic readers made fewer visual-recall errors than did the dysphonetic and alexic groups.

Obrzut concluded that these findings appear to indicate that dyseidetic dyslexics who can blend sounds and syllables and who have better auditory memory and phonetic analysis skills are not as deficient as are the dysphonetic and alexic subgroups who are lacking in these higher-order skills. Obrzut proposed, in addition, that dysphonetic readers who attempt to read

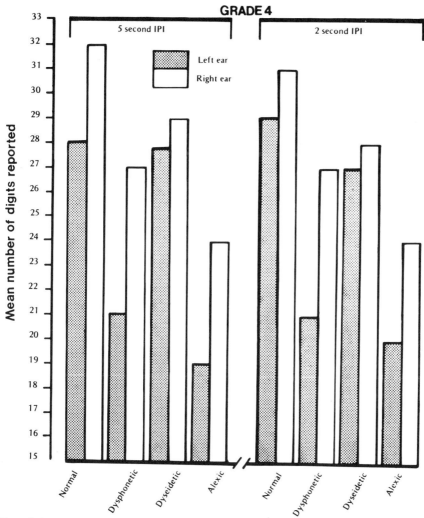

Fig. 6-4. Mean number of digits recalled by reader groups. A total score of 36 was possible for each ear. [From Obrzut, JE. Dichotic listening and bisensory memory skills in qualitatively diverse dyslexic readers. *Journal of Learning Disabilities,* 1979, *12,* 304–314. With permission.]

by sight and who display difficulty in analyzing, blending, and integrating speech sounds to the visual symbol may be reflecting a problem specific to the left hemisphere. Dyseidetic readers who attempt to read by ear and who display difficulty with nonphonetic words, in contrast, may be reflecting a problem specific to the right hemisphere.

Dalby and Gibson (1981) also employed the Boder (1971, 1973a, 1973 b) classification system and administered a hemispheric timesharing task, a conjugate lateral eye-movements task, and a tactile direction perception task as a means of assessing both left- and right-hemispheric lateralization in Boder's three subgroups of dyslexic readers as well as in a matched normal-reader control group. From a pool of 112 disabled readers, 45 dyslexic male readers (15 nonspecific, 15 dysphonetic, and 15 dyseidetic) were selected for the study. Additionally, from a pool of 26 subjects, 15 age-matched normal readers were selected. All subjects were right-handed, were between the ages of 9 to 12 years (mean age = 11.3), and were of normal intelligence. The dyslexic readers, in addition, were reading 1.5 or more years below their present grade placement, with borderline cases being excluded from consideration.

On the hemispheric timesharing task, the children engaged in a manual finger-tapping exercise (recorded on an electric typewriter) over six different conditions. These conditions were: a right-handed control condition with no concurrent task; a left-handed control condition; a right-handed condition while reciting animal names (dog, rabbit, horse, buffalo); a left-handed condition while solving spatial problems (items 7–12 from the Raven's Coloured Progressive Matrices Test); and, a left-handed condition while solving spatial problems.

It should be noted that the third and fourth conditions were thought to require left-hemispheric processing, while the last two conditions load heavily on right-hemispheric processing. An analysis of the percentage of reduction of correct manual responses across these conditions indicated that the control children showed left hemisphere lateralization of language and right hemisphere lateralization of spatial functions; the nonspecific-reader group demonstrated a left hemisphere language lateralization and bilateral spatial representation; the dysphonetic-reader group showed bilateral representation of both verbal and spatial functions; and, the dyseidetic group demonstrated bilateral verbal representation and right-hemispheric lateralization of spatial functions.

On the conjugate lateral eye-movements task, the direction of eye movements in response to ten verbal and ten spatial questions was recorded for each child, using a biometrics eye-movement monitor. Due to the fact that analyses of these measurements for the control group failed to reveal the expected theoretical relationship between lateral eye movement and hemispheric activity (leftward gaze shift when solving spatial questions and rightward gaze shift for verbal questions), the authors correctly chose to disregard the data for the disabled-reader group.

The tactile directional-perception task required the children to match the directional orientation of a stimulus rod (glued to the top of a wooden block in one of nine different directional orientations) with one of nine rods in a multiple choice array. The children were allowed to explore the materials tactually but not visually, and then were directed to move their hand over the response array, choosing the match. Nine trials were given to each hand. It should be noted that the typical left-hand superiority found on this task has been previously interpreted as evidence of greater right hemisphere involvement. The results indicated that both the control and dyseidetic children performed significantly better with the left hand, while the nonspecific and dysphonetic group showed no differences across hands on this task. While the control and dyseidetic children thus showed the typical right-hemispheric lateralization for this task, the nonspecific and dysphonetic children appeared to show bilateral cerebral representation of spatial functions. The authors pointed out that these results were consistent with the findings from the hemispheric time-sharing task.

Dalby and Gibson (1981) concluded by saying that although the results of the study showed that patterns of cerebral organization do, in fact, vary across types of reading disability, it should be emphasized that the findings reflected group performances and that the extent to which individuals conform to the group pattern varies across groups and across functions. Simply stated, significant variability thus existed within each group of subjects. The authors went on to support the contention of Pirozzolo and Rayner (1979), which stated that the differences in findings across the laterality studies were a function of the type of subjects used, for example, a heterogeneous population of dyslexic children.

Finally, Fried and a group of co-workers (Fried, Tanguay, Boder, Doubleday, and Greensite, 1981) at the UCLA Neuropsychiatric Institute also employed the Boder (1971, 1973a, 1973b) classification system and event-related potential (ERP) techniques in order to study information processing in the left and right hemispheres of dyslexics, who were classified according to subgroup, and that processing in normal readers. More specifically, the authors were interested in finding out if cortical activity, in the form of waveform differences between auditory-evoked responses to word and to musical-chord stimuli would be quantitatively different between dyslexic subgroups as a function of the side of the scalp from which the recordings were made. Subjects for the study consisted of 13 dyslexic boys (five dysphonetic, six dyseidetic, and two alexic) ranging in age from 8 to 12 years, all but one of whom were right-handed. The dyslexic children were, in addition, all of normal intelligence; were free from gross neurological defect, primary psychiatric disorder, and sensory impairment; and were at least two years retarded in reading and in spelling. They were matched for age and sex with 13 normal-reader controls, all of whom were right-handed and were reading and spelling on or above grade level.

Electrophysiological recordings were accomplished by placing Ag/AgCl disk electrodes at left and right frontal locations (F_7, F_8) and at left and right temporoparietal sites (midway between T_5 and C_3, and midway between T_6 and C_4) according to the international 10–20 system (Jasper, 1958). The EEG data and stimulus markers representing the onset of word or musical-chord stimuli were recorded on magnetic tape and were also continuously monitored by paper write-out to ensure that the subjects remained relaxed and alert. Initially, each subject was administered a standard dichotic listening test followed by the word and musical-chord presentation, which was delivered binaurally in groups of 50 stimuli (25 word and 25 musical-chord stimuli randomly arranged), with each subject receiving a total of 150 word and 150 musical-chord stimuli. Event-recorded potentials (ERPs) were averaged off-line using a PDP-11 computer, and waveform differences were estimated through a cross-correlational analysis in which interstimulus latency differences in ERPs were minimized by lagging word or musical chord to the point at which a maximum correlation was obtained.

Results indicated that normal readers and dyseidetic dyslexics, whose reading handicaps involved visual-spatial processing deficits, had greater word versus musical-chord ERP waveform differences (maximum "r" values were significantly smaller) over the left hemisphere, as compared with the right hemisphere (Fig. 6–5). Dysphonetic dyslexics, whose reading difficulties were related to auditory-verbal processing deficits, did not exhibit any significant interhemispheric differences.

The authors interpreted the lack of greater word–musical-chord ERP waveform differences over the left hemisphere in the dysphonetic group as evidence in support of the theory that suggests that the left hemisphere of dysphonetic dyslexics may not have fully developed the capacity to process auditory information in a normal manner. The dyseidetic dyslexics, in contrast, who all possessed the capacity to phonemically decode and encode reading materials fairly well, were found to exhibit a normal pattern of left-waveform greater than right waveform differences. While the dyseidetic dyslexics exhibited the same waveform pattern as normal readers, they did differ from normal readers with respect to the magnitude of latency and amplitude differences between word and musical-chord ERPs. The authors attributed this result to attentional factors between the groups, thus supporting claims made by researchers using learning-disabled populations (Hynd et al., 1979; Hynd & Obrzut, 1981). The authors concluded by saying that the question as to whether visual-spatial difficulties in reading exhibited by the dyseidetic dyslexics can be attributed to a right hemisphere dysfunction remains for future research using visual stimuli.

In the final study to be presented here, Bauserman and Obrzut (in press) used the Boder (1971, 1973a, 1973b) classification system in order to compare normal readers and subgroups of dyslexic readers on a task of intrasensory integration. This task required the subjects to match (same-

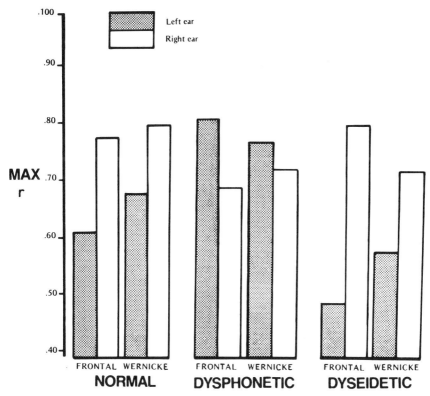

Fig. 6-5. Waveform differences between word and musical-chord ERPs as a function of electrode location and side of head. Waveform differences were estimated through a cross-correlational analysis in which interstimulus latency differences in ERPs were minimized by lagging word on musical chord to the point at which a maximum correlation (max r) was obtained. Waveform differences were significantly greater over the left hemisphere in the normal and dyseidetic subects, but were not in the dysphonetic group. [From Fried, I, Tanguay, PE, Boder, E, Doubleday, C, & Greensite, M. Developmental dyslexia: Electrophysiological evidence of clinical subgroups. *Brain and Language*, 1981, *12*, 14–22. With permission.]

different) temporal (T) stimuli (light flashes) to spatial (S) stimuli (printed rows of dot patterns) in four separate conditions: S-S, S-T, T-S, and T-T. Subjects came from the fifth grade of a middle class school, had normal intelligence, and were free from sensory, emotional or physical handicaps. The dyslexic readers, as noted above, were further classified into either the dysphonic, dyseidetic, or alexic group.

The results indicated that differences between the reader groups were found only when they were required to perform T-S and T-T matches, with average readers being superior to dyslexic readers in each case. When the four reader groups were analyzed separately for order of difficulty, the following patterns were observed: average readers found the S-S task easier than the S-T, T-S, and T-T tasks, which were all found to be approximately equal in difficulty. The dyseidetic-reader group displayed an identical pattern across tasks, differing from the normal readers in the greater number of errors made. The dysphonetic and alexic groups, in contrast, exhibited an order of difficulty characterized by an increasing progression of errors from S-S to T-T, with no difference found between T-S and T-T tasks. The only difference between these two groups was in the number of errors made, with the dysphonetic group performing better than the alexic group. When compared with the normal reader, the dysphonetic and alexic groups were found to be significantly below the level of the normal-reader group on T-S and T-T matching.

Based on the results of this study, Bauserman and Obrzut (in press) concluded that it appears that matching tasks that begin with temporal information (T-S, T-T) represent the most difficult tasks and therefore diminish the importance of integration as the crucial deficit underlying developmental dyslexia. Also, they felt that based on this result and on the finding that dysphonetic and alexic readers differed significantly from normal readers on the T-S and T-T tasks, it would seem that a deficit in the memory's capacity to order information sequentially may be at the root of their problem, whereas the dyseidetics demonstrate deficits in Gestalt and spatial processing. Third, severely disabled readers demonstrate qualitatively and quantitatively different deficiencies, depending on the nature of the disability; and lastly, the results of this study appear to be consistent with the contention of Obrzut (1979) that dysphonetic readers may be reflecting a neurological problem specific to the left hemisphere, while dyseidetic readers may be reflecting problems specific to the right hemisphere.

CONCLUSIONS

Within the last 20 years more progress has been made in understanding the neuropsychological processes involved in developmental dyslexia than in the previous century. The work of Kinsbourne and Warrington (1963), Bannatyne (1966a, 1966b), Boder (1970, 1971, 1973a, 1973b), Mattis et al. (1975), and Pirozzolo (1979) stand out as truly significant in reshaping our conceptualization of cognitive processes and related brain functioning in dyslexic children. Their research has been characterized by meaningful clinical insights coupled with soundly designed research paradigms. Based on their contributions the following conclusions seem warranted.

The major implication of the single factor research presented in Chapters 4 and 5 is that dyslexic readers as a group have been shown to be deficient in a wide variety of skills necessary for the development of adequate reading ability. Coupled with the findings of the subgroup research, it appears reasonable to conclude that there exists a heterogeneous population of dyslexic children comprised of independent subgroups of dyslexic readers, each with a distinct deficit or cluster of deficits of neurological origin.

The evidence depicting dyslexic children as deficient in various psycholinguistic abilities would thus lend support to the view that at least one relatively common subtype of developmental dyslexia is associated with disordered functioning of the left (dominant) hemisphere. Evidence also exists to support another group of dyslexic children who exhibit fairly intact psycholinguistic skills but in whom visual-spatial or visual-motor skills are lacking. These children have difficulty in sight-word recognition and may be deficient in right-hemispheric functioning. A third, less well-differentiated subtype of dyslexic child also appears to exist, and the available evidence indicates that this child is experiencing deficits in the skill areas thought to be subserved by both hemispheres.

In terms of neuropsychological or clinical diagnosis, it may no longer be considered acceptable to simply diagnose a child as dyslexic. The evidence in favor of differential diagnosis is too strong, and good clinical practice demands more rigorous assessment practices. If differential diagnosis is possible, then so is differential treatment. It appears that the heterogeneity of the dyslexic population has led to confusion regarding appropriate remedial strategies. One must know the source of an infection to treat it successfully and, likewise, differential diagnosis is a necessary prerequisite for success in differential treatment of the dyslexic. For these reasons the remainder of this volume will deal with these important topics.

PART III

Clinical Differentiation and Intervention

———Chapter 7———
Neuropsychological Assessment of the Dyslexic Child

Considering the relatively detailed definitions of dyslexia now usually accepted, it seems surprising that a resistance still exists to diagnosing a child as being dyslexic. It is the experience of the authors that it is not the diagnosis or identification of severe reading problems that is necessarily at issue. Since the term dyslexia arises from the medical literature, a resistance exists instead in applying the label to a child evidencing a severe reading disability in concert with soft neurological signs. This is despite the fact that dyslexia is specifically mentioned as falling under the broader term of learning disabilities (Federal Register, 1976). From a diagnostic standpoint, educators or psychologists working in an educational environment should thus feel it is indeed appropriate to apply the label of dyslexia to a child evidencing the characteristics of what constitutes dyslexia as noted in our discussion in Chapter 1.

It is often the case that a child will demonstrate some "soft" neurological signs during an evaluation of a severe reading disability. Assuming that there may be a possible neurological basis to the reading disability, it is not uncommon to see the child referred to a neurologist for a formal neurological evaluation. Perhaps due to the confusion over what constitutes "hard" versus "soft" neurological signs, and due to a lack of clear understanding as to what comprises a neurological examination and what a neurologist can or cannot offer, it is more often the case that the report derived from a neurologist's evaluation will prove to be of little or no value from an educational or psychological standpoint. Prior to our discussion as to some important issues regarding this perspective on assessment and what may be appropriate in clinical neuropsychological differentiation of dyslexic subtypes, it is worthwhile to consider the role of the neurological evaluation in clinical medicine. A better understanding of the role of the neurologist and of what comprises the typical neurological evaluation may assist the clinician and remedial educator in knowing when to refer to a neurologist, what to expect from the evaluation, and in what capacity the neurological evaluation should be considered in differential diagnosis.

THE NEUROLOGIC EXAMINATION

The neurologic examination is a relatively costly procedure when compared with services offered within the public schools for no charge. It is therefore important to be familiar with the three main situations in which the diagnostic neurologic examination is performed (Oppé, 1979). First, when a child is suspected of suffering a neurologic disease, the neurologist sees the child primarily to locate and define the pathologic processes. It is important to recognize this function with school-age children, since some neurologic disease processes may present first as referrals for learning problems. Disorders such as Duchenne's muscular dystrophy may first manifest itself as deterioration in intellectual ability or as a decline in levels of achievement. A second situation in which the neurologic examination is appropriate is when there are no obvious neurological difficulties but the pattern of behavior suggests some possible pathology of the central nervous system. A child who blinks rapidly, seems to stare off into space, and fails to comprehend momentarily may indeed suffer a petit mal (absence) seizure. This child should be suspect and it is obviously appropriate to request a neurological examination. Finally, the neurologic examination may be useful as a screening to sort out childhood difficulties that have a neurologic basis from those that do not. It is important to identify the child whose reading failure is the result of neurologic factors from the child who simply has failed to profit from instruction. As Oppé (1979) has pointed out, this screening function of the neurologic examination may be of less value than other approaches in differentiating these children. It will be argued, in fact, that the neuropsychological examination will be of more value than separate neurological, psychological, and educational evaluations. First, however, it is important to understand what the typical neurologic exam entails.

Format of the Neurological Examination

The neurological examination has evolved considerably over many decades of clinical experience. To a psychologist or educator used to the standardized and norm-referenced approach of measurement, the neurological examination may seem uncommonly qualitative and subjective. It is qualitative and subjective, indeed, but it does lead to reliable and valid estimates of neurological status.

Within the past decades, the neurologic examination has become more closely tied to psychophysiological measures of neurological integrity. The clinical utilizations of the electroencephalograph, evoked potential apparatus, visual half-field and dichotic listening techniques, and CT scans are all valuable in assisting the neurologist in the examination. The following standard instruments, however, are typically used in the developmental neurological examination: tape measure, ophthalmoscope, torch, reflex hammer, spatula, sharp object, colored wooden cubes, a bell or rattle, crayons, and possibly, several small toys. Depending on the developmental level of the child, the child's cooperation, and the time available, the examination will usually focus on the following:

1. Test of Cerebral Function
   Language usage
   Level of consciousness
   Intellectual abilities
   Orientation
   Emotional status
2. Tests for Cranial Nerves
   General (hearing, vision, and speech)
   Specific
     Olfactory
     Optic
     Oculomotor
     Trochlear
     Abducent
     Trigeminal
     Facial
     Acoustic
     Glossopharyngeal
     Vagus
     Spinal Accessory
     Hypoglossal
3. Tests for Cerebellar Functions
   Finger-to-nose-to-finger
   Rapid alternating movements
   Heel-to-toe walking
   Standing—eyes open
   Standing—eyes closed

4. Motor Functioning
    Muscle size
    Muscle tone
    Coordination
    Reflexes
5. Tests of Sensory System Function
    Superficial tactile sensation
    Superficial pain
    Proprioceptive sensation
    Stereognosis

It should be recognized that the listing of the very basics of a neurological examination may lead to the wrong impression that the evaluation is terribly structured and not sensitive to the needs or to the unique problems of the child. This is simply not the case, as the complete neurological examination is an involved and individualized process that may take a considerable amount of time and employ many, if not more, of the tasks noted above (as well as the various psychophysiologic measures noted earlier).

There are, however, several points to glean from the previous brief overview of the purpose and content of the neurological examination. First, the concentration on the neurological examination is on the central nervous system. In educational circles it is an often overlooked fact that the central nervous system incorporates much more than just the cerebral cortex. The brain stem, cerebellum, and cranial nerves as well as the peripheral nervous system are very important to the neurologist and, as can be seen from our brief outline of the neurological examination, are the focus of considerable attention.

A second point that needs to be made is that that portion of the neurological examination that deals with mentation, or cognitive functioning, is relatively brief and is based primarily on subjective clinical judgment as to whether a child's cognitive process are normal or are impaired. This is not to say that some neurologists or pediatric neurologists do not make use of psychological or educational test data. Many neurologists work closely with professionals in psychology and education; however, they usually have less data on which to base their judgments of a child's cognitive ability than do teachers or psychologists. In fact, the soft signs (neurologic signs that are often difficult to elicit and are thought to differentiate between normal and pathological children, e.g., rotating a design when copied) that are associated with dyslexic children are more evident on the psychological evaluation than in the neurological evaluation. This is because these indices of neurologic dysfunction are associated with higher cortical areas and therefore do not become evident in the evaluation of subcortical function.

If much of the neurological evaluation has as its focus subcortical functioning that is not relative to the severe failure in reading and, if that aspect of the examination that does focus on cognitive functioning is not complete, of what value is the neurological examination of the dyslexic child? In most cases the neurological examination of a child with severe reading failure is not warranted unless there are specific questions that can only be answered by a neurologist.

When is a Neurological Examination Appropriate?

As indicated previously, the soft neurological signs often associated with dyslexia can usually be observed on the psychological evaluation. As Lezak (1976) points out, clinical neuropsychology has as its major goal the assessment of behavior as it relates to neurological status. The framework provided by neuropsychological assessment thus is usually adequate in identifying the neuropsychological (neurological-cognitive) basis of severe reading failure.

The questions that cannot be answered or addressed adequately through neuropsychological evaluation focus primarily on the issue as to whether the observed behavioral difficulties are related to a deteriorating or to a progressive neurological disease process. If a child appears normal in every aspect in kindergarten and in first grade and makes normal progress until the fifth grade, when he seems to begin a slow course of academic deterioration, a question of possible disease processes exists. A referral should be made.

It is also appropriate to refer to a neurologist if other neurological signs seem evident when the dyslexic child is first administered a neuropsychological evaluation. If during an evaluation, for example, a child mentions being awakened by sudden and severe nocturnal headaches, a referral to a neurologist is certainly warranted.

It would also be appropriate to seek out the services of a cooperating neurologist should the expertise of a well-trained neuropsychologist not be available. A well-trained psychologist working in concert with a neurologist who is interested in dyslexic children should be able to concur from their separate evaluations as to whether the severe reading failure is due to neurodevelopmental factors.

It may seem inconsistent to recommend discrete use of the neurological examination while recognizing that dyslexia does have a neurological basis. Since dyslexia is not a life-threatening disorder, is characterized by performance on neuropsychological measures, and cannot be treated from a medical perspective, it would seem a wise use of professional expertise to refer only when it is clearly appropriate.

NEUROPSYCHOLOGICAL EVALUATION:
PERSPECTIVES

The neuropsychological evaluation of the dyslexic child is based on the assumption that to truly understand the exact nature of the reading failure one must relate the unique aspects of the problems in reading to cognitive and neurological functioning. It should be stated at the beginning that to be labeled dyslexic a child should meet the criteria discussed in Chapter 1. That is to say, a significant reading disability should exist (probably greater than a discrepancy of two years between actual achievement and current grade placement), there should be adequate intellectual ability (IQ > 85), the discrepancy should not be attributable to secondary factors, and perhaps most importantly, evidence should exist that the severe reading failure is attributable to central nervous system dysfunction. If no evidence as to central nervous system dysfunction exists, then it is inappropriate from our perspective to diagnose the condition of severe reading failure as dyslexia. Intervention and remedial programming for the child who evidences no neurologic indicators is different in focus from that for the dyslexic child. This important implication of diagnosis is discussed in the following chapter.

Neuropsychological Test Batteries

Since it is imperative to diagnose or at least to identify patterns of behavior that are consistent with central nervous system dysfunction, one might assume that recognized neuropsychological assessment batteries would be most appropriate for use with the dyslexic reader. This is a reasonable assumption because some neuropsychological test batteries have been in clinical use for many years, evidence exists as to the tests' reliability and validity for children with learning disorders, and some of the subtests have been shown to be very accurate in discriminating between neuropsychologically based disorders and those that are due to secondary factors.

Essentially, three neuropsychological test batteries exist for school-age children. For children in the 5 to 8-year-old range there is the Reitan-Indiana Neuropsychological Test Battery for Children. The Halstead Neuropsychological Test Battery is appropriate for use with children in the 9- to 14-year-old range. Finally, there exists the Luria-Nebraska Children's Battery for children in the 8- to 12-year-old range. The various subtests and tests associated with each of these neuropsychological test batteries are noted in Table 7-1.

The true genesis of these test batteries was the work of Halstead, who in the 1930s and 1940s developed and validated tests that were sensitive to the psychological and behavioral manifestations of brain lesions in adults.

Table 7-1
Tests and Subtests Associated With Neuropsychological Batteries for Children

Reitan-Indiana * (5–8 years)	Halstead Test Battery † (9–14 years)	Luria-Nebraska (8–12 years)
Category Test	Category Test	Motor Skills
Tactile Performance Test	Tactile Performance Test	Rhythm
Finger Tapping Test	Seashore Rhythm Test	Tactile
Sensory-Perceptual Measures	Speech Sounds Perception	Visual
Aphasia Screening Test	Test	Receptive Speech
Grip Strength Test	Finger Tapping Test	Expressive Speech
Lateral Dominance Examination	Tactile Auditory and Visual	Writing
Color Form Test	Imperception Test	Reading
Progressive Figures Test	Finger Recognition Test	Arithmetic
Matching Pictures Test	Finger-tip Number Writing	Memory
Target Test	Tactile Form Recognition	Intelligence
Individual Performance Test	Aphasia Screening Test	
Marching Test	Grip Strength Test	
	Trail Making Test	
	Lateral Dominance Exam	

*The Reitan-Indiana is usually administered along with the Wechsler Preschool and Primary Scale of Intelligence (WPPSI) and Wide Range Achievement Test (WRAT).
†For the Halstead Test Battery, the child is administered the Wechsler Intelligence Scale for Children-Revised (WISC-R) and the WRAT.

It was Reitan, however, who conceptualized the contribution that a standardized battery could make in clinical practice. Reitan's work over the past three decades has provided neuropsychologists with a validated battery of tests that have been shown to be sensitive to the effects of brain dysfunction. For a comprehensive overview of the batteries developed by Halstead and Reitan the interested reader is referred to Selz (1981).

It should be pointed out that the neuropsychological test batteries developed and refined by Reitan are based on the notion that function is both well distributed and relatively well localized in the brain and that to adequately assess brain-behavior relations, a battery must include tests that are discretely sensitive to different regions of the cortex as well as to global functioning. In part, many of the validating studies on these batteries bear out this assumption.

A somewhat different approach has been offered by Luria (1980), who, as discussed previously, sought to apply the concept of "functional systems" to his conceptualization of brain-behavior relationships. Assessment from this perspective would thus focus on the evaluation of various components found to be common to many functional systems. Through a rather dynamic process of assessment, which relies heavily on clinical experience, cognitive abilities are identified that are deficient and that are thus disrupting the integrity of one or more functional systems.

Based on Luria's concepts, Golden (1981) has articulated his standardization of such a uniquely different assessment perspective. As can be seen in comparing the subtests (Table 7-1) incorporated in the Reitan-Indiana and in the Halstead Neuropsychological Test Battery, they differ significantly in focus from the rather broad subtests listed under the Luria-Nebraska.

A complete overview of these specific neuropsychological test batteries or even other alternate approaches is beyond the scope of this chapter. For a more thorough overview of these batteries, the interested reader is referred to Hynd and Obrzut (1981). It is proposed that these neuropsychological test batteries are not necessary or even appropriate for the evaluation of the dyslexic child. Conceptual as well as practical issues support this conclusion. Consider, for example, one neuropsychologist's view as to the purpose of a neuropsychological test battery:

> For a neuropsychological test battery to be maximally useful, it needs to be capable of diagnosing the location and approximate size of a lesion, the probable cause of the lesion, and the severity of impairment incurred. Such a battery should include tests that are sensitive to the general adequacy of brain functions as well as the integrity of specific parts of the brain. A broad range of psychological functions subserved by the brain would need to be assessed. (Selz, 1981, p. 196)

Considering that neuropsychological theory and practice have, in large part, originated from clinical practice with brain-damaged adults, the focus and purpose noted by Selz (1981) seem most appropriate. One must, however, question the relevance of this purpose with school-age children, particularly in relation to questions such as localizing the site and size of a lesion, or its probable cause.

Purpose of Neuropsychological Assessment with Dyslexic Children

If it is presumed that dyslexia is related to neurodevelopmental factors (as so strongly suggested by the evidence cited in this volume) then the neuropsychological evaluation of the child with severe reading failure must have as a priority the determination as to the possible neuropsychological nature of the disorder. The location and size of the lesion (or developmental anomaly) thus is not nearly as important as whether there is evidence of neuropsychological factors associated with the reading failure.

In a clinical or hospital setting, it is often known whether a patient has neurological damage. The symptomatology of a cerebral vascular accident (CVA) is rather straightforward, and the focus of the examination is to articulate the extent of the lesion and the prognosis for the patient. In an educational setting this is clearly not appropriate.

We would emphasize, in fact, that hypothesizing as to the site of the neurological dysfunction in the child's brain is a clearly inappropriate practice in work with school-age children with severe reading failure. This notion is supported by others (Gaddes, 1980) who suggest that neuropsychological data be used to develop working hypotheses as to how particular children utilize the abilities available to them. Strengths and weaknesses should be addressed in the report and recommendations, as is traditionally the case. For the child whose neuropsychological test profile suggests an organic basis to the severe reading failure, however, the focus of the recommendations should be on capitalizing on available strengths rather than focusing the remedial process on tasks already proven to be nonproductive in helping the child (Reynolds, 1981).

It could be argued that if the purpose of neuropsychological assessment is not to localize the site of the lesion, then of what value is neuropsychological assessment? Reschly (1982) has stated that neuropsychological assessment with school-age children represents application of high inferential thinking in reaching a diagnostic conclusion. It would be much better, he argues, to simply assess what the child can and cannot do, thereby avoiding the problem of inferring observed behavior back to hypothetical constructs. Hynd (1982) has argued that by just using strict behavioral measures to determine areas of possible remedial focus, the psychologist ignores the fact that deficits in behavior may be the direct result of cortical dysfunction. It is for this reason that the neuropsychological evaluation is so critical, because it will determine whether the problem is merely behavioral (from an operant perspective) or is the result of neurological dysfunction. Both behavioral approaches and neuropsychological perspectives to assessment, in fact, should not be viewed as inconsistent from a theoretical standpoint.

Integration of Behavioral and Neuropsychological Paradigms

It is proposed that the typically behavioral approach in assessment as used by teachers (behavior checklists, rating scales, criterion-referenced measurement) is compatible with data derived from neuropsychological assessment. From the perspective of what has been termed behavioral neuropsychology it is assumed that data generated from neuropsychological assessment accurately describes brain-behavior relationships and serves to pinpoint the direction in which behavioral intervention should proceed (Horton, 1981).

The schism so apparent in our thinking about the appropriateness of behavioral versus neuropsychological assessment may be traced in large part directly to B. F. Skinner (1938) who proposed the following:

> There are two independent subject matters (behavior and the nervous system) which must have their own techniques and methods and yield their own respective data . . . I am asserting, then, not only a science of behavior is independent of neurology but that it must be established as a separate discipline whether or not a rapprochement with neurology is ever attempted. (cited by Gaddes, 1980)

The traditional behavioral model has made the assumption that all actions can be accounted for in a stimulus-response paradigm (Skinner, 1938). Unobserved or inferred variables are to be ignored as irrelevant. Behavior therapy and its direct implications for educational intervention, however, offers a different theoretical construct in that inferred behavioral variables may be relevant in remedial intervention. If neuropsychological data are viewed as a hypothetical construct (i.e., it represents an actual, observable physical state) then it can be said that a behavioral perspective to neuropsychology and its hypothetical constructs regarding important brain-behavior relationships is consistent from a theoretical standpoint.

While many might argue about the role of cognitive factors in a behavioral framework (Beck & Mahoney, 1979; Ellis, 1979; Lazarus, 1979; Wolpe, 1978), it does seem that if one treats data from the neuropsychological examination as evidence of a contruct amenable to behavior therapy the "rapprochement" mentioned by Skinner (1938) may indeed be possible. In summation, it might be said that since a neuropsychological and behavioral paradigm are consistent from this theoretical perspective, then the neuropsychological evaluation must consider indices of overt behavior, and, in those in whom it is determined that cortical dysfunction does exist, recommend behavioral approaches in using those principles as outlined in Chapter 8.

NEUROPSYCHOLOGICAL EVALUATION: CONCEPTUAL FRAMEWORK

It should go without saying that children represent a considerably different challenge in neuropsychological evaluation than do adults. First, differential utilization of various cognitive functions may occur not only with developmental age but also according to proficiency in completing the task at hand. Children may do poorly on the Similarities subtest of the Wechsler Intelligence Scale for Children-Revised (WISC-R), for example, because they are developmentally immature (are not able to conceptualize how two concepts are similar) or because they have not had enough experience in verbally expressing themselves. Because of the developmental nature of neuropsychological assessment with school-age children, one also encounters the problem of finding tasks or tests that have an adequate floor and ceiling. Due to the greater variability of measures at younger age levels, conclusions need also to be stated more cautiously since it is quite possible that considerable change in performance can occur over repeated evaluations. This variability, however, is less likely on straightforward neurological tests. For these reasons, as well as others, it becomes very important to identify patterns of consistent performance that relate to the conceptual framework associated with dyslexia and dyslexic subtypes. More on this topic will be addressed later in the chapter. Other potential issues in neuropsychological assessment (e.g., premorbid level of intelligence, organicity and old age, complicating illness such as alcoholism, etc.) that are pertinent to an adult population may have little impact on assessment of the dyslexic child.

J. Obrzut (1981b) has provided us with a potentially valuable framework for conceptualizing neuropsychological assessment with the school-age child who has been referred for an evaluation of a severe reading disability. He proposed that learning may be viewed as a hierarchy of information processing. As outlined by Johnson and Myklebust (1967) this hierarchy involves sensation, perception, memory, symbolization, and conceptualization. To this framework one might add motor functioning to perception since, for example, motoric ability provides kinesthetic feedback and serves as a basis for perceptual learning. Within this context it is important to realize that being hierarchic in nature, any deficit or disability acquired at one level will affect development of abilities at other, higher levels of cognitive functioning. Deficient performance on perceptual tasks will thus likely affect memory, symbolization, and conceptualization.

It is within this framework that neuropsychological assessment with the school-age child might best be conceptualized. Recognized and validated clinical assessment procedures pertinent to abilities and skills within each of these hierarchic levels of information processing can be incorporated within the clinical assessment. In this manner the clinician is not tied to a set neuropsychological battery that may be inappropriate for a particular child; instead, the clinician may utilize assessment instruments both pertinent to the particular child and to the child's other needs, and use tests that the clinician has found especially useful. The complete neuropsychological evaluation will still take between six to twelve hours, usually covering at least one to two complete days. Needless to say, the amount of time any particular evaluation takes will depend greatly on the extent of the evaluation, on the expertise of the examiner, on the cooperation of the child, and, of course, on the time available to work with the child.

So that the possible context for the neuropsychological evaluation of the child with severe reading failure can be determined, the following discussion will focus on the hierarchy of information processing noted earlier, along with possible tests that are appropriate to tap abilities at each level. The various tasks or tests suggested are only recommended. At least two points should be kept in mind. First, abilities at each level should be adequately assessed using at least two, if not more, correlated measures. In this fashion the probability of making errors in clinical judgment (i.e., diagnosing neuropsychological deficits when none exist) will be greatly reduced. If deficit performance on one task cannot be supported by equally deficient performance on some related (correlated) task, then a judgment regarding neuropsychological deficit should probably not be made. A child, for example, may evidence a relative difficulty in naming familiar objects (anomia—a symptom often associated with receptive aphasia). Referring back to Table 6-1, it will be seen that this is a symptom often associated with the language-disordered dyslexic subtype described by Mattis et al. (1975). This is also noted by Pirozzolo (1981), as can be seen under his description of the deficits associated with his auditory-linguistic subtype (see Table 6-2). Simply because some children seem to possess a deficit in object naming does not qualify them as being dyslexic. Other correlated deficits must also appear, and Mattis et al. (1975) list several that may be considered correlated deficits. A second and obviously related point to consider is that the subtypes discussed in this volume are not all-inclusive. The subtype literature discussed in some detail in Chapter 6, coupled with the articulation of the functional system involved in reading and in associated neurodevelopmental abnormalities in the dyslexic child (Drake, 1968; Galaburda & Kemper, 1979), argues strongly that the pattern of deficits found in each dyslexic child will be relatively unique. Considerable clinical expertise in neuropsychological assessment and diagnosis is therefore required to adequately conceptualize and describe the unique pattern of deficits found in each child evaluated. The subtype literature merely points the way in which generalized patterns of deficits may be manifested from a clinical-psychometric standpoint. With these points in mind, it is now appropriate to discuss the framework for the neuropsychological battery pertinent to the dyslexic child.

Sensation and Sensory Recognition

Sensation refers to the lowest possible aspect of behavior in that sensory mechanisms appear to activate appropriately to stimulation. In many respects, it is difficult to differentiate sensation from perception since the two mechanisms are so closely tied. For our purpose we will consider lower levels of perception tied to sensory abilities.

In this framework, it is imperative to attend to two basic processes associated with sensory abilities: acuity and recognition of sensation. The complete developmental and health history of the dyslexic child is obviously important in that early deficits in the acuity of sensation may be reported. A child who seems unresponsive to loud noise as an infant and who has a history of early otitis media may well be evidencing auditory sensory deficits. These behaviors are often associated with impaired speech and language (Katz, 1978; Needleman, 1977), behavioral problems (Hersher, 1978), and various learning disorders (Downs, 1977; Howie, 1977; Zinkus, Gottlieb, & Shapiro, 1978). Visual difficulties may similarly be manifested at an early age, thus making the careful taking of a developmental and health history even more important. It also should not be assumed that the child has adequate visual or auditory acuity simply because there is no history of problems suggestive of this. While the schools should provide every child with a vision and hearing screening, it is an unfortunate fact that many do not. Unless, therefore, there is evidence that hearing and vision have been checked, each child should receive a vision and hearing evaluation prior to the more formalized neuropsychological assessment.

At a somewhat higher level of functioning is sensory recognition, which admittedly involves basic perceptual processes. These basic perceptual processes, however, are at such a low level that their inclusion is appropriate. It is here that basic recognition and awareness of sensory stimulation becomes apparent. As can be seen in Table 7-2 such tasks as Fingertip Number Writing, the Single and Double Simultaneous (Face-Hand) Stimulation Test (Centofanti & Smith, 1978), and the Tactile Form Recognition Test would be appropriate measures of sensory recognition. The Finger Agnosia Test (Gerstmann, 1924, 1930) has been controversial (Benton, 1955) but in many reports also seems to be sensitive to sensory dysfunction in reading-disabled children (Hermann, 1964; Kinsbourne & Warrington, 1963; Lindgren, 1978; Satz & Friel, 1973, 1974). In fact, in the study reported by Lindgren (1978) in which 100 kindergarten children were administered a test battery at the beginning of kindergarten and later, at the end of first grade, assessed as to reading ability, it was concluded that in classifying the "sample of children as poor readers or as adequate readers [at the end of first grade] on the basis of FL [finger localization] performance alone results in correct classification for three out of four children" (p. 97). It is the complex nature of the finger agnosia task in terms of the functional cortex involved in sensory recognition that makes it such a potentially sensitive measure in reflecting significant neuropsychological deficit.

There are at least two considerations that should be pointed out. First, performance on the ability to localize which finger was touched by the examiner, as on the Finger Agnosia Test, should be considered in light of right-sided–left-sided differences. Consistently poor right-sided performance on Finger Agnosia, on Tactile Form Recognition, or on the Single and Double Simultaneous (Face-Hand) Stimulation Test usually indicates cortical dysfunction on the contralateral side. A child with consistently poor

Table 7-2
Conceptual Hierarchy and some Associated Tests for
the Neuropsychological Assessment of
the Dyslexic Child*

Sensation and Sensory recognition

Acuity
　Visual Acuity
　Auditory Acuity
　Developmental and Health History

Recognition
　Finger Agnosia (Finger Localization)
　Finger-tip Number Writing
　Single and Double Simultaneous (Face-Hand) Stimulation Test
　Tactile Form Recognition Test

Perception

Auditory
　Speech Sounds Perception Test
　Seashore Rhythm Test
　Wepman Auditory Discrimination Test

Visual
　Bender Gestalt Test
　Berry Visual Motor Integration Test (VMI)
　Benton Visual Retention Test

Tactile-Kinesthetic
　Tactual Performance Test (TPT)
　Tactile Form Recognition

Motor

Cerebellar Screening
　Tandem Walking (heel-to-toe)
　Finger to Nose to Examiner's Finger
　Tests for Dysarthria
　Tests for Nystagmus
　Evaluation for Hypotonia

Lateral Dominance—Motor Only
　Grip Strength
　Edinburgh Inventory
　Halstead-Reitan Lateral Dominance Examination
　Finger Oscillation (Finger-Tapping) Test

Psycholinguistic

Screening Measures
　Aphasia Screening Test

Fluency Test
Peabody Picture Vocabulary Test—Revised (PPVT-R)

Formal Batteries
Boston Diagnostic Aphasia Examination
Orzeck Aphasia Evaluation
Illinois Test of Psycholinguistic Ability (ITPA)
Northwestern Syntax Test

Language Asymmetries
Dichotic Listening Task
Visual Half-Field Technique

Academic (Reading)

Informal Batteries
Clinical Interview
Attitudes
Interests
Socialization
Self Concept
Test for Phonetic Sounds (nonsense words)
Test for Vowel Principles (nonsense words)
Syllabication (nonsense words)
Informal Reading Inventory
Writing Sample
Spelling Test
Try-outs—Diagnostic Teaching

Formal Batteries
Learning Modalities
Mills Learning Methods Test
Detroit Tests of Learning Aptitude
Illinois Test of Psycholinguistic Ability (ITPA)
Durrell Analysis of Reading Difficulties
Gates-McKillop Reading Diagnostic Test
Woodcock Reading Mastery Tests
Wide Range Achievement Test
Boder Diagnostic Reading-Spelling Test

Cognitive—Intellectual

Category Test
Raven's Coloured Progressive Matrices Test
Kaufman Assessment Battery for Children (K-ABC)
McCarthy Scales of Children's Abilities (MSCA)
Wechsler Intelligence Scale of Intelligence—Revised (WISC-R)
Wechsler Preschool and Primary Scales of Intelligence

---

* It should be emphasized that this conceptual hierarchy and the suggested assessment procedures are not meant to be all inclusive. The knowledgeable clinician should use their professional expertise in designing a comprehensive and individually appropriate neuropsychological battery in keeping with each child's unique needs.

right-sided sensory performance may well turn out to have neuropsychological deficits associated with higher cognitive processes important in reading acquisition, which we know in most individuals are also lateralized to the left cerebral cortex.

A second consideration relates to in which modality the associated deficit manifests itself. Are only tactile-kinesthetic abilities affected or are basic auditory deficits also present? If the deficits appear only in the tactile-kinesthetic domain one might suspect more parietal lobe dysfunction and, thus, look for other correlates of parietal lobe dysfunction that may be associated with poor reading disability (e.g., inability to copy or to recognize geometric shapes, an ability obviously important in letter or word recognition). The fact that isolated deficits may appear is again relatively meaningless unless the deficits can be correlated in a meaningful fashion with other test data as the data relates to our conceptualization of the processes involved in the functional system of reading. It is for this reason that an in-depth understanding of the material presented in Chapters 2 and 3 is so critical. It is also for this reason that so many measures are typically administered in a comprehensive neuropsychological examination.

Perceptual Processes

Basic brain-behavior relations begin with perception, which involves the organization and integration of basic sensory stimulation (J. Obrzut, 1981b). As with basic sensation, visual, auditory, and tactile-kinesthetic modalities are involved in the perceptual processes. Auditory, visual, and tactile-kinesthetic memory may also be involved in perceptual learning.

In the auditory domain, the Seashore Rhythm Test (Knights & Norwood, 1979) is a popular measure of the ability to differentiate like from dissimiliar pairs of sounds. The test requires the ability to sustain attention, remain alert to incoming auditory stimuli, and make comparative judgments regarding competing rhythmic sequences.

Visual perception has typically received more attention in the neuropsychological examination than has assessment of auditory perception. This is probably due to the emphasis placed on higher levels of language processes in the information processing hierarchy. In large part, the relative neglect of the assessment of formal auditory-perceptual processes at the lower levels is due to the fact that basic processes that are affected by auditory-perceptual processes will later be associated with performance at higher levels of information processing.

The Bender Gestalt Test is one of the most frequently administered tests by neuropsychologists (Craig, 1979) as well as by psychologists who work within the school system (Goh, Teslow, & Fuller, 1980). The ability to correctly copy the designs presented on stimuli cards seems to assess the integrity of the visual-spatial perceptual system in integrating and organizing stimuli. Poor performance on the Bender Gestalt may relate to developmental immaturity or may indicate subjects with parietal lobe dysfunction (Garron & Cheifetz, 1965), which is usually right parietal lobe damage (Diller, Ben-Yishay, Gerstmann, Goodkin, Gordon, & Weinberg, 1974; Hirschenfang, 1960). Poor performance on the Bender can either be indicative of developmental delay or be due to cerebral dysfunction, and it is for this reason that one must be familiar with appropriate norms (Koppitz, 1963) and performance indicative of cortical pathology. Usually, the older the child, the fewer errors that could occur. For a 12-year-old boy referred for evaluation of severe reading difficulties, ten errors would thus be truly significant. Qualitative analysis of performance is also necessary in clinical diagnosis, as some copying errors are more indicative of cerebral dysfunction than are others.

Another test that has been popular and is frequently used with school-age children is the Developmental Test of Visual Motor Integration (VMI) (Berry, 1974). Designed for preschool and elementary school children, the Berry VMI has been found to discriminate reasonably well between children who become fluent readers from those who later evidence reading problems (Lindgren, 1978). This test simply requires a child to copy a series of progressively more difficult geometric designs. Developmental aspects affecting performance again need to be considered along with possible indices of cortical dysfunction.

Within the tactile-kinesthetic realm, two measures seem particularly useful for assessment of the child with severe reading failure. The Tactual Performance Test (TPT) is a modification of the Seguin-Goddard Formboard. Six forms are to be placed on a board by the child. The children are blindfolded prior to being administered the test, the children's hands are run over the form outlines on the board, and the children are told to fit the forms in the proper spaces using only their preferred hand. They then perform this task a second time using their non-preferred hand and, finally, a third time using both hands. The time required to complete the task with each hand may provide a good indicator of right-sided–left-sided performance. After the TPT board has been removed from sight, the children are asked to draw a diagram of the board, noting the proper location of each form. Three scores are considered in evaluating the TPT results: Time, Memory, and Localization. In addition to providing some data on right-left differences, the TPT assesses tactile-kinesthetic form discrimination, incidental spatial memory, spatial visualization, and tactile memory (Selz, 1981).

The Tactile Form Recognition Test is another relatively simple task to administer to a child. Four plastic forms (circle, square, triangle, and cross) are placed in the child's hand and must be matched against forms visually presented. Both errors and response time are recorded. This test can provide a good measure of parietal lobe functioning as well as data pertinent to right-sided–left-sided comparisons.

When using these measures, it would not be surprising for one to find a child with characteristics similar to the dyseidetic dyslexic (see Chapter 6), who evidenced deficit performance on the Bender Gestalt, a significant number of errors on left-handed performance on the Tactile Form Recognition Test, and equally deficient performance on the left-handed Fingertip Number Writing Task. Coupled with spelling and reading patterns typical of performance of the dyseidetic, it would be appropriate to conceptualize the deficits of this particular child as reflective of right parietal-lobe dysfunction.

As indicated earlier, however, it is absolutely inappropriate to suggest in a neuropsychological evaluation, which is intended for use by educators for programmatic purposes, that a school-age child suffers right parietal-lobe dysfunction. This is a meaningless conclusion from an intervention standpoint. What is appropriate is to conclude that the child has neuropsychological deficits that are associated with the utilization of visual-perceptual and tactile-kinesthetic abilities. The most probable course for successful intervention for this child, assuming other abilities are intact, is through auditory-linguistic approaches focusing on phonetic analysis. The notion, of course, is to focus intervention on available strengths and away from abilities not fully developed that are most likely due to cerebral dysfunction (Reynolds, 1981). The report thus directs attention toward cognitive abilities that are intact, avoids the use of terms not usually accepted in the educational community (e.g., brain damage, parietal lobe dysfunction), and points the way toward the intervention approach that is most likely to succeed either through direct behavioral intervention or through more traditional curriculum approaches as discussed in Chapter 8.

Motoric Evaluation

Conceptualization of the evaluation of the motor system should entail screening of cerebellar and motoric functioning, and an evaluation of lateral motor dominance. The first component of the evaluation should be considered as a screening for neurological integrity. If significant deficits are suspected, it may then be appropriate to refer to a neurologist. The same applies should a suspicion exist that deterioration or cerebellar disease may be present. The second aspect of the motoric evaluation is to determine both the preferences and the levels of lateralized motor performance. Such an evaluation can indicate contralateral cortical dysfunction or weak preference patterns that may be identified in the dyslexic child.

Cerebellar Functioning

DeMeyer (1974) has noted that there are many misunderstandings regarding what the cerebellum actually does. He quotes Laurence Sterne

(1713–1768), who satirized the "speculative neurophysiology" that was popular in the 18th century.

> But how great was his apprehension, when he farther understood, that (the force of Paturition) acting upon the very vertex of the head, not only injured the brain itself, or cerebrum,—but that it necessarily squeezed and propelled the cerebrum towards the cerebellum, which was the immediate seat of the understanding!—Angels and ministers of grace defend us! cried my father,—can any soul withstand this shock?—No wonder the intellectual web is so rent and tattered as we see it; and that so many of our best heads are no better than a puzzled skein of silk,—all perplexity,—all confusion within-side. (From *The Life and Opinions of Tristain Shandy Gentleman*, as quoted by De-Meyer, 1974, p. 237)

As was discussed in Chapter 2, the cerebellum working in concert with the pons coordinates posture, muscle movement sense, and controls and refines motor movements. Unfortunately, it is not the "seat of understanding!" Dystaxia, dysarthria, nystagmus, and hypotonia are considered to be clinical signs of cerebellar dysfunction. Children or adults who manifest clinical signs of dystaxia resemble a person who is intoxicated. They typically have difficulty standing on one foot and sway and stagger when walking. Tandem walking (or walking heel-to-toe) often elicits dystaxic behavior. Dystaxia–dysmetria of the arm can also be elicited by asking the child to touch his nose and then touch the examiner's finger, which is moving in an arc approximately one foot from the face of the child. A child who evidences dysmetria often undershoots or overshoots the target and thus, poorly estimates the distance and arc between his nose and the examiner's finger. This performance results from dysequilibrium of contractions of the muscles or, as DeMeyer (1974) states, "the agonist-antagonist contractions which arrest movement" (p. 244).

Dysarthria can be elicited or noted on tests of higher cognitive functions and should be apparent on the Aphasia Screening Test, or more comprehensive aphasia diagnostic exams (e.g., Boston Diagnostic Aphasia Examination, Orzeck Aphasia Evaluation), or on oral reading tests in which slurred speech may be evident. Nystagmus, or jerky eye movements, may be associated with cerebellar dysfunction or may be due to the close relationship the pathways have to other brain stem structures. Nystagmus may result from lesions of the eye, vestibular system, or other brainstem lesions. They can be elicited by asking the child to slowly follow the examiner's finger with his eyes. The child's head should remain stationary while this task is executed. The faulty eye movements noted by Pirozzolo (1981) in Table 6-2 may be associated with the visual-spatial dyslexic. If nystagmus is found in screening, there is no reason to refer to a neurologist unless the symptoms have an acute onset, are associated with nausea (with or without vomiting), vertigo is experienced, and/or oscillopsia (oscillating vision) is present. The congenital nystagmus that are often found in dyslexic children (or children with other learning disabilities) are usually asymptomatic (DeMeyer, 1974).

The child evidencing hypotonia gives the impression of being like a rag doll. The arms and feet seem floppy and he may look somewhat out of control when he walks. Passive movement of the arms or legs will reveal poor muscle tone for the child's age.

Lateral Dominance

In this component of the neuropsychological examination, it is important to evaluate performance in at least two dimensions. First, the level of performance itself is important since the implications on some tests of depressed bilateral performance are different from that of unilaterally depressed performance. In concert with this notion is the idea of comparing right-sided versus left-sided performance.

The Grip Strength Test simply assesses the child's grip strength as evidenced on a dynamometer. Using the Smedly Hand Dynamometer, a child is allowed two trials for each hand. Grip strength is measured in kilograms and the score is the average of the two trials per hand. As with Finger Oscillation (Finger-Tapping), Finger Localization, and Finger-tip Number Writing, normative data are provided for males and females, aged 6 through 14. The vast majority of children should show a strong right-sided preference. Unilaterally, poor performance is usually associated with cortical dysfunction in the contralateral cerebral hemisphere.

The Finger Oscillation Test assesses motor speed on a manual finger tapper. The child rests his or her hand on a board and taps the tapper key as fast as possible for ten seconds. Five ten-second trials are given for each hand, using the index finger to depress the key. The score reported is the average number of taps for each hand over the ten-second trials. Similar to the Grip Strength Test, finger oscillation provides a good indication of the contralateral motor cortex for the child.

The Edinburgh Inventory (Oldfield, 1971) and the Halstead-Reitan Lateral Dominance Examination provide a good indication of a child's preferences on lateral motor tasks. It is a widely accepted fact that many dyslexics do suffer deficits in lateralized motor performance. Simply stated, mixed or weak preferences on lateralized tasks are often found in children who have learning problems but they are not correlated directly with academic or intellectual abilities (Hynd, Obrzut, & Obrzut, 1981). It is important, thus, to assess lateral dominance; but, since it represents an ability that may or may not be involved in the neuropsychological profile of reading failure for a specific child, one should be cautious about drawing conclusions regarding cognitive functioning. It may be helpful at this point to go back and review the distinction drawn in Chapter 5 regarding lateralized performance on motor tasks versus central-perceptual asymmetries, the latter being more related to cognitive processes involved in reading (e.g., dichotic listening or visual half-field techniques).

To this point we have discussed, in rather specific terms, various tests or tasks associated with the assessment of basic sensory, perceptual, and motor abilities that serve as a foundation for the development of higher cognitive functioning. It has been proposed that there is a great likelihood that deficits or dysfunctional abilities at these lower levels may adversely affect learning and performance on such tasks as reading. This proposal is not absolute as it is easy to find children with mild cerebral palsy who suffer only motor dysfunction and who seem to have more than adequate cognitive abilities. The probability that deficits associated with audition and vision will affect language learning or reading, however, is greater than with deficits in the motor systems since these two basic sensory/perceptual processes are directly involved in most higher cognitive functions. It is once again stressed that differential diagnosis must involve the articulation of indices of cortical dysfunction with the pattern of deficits on cognitive tasks as they relate to our understanding of the functional system of reading.

Since memory, symbolization, and conceptualization, the last three aspects of our information processing hierarchy, are so closely intertwined, they will be considered within the context of recognized components of assessment of higher cortical function as pertinent to the evaluation of the dyslexic child. The following discussion will be organized into three broad categories: evaluation of psycholinguistic functioning, assessment of reading abilities, and evaluation of cognitive intellectual processing abilities.

Psycholinguistic Functioning

As used in the context of this volume, an assessment of psycholinguistic functioning entails more than simply the ability to use speech and language. It encompasses the ability to use speech and language in a meaningful and socially acceptable fashion; it relates speech and language to the psychological processes that are inherent in articulating meaningful concepts. Psycholinguistic evaluation should thus examine not only the very basic abilities associated with language but also should qualitatively relate speech and language capabilities to age-appropriate behavior.

The Aphasia Screening Test and the Fluency Test provide good screening measures that may indicate whether more thorough in-depth evaluations are in order. More often than not, a formalized assessment of psycholinguistic abilities should be carried out with a dyslexic subject unless it is believed other measures associated with academic and cognitive assessment will reveal similar information. The Aphasia Screening Test resulted from Reitan's revision of the Halstead-Wepman Aphasia Screening Test (Halstead & Wepman, 1949). Its primary purpose is to identify language-based disorders that may be manifested on spelling, reading, arithmetic, articulation, and orientation tasks (Selz, 1981). The Fluency Test simply requires the child to name as many words as possible in 60 seconds. For more fluent individuals (such as older adolescents or adults) the task can be made more difficult by asking them to name as many words as they can that begin with a specific letter, such as "e," in 60 seconds. The Peabody Picture Vocabulary Test-Revised (PPVT-R) has been shown to be especially useful with children suspected of having receptive language difficulties (Zaidel, 1976).

The various aphasia test batteries, such as the Boston Diagnostic Aphasia Examination (Lea & Febiger, 1972) or the Orzeck Aphasia Evaluation (Orzeck, 1966), are more appropriate for older adolescents who suffer significant speech and language difficulties. These batteries typically assess for fluency, naming, repetition, paraphasias, and other characteristics often associated with aphasia. An important factor to consider is that since these batteries are so complete the results can be useful in conceptualizing cognitive deficits in the functional system that are believed to be associated with reading. Many of the tasks included on these batteries have been shown to correlate well with deficient left temporal and parietal lobe functioning (Frisch & Handler, 1974; McFie, 1960; Swiercinsky, 1979).

Probably of more relevance to neuropsychological assessment of school-age children considered as dyslexic is the Illinois Test of Psycholinguistic Ability (ITPA). The conceptual framework on which this particular test was developed seems sound enough (Kirk, 1972; Kirk, McCarthy, & Kirk, 1968). It is, however, the application of this framework in designing remedial programs that focus on improving deficit psycholinguistic skills that is questionable. An overview of the controversy of the remedial program of the ITPA follows in Chapter 8. Basically, the ITPA assesses psycholinguistic processes related to perception, association, and expression in both the visual and auditory channels. Six subtests each appear at the representational level of organization and at the automatic level. Pirozzolo and Hess (1976) found the ITPA especially useful in differentiating between the two dyslexic subtypes later detailed by Pirozzolo (1981).

It is definitely important to assess psycholinguistic functioning in the child referred for severe reading failure. Behaviors such as agrammatism or anomia (word-finding difficulty) seem to be associated with dyslexic children who have a deficient language processer (Mattis et al., 1975; Pirozzolo, 1981). Only through an in-depth analysis of psycholinguistic functioning may these deficiences become apparent.

It is at this point in the evaluation in which it may be meaningful to look at the relationship psycholinguistic functioning has to measures of language asymmetry. The dichotic listening and visual half-field paradigms may reveal important data about asymmetries in language processing (i.e., Does a strong right-ear effect exist? Do normal visual half-field asymmetries exist?) as well as revealing how efficient the language processer is in relation to indices of psycholinguistic abilities. For a child who has evidenced expressive and receptive speech deficits including poor oral fluency, anomia, and deficit phonetic analysis of unknown words, for example, it would not be unusual to find overall depressed dichotic listening performance in both ears or, more typically, poor recognition of dichotically presented stimuli to the right ear. It will be recalled that a right-ear effect on a dichotic task indicates left-cerebral hemispheric dominance for language. Since the dichotic listening task and visual half-field paradigms involve rather complex theoretical as well as practical issues, the reader may wish to refer to Satz et al. (1976), Kinsbourne and Hiscock (1981), or Hynd and Obrzut (1981) for a detailed discussion.

In concluding this brief section on the psycholinguistic assessment as part of a comprehensive neuropsychological evaluation of the dyslexic reader, a few points need to be made. First, the relatively subtle deficits that children with dyslexia may make on these possible evaluation instruments argues strongly that one should not attempt to localize a lesion site. This makes not only good clinical sense but is also dictated by a knowledge of the aphasia literature. It has been realized over time, that many subtypes of aphasia exist that are equally as difficult to diagnose as are the subtypes of dyslexia. It is known, furthermore, that the localization of expressive and receptive language deficits may occasionally involve the "minor" hemisphere in some cases and various subcortical structures in still others (April & Han, 1980; Kirshner & Kistler, 1982; Naeser, Alexander, Helm-Estabrooks, Levine, Laughlin, & Geschwind, 1982; Silverberg & Gordon, 1979). It should also be realized that if neuroanatomical deficits do exist (as strongly supported by the research of Duffy [1980a] and Galaburda [1979]), the nature of the cytoarchitectonic abnormalities may be widely distributed throughout one hemisphere or, possibly, even throughout both hemispheres. If this is indeed the case, the focus of the neuropsychological examination at this level should be on identifying disrupted systems of communication that are not on possible localized cortical lesions. The previously noted cortical abnormalities revealed by Galaburda and Kemper (1979) were discrete but well distributed throughout the left hemisphere. The localization of all of these discrete lesion sites would have been almost impossible even through an exceptionally comprehensive neuropsychological assessment. Certainly some of the deficits would have been identified, but not all of them. What is important is that the functional system of reading (and language) was disrupted, and these deficits were manifested on the test profile. Further verification through assessment of academic achievement and cognitive abilities, however, is needed.

Academic Achievement

Many of the readers of this volume will be most familiar with the realm of the assessment of academic and cognitive intellectual functioning. Studies have consistently shown that these domains are more frequently evaluated by diagnostic specialists working with children (Goh et al., 1980). For this reason, not every possible assessment technique or evaluation method noted in Table 7-2 will be discussed in detail. The focus will instead be on discussing those techniques that are often overlooked or those that are less frequently used as part of the clinical assessment.

Informal Evaluation

The clinical interview can be one of the most productive encounters between the examiner and child. It is during the interview that the examiner can follow up on tentative hypotheses developed from reading the referral, from reading the developmental/health history, or from discussing the child with the parent. It is often productive to first interview the parent(s) and the child together so that the child is able to know with certainty some of the perceptions of the parent(s) prior to being interviewed separately. When the child is interviewed alone, it is critical to gain some understanding as to how the child perceives himself and his reading problem, to determine his attitudes and interests, to determine his feelings toward peers, and to gain an overall picture as to his self-concept.

An understanding of the child's interests and attitudes is obviously important. First, it is vital to determine if a more formalized evaluation of emotionality and behavior needs to be conducted. Formalized personality evaluation by a qualified psychologist is essential if emotional problems are even suspected. It will be recalled in the definitions discussed in Chapter 1 that the severe reading disability must be primary; that is, it cannot be due to variables such as emotional factors, or sociocultural differences. A severe reading disability may exist concurrently with a behavioral disorder, but from a definitional standpoint the reading difficulty must be primary to be termed dyslexia. If emotional problems are even suspected, a thorough evaluation must be conducted. A second reason for such an in-depth examination (more formal tests might well be used) of attitudes and interests is to determine what reading matter might be of greatest interest to the child during the intervention phase. Obviously, one wants to maximize motivation.

Informal assessment has as its goal the determination of how the child actually reads by observing the child reading. The Slosson Oral Reading Test or Dolch Word List may be used, for example, in determining an appropriate entry level for the administration of an Informal Reading Inventory, which can be used to measure oral-reading competency and silent and oral comprehension. Observation of the error patterns on tests for phonetic sounds and vowel principles using nonsense words (to avoid the confounding effect of previous learning) as well as a qualitative evaluation of errors on a free-writing sample or on a spelling test can reveal a great deal regarding the nature and patterns of reading errors. Diagnostic teaching or try-outs may assist greatly in matching a child's ability to read with proper instructional strategies as well as with appropriate curriculum materials. This is an often overlooked aspect of clinical evaluation, especially when conducted by a psychologist or some other diagnostic specialist who may not have knowledge or skills in curriculum materials and remedial programming. It is for this reason that a comprehensive neuropsychological evaluation that encompasses a detailed academic assessment might best be conducted by a multidisciplinary team. In this fashion, neuropsychological knowledge might be more closely matched with principles and practices of educational diagnosis and intervention.

Formal Batteries

The formal assessment tests or batteries offer potentially less specific clinical information on how the child actually does read, but they do have the advantage of examining recognized components of the reading process. Items such as word and letter recognition, sight vocabulary, word-attack skills, reading comprehension, and use of contextual cues can be assessed in a quantitative manner such that a child's performance can be compared to either local norms or to the performance of some other, more general reference group. The standard scores, percentiles, grade equivalent scores, and derived stanine scores all can be useful in charting a child's profile of reading abilities. The Durrell Analysis of Reading Difficulties, Gates-McKillop Reading Diagnostic Test, and Woodcock Reading Mastery Tests can be especially valuable in pinpointing specific areas of strength or weaknesses in reading.

The evaluation of preferred learning modalities is critical if one is to adequately match aptitudes and treatments (Reynolds, 1981). The Mills Learning Methods Test, the Detroit Tests of Learning Aptitude, and even the ITPA can be very useful in this regard. Strengths in visual or auditory channels or even the tactile channel as measured by the Mills Learning Methods Test can be useful in helping maximize potential achievement. This seems particularly important in assisting the severely handicapped child (Wilson, 1981). Since the process of reading and, especially, the learning-to-read aspect may involve the differential use of preferred modalities (Bakker, 1981), clinicians need to be cautious in their conclusions and, due to the developmental nature of variations in preferred learning modalities, a constant monitoring should take place to ensure accurate conclusions regarding preferred learning modalities.

The Boder Diagnostic Reading-Spelling Test is a recently published elaboration of her diagnostic approach discussed in Chapter 6. Essentially, this screening test measures the child's ability to read and to spell known and unknown phonetic and nonphonetic words. Ten lists of 20 words each are available, graded from the preprimer level through 12th grade. The evaluation of the performance of the child allows one (according to a decision key) to diagnose a child into one of five categories (normal, retarded reader, dyseidetic, dysphonetic, and alexic or combined). The work of Bauserman and Obrzut (in press), Dalby and Gibson (1981), Fried et al. (1981), and Obrzut (1979) as discussed in Chapter 6 seem to substantiate the basic validity of the system of classification described by Boder (1982).

Caution in using any classification system for subtypes needs to be urged, however. If the conclusions based on Boder's test cannot be substantiated through the other assessment techniques employed, then her classification criteria and labels should not be applied. If, on the basis of Boder's system a child can be classified as dysphonetic, evidences severe difficulties in syllabication, does poorly on tests for phonetic sounds and vowel principles, has a verbal IQ significantly less then his performance IQ, and achieves poorly on standardized batteries assessing components of reading, then the label dysphonetic would be appropriate. It is the global picture of the results that leads one to conclusions regarding the subtype of dyslexia, and only a knowledge of the clinical and experimental literature will provide the appropriate conceptual framework for decisions. As Satz and Morris (1981) have noted,

> Whereas Boder's (1973) subtypes have an intuitive appeal and "resemblance" to reports in the clinical literature, they must be viewed with caution until the rules for subtype classification are more clearly operationalized and validated against external criteria. For example, are there differences or similarities in the phonetic analysis skills of dysphonetic and dyseidetic dyslexics (Group III)? If differences, are they in terms of levels or patterns? Are the differences scalar? . . . One might also ask whether the subtypes vary by age, IQ, sex, neurological status, or performance on nonreading measures of ability. (p. 121)

Cognitive–Intellectual Processes

The evaluation of higher cognitive processes from a neuropsychological standpoint represents one of the greatest challenges and potential pitfalls if one is attempting to relate recognized cognitive processes to functional neuroanatomy. It will be recalled that Gall believed intelligence was localized to the frontal lobes, based primarily on his observations of his students (Pirozzolo, 1979). Since we know that basic life-sustaining functions, basic perceptual processes, and even expressive speech are relatively localized within the functional geography of the brain, it is tempting to relate and project our perceptions in this regard on higher mental processes. The localization of intellectual processes is unfortunately not a reality that can usually be said to exist. Luria's concept of a functional system is most relevant to our discussion here (Luria, 1980, pp. 32–33; Ukhtomskii, 1945).

> If the higher mental functions are complex, organized functional systems that are social in origin, any attempt to localize them in special circumscribed areas ("centers") of the cerebral cortex is even less justifiable than the attempt to seek narrow circumscribed "centers" for biological functional systems. The modern view regarding the possible localization of the higher mental functions is that they have a wide, dynamic representation throughout the cerebral cortex based on constellations of territorially scattered groups of "synchronously working ganglion cells, mutually exciting one another" (Ukhtomskii, 1945). . . . We therefore suggest that *the material basis of the higher nervous processes is the brain as a whole* but that *the brain is a highly differentiated system whose parts are responsible for different aspects of the unified whole.* (Italics original, pp. 32–33)

In the assessment of higher cortical functions in school-age children, especially children with reading or learning problems, the developmental characteristics of intellectual processes compound the notion of differential cortical localization even further. Luria (1980) elaborates on this notion:

> The structural variation of the higher mental functions at different stages of ontogenetic (and, in some cases, functional) development means that their cortical organization likewise does not remain unchanged and that at different stages of development they are carried out by different constellations of cortical zones. (pp. 34–35)

Thus,

> *The character of the cortical intercentral relationships does not remain the same at different stages of development of a function and that the effects of a lesion of a particular part of the brain will differ at different stages of functional development.* (Italics original, pp. 34–35)

These quotes have been cited because they underscore the naiveté of those who suggest that IQ measures can be used to differentiate "right-versus left-brained thinkers" or, for example, that performance on one subtest on the WISC-R can definitively reveal deficits in right parietal lobe function. It is not argued that correlations or relationships may exist between performance on various subtests of IQ tests and cortical deficits, but that due to psychometric issues (Kaufman, 1979), conceptual problems, and a basic understanding of Luria's theory, it is best to use IQ tests and other tests of higher cortical functioning as overall measures of the intactness of higher mental processes. Coupled with information gleaned from other sources and from assessing different aspects of lower-level functioning, it may be appropriate to hypothesize about the site of cortical lesions in adults or in cases in which children are known to suffer brain damage. With school-age children referred for an in-depth neuropsychological evaluation of severe reading failure, however, it is again argued that it is inappropriate to attempt a diagnosis of the site of cortical dysfunction. The cortically based processes that can be attributed to neuropsychological dysfunction serve as the basis for remedial programming, focusing on available strengths.

The Category Test (from the Halstead Battery) consists of 168 consecutively presented slides. The slides are projected on an opaque screen and four numbered levers appear below the screen. The child looks at the stimulus projected onto the screen and depresses one of the four numbered levers. Immediate feedback is provided to the child. A bell indicates the selection of a correct choice, while a buzzer indicates an incorrect choice. The next slide automatically appears on the screen after the feedback. Six groups of slides exist, each group having an underlying principle governing the correct response. It is the child's task to learn the principles based on their experience. The Category Test is believed to assess the ability to reason abstractly and form concepts. It also measures the child's ability to learn from experience and shift conceptual sets. It is believed, overall, to be a good measure of intellectual and cognitive ability.

The Raven's Coloured Progressive Matrices Test, originally conceived of and developed in England, is a multiple-choice paper and pencil test for children 5 to 11 years of age. Similar to the Category Test, it is believed to be more culturally fair than are many traditional intelligence tests (e.g., Stanford-Binet, WISC-R). It takes about 45 minutes and simply requires the child to match a nonrepresentational colored pattern with a correct choice. While the Raven's Coloured Progressive Matrices Test seems to be a relatively good measure of overall ability, it does correlate with educational level and has nonstratified norms. While this test may be a good general measure of simple and complex reasoning skills, it thus should probably only be used as an adjunct measure of ability.

By far, the test of intellectual ability that has received the greatest attention has been the WISC-R. Divided into two subscales, the subtests of the WISC-R provide a verbal intelligence and performance intelligence quotient as well as providing a Full-Scale IQ score. While there appears to be a great amount of research relating performance on the Wechsler Intelligence Scale for Adults (WAIS) to localized brain dysfunction, little has been done along this line with the WISC-R. Evidence does exist, as discussed previously in this volume, that the left hemisphere is responsible for analytic, sequential, and language processing. The right cerebral hemisphere seems more responsible for gestalt propositional processing (Bogen, 1969a, 1969b, 1975; Gazzaniga, 1975). It therefore seems a reasonable assumption that the Verbal-Scale IQ score should reflect left-hemisphere functioning while the Performance-Scale IQ should reflect the integrity of the right cerebral hemisphere. While there is certainly some correlative evidence that suggests this may be the case (Fedio & Mirsky, 1969; Rourke, Young, & Flewelling, 1971), the fact is that the difficulty in finding children with circumscribed lateralized lesions has precluded any definitive statements in this regard (Reed, 1976). Once again, it thus seems prudent to consider the preferred mode of processing information as being diagnostically more meaningful. Bannatyne (1971, 1974) originally proposed a recategorization of the WISC-R subtests into a more meaningful framework. Using his categorization scheme, children with severe reading failure did best on subtests assessing spatial ability while they did poorest on subtests assessing sequencing skills (Arithmetic, Digit Span, and Coding) (Rugel, 1974; Smith, Coleman, Dokecki, & Davis, 1977).

Based on the seminal work of Luria (1980), some authors have advanced evidence that two distinct modes of information processing exist (Das, Kirby, & Jarman, 1975). Successive processing is exactly what it implies. Information is processed temporally and may be affected by damage to the frontal and temporal lobes. Simultaneous processing, on the other hand, involves gestalt-like processing in which information is processed as a whole. Occipitoparietal dysfunction may disrupt simultaneous processing. As J. Obrzut (1981b) notes, the nature of the stimuli may be unrelated to the processing whereas, "verbal processing [is] . . . not necessarily associated with successive processing, and visual-spatial stimuli do not automatically demand simultaneous processing" (p. 261). Related to the WISC-R, simultaneous processing would be assessed by performance on the Picture Completion, Block Design, and Object Assembly subtests. Successive processing, on the other hand, could be inferred through a subject's performance on Picture Arrangement, Coding, and Mazes subtests. No matter what perspective is used in attempting to analyze WISC-R performance, the reader should focus on processing strategies that seem to relate to other neuropsychological test data and avoid the temptation to localize dysfunction based on WISC-R performance.

Other potentially useful measures of cognitive-intellectual functioning include the McCarthy Scales of Children's Abilities (limited for use with younger dyslexics due to the low ceiling) and the recently published Kaufman Assessment Battery for Children (K-ABC). Research conducted by Kaufman, Kaufman, Kamphaus, and Naglieri (1982) and by Kamphaus, Kaufman, and Kaufman (1982) seem to support two robust factors, simultaneous and successive from age 2.5 years through 12.5 years. This test could potentially have the impact on pediatric neuropsychology as Wechsler's measures did on psychology if future research with normal and brain-damaged children provides further evidence as to the K-ABC's construct validity and reliability. In one study (Hooper & Hynd, 1982) the K-ABC Scales provided excellent discrimination between normal and dyslexic children but the discriminative ability of the test was poor in differentiating between subgroups described by Boder (1971, 1973a, 1973b). Considering the reservations expressed by Satz and Morris (1981) regarding Boder's clinical procedures, this result may tell us more about Boder's clinical techniques than the K-ABC will in differential diagnosis of dyslexic subtypes.

This relatively brief overview of potentially meaningful measures of sensation, perception, motor, psycholinguistic, and cognitive-intellectual development was intended to orient the reader in viewing assessment techniques from a neuropsychological perspective. More detailed descriptions of appropriate neuropsychological procedures exist elsewhere (Hynd & Obrzut, 1981; Lezak, 1976). It is only through a well-thought-out analysis and assessment of a child's abilities at all levels of this information processing hierarchy that a reasonably clear picture should emerge. Prior to presenting illustrative case reports, it might be helpful to briefly review some potential pitfalls that may be encountered in clinical neuropsychological assessment.

NEUROPSYCHOLOGICAL EVALUATION: PITFALLS

The most obvious pitfall in applying the principles of neuropsychological assessment to school-age children is related to the qualifications of the examiner. Other potential pitfalls include overgeneralizations based on insufficient data and overstepping professional boundaries.

Poorly Qualified Examiners

The qualification of neuropsychologists or psychologists who adopt a neuropsychological perspective has always been a concern of those who advocate this approach in working with children with severe learning problems (Gaddes, 1980; Hynd, 1981). Rourke (1976) has proposed at least a year of intensely supervised neuropsychological assessment experience as minimal. Meier (1981) and Hynd (1981) have discussed respectively appropriate training experiences for competency assurance for doctoral level neuropsychologists and for school psychologists interested in specializing in providing neuropsychological services to school-age children. Standards provided by the American Psychological Association (APA) would usually require the completion of a recognized program in neuropsychology for someone wishing to switch fields of expertise. The most recent survey on this matter, however, shows that the preferred manner in which neuropsychologists have received training is through workshops conducted by Reitan (Craig, 1979). The situation will undoubtedly change, and the neuropsychological perspective and services proposed in this book should not be offered by inadequately trained or poorly supervised personnel.

Overgeneralization Based on Insufficient Data

No knowledgeable neuropsychologist would dare diagnose constructional apraxia on the basis of poor performance on the Bender Gestalt Test. It has been our experience, however, that psychologists suspecting brain damage because of poor Bender performance may refer their clients to a neurologist for an extensive evaluation. Inexperience is obviously at work here. As Wilson (1981) notes, overgeneralization refers to the following:

> The tendency to use total test scores without examination of the pattern of test scores; the tendency to draw conclusions before all facts are in; the tendency to rely upon the first significant symptom, and the tendency to hazard guesses outside the professional field. (p. 187)

It makes a great amount of sense to avoid making any statement unless at least two, if not three or more, separately elicited behaviors correlate. Simply put, it is better to say nothing or state something cautiously than to overgeneralize.

Overstepping Professional Boundaries

To anyone who has completed clinical training in a hospital setting, it is known that while the roles of the physician, psychologist, or educational specialist are clearly defined, they can easily become obscured on occasion. It is not unusual to find a psychologist knowledgeable about psychopharmacology consulting with physicians about drug dosages. Physicians knowledgeable about psychological testing frequently administer tasks designed to elicit information about a patient's mental status. In applying neuropsychological knowledge to school-age children one must relate psychological and neurological knowledge to the problem at hand. Neurological screening, however, even when applied in the comprehensive neuropsychological examination, is exactly what it implies. If serious neurological problems are suspected on the basis of the screening tasks recommended in this chapter, the child should see a neurologist. Most psychologists also do not have a great deal of expertise in curriculum design. The recommendations of the report, therefore, should set the broad focus of educational intervention, and it should remain the responsibility of the educator or the remedial specialist to select the most relevant remedial procedures. By a careful respect and delineation of professional roles, the potential effectiveness of the multidisciplinary effort will be enhanced.

CONCLUSIONS

The goal of this chapter has been to provide an overview as to a number of important topics relative to the neuropsychological evaluation of the dyslexic child. Considerations that were discussed include what comprise the neurological examination, when to refer to a neurologist, the usefulness of commercially available neuropsychological assessment batteries with dyslexic children, the purpose of the neuropsychological examination with school-age children, and how behavioral and neuropsychological assessment paradigms may be theoretically compatible. The major focus of the chapter has been, however, to provide a conceptual framework for neuropsychological evaluation of dyslexic children. The foundation for this conceptualization comes from the work of Johnson and Myklebust (1967) as well as the work of J. Obrzut (1981a, 1981b), in which a hierarchy of information processing is central. Finally, this chapter concluded with a brief overview of potential pitfalls associated with the administration and interpretation of the neuropsychological assessment battery. These potential pitfalls pertain to the qualifications of the examiner, overgeneralizations derived from insufficient data, and overstepping professional boundaries (Wilson, 1981). The material presented in this chapter allows for the following conclusions.

Referrals to a neurologist for an evaluation of a child suspected of being dyslexic may not be warranted in most cases. The neuropsychological evaluation of the cognitive deficits most often associated with dyslexia will usually be more complete than that derived from the neurological examination. If, however, significant neurologic dysfunction exists, as manifested on the screening tests employed in the neuropsychological examination, it may indeed be appropriate to refer. If the learning or behavioral condition seems to be deteriorating or obvious neurological signs are also evident (e.g., nocturnal headaches, projectile vomiting, etc.), a referral is definitely indicated.

Since it is presumed that dyslexia is due to neurological dysfunction, as indicated in various definitions of dyslexia, no child should be diagnosed as dyslexic if the severe reading failure is not accompanied by identifiable signs of neuropsychologically based deficits. This fact argues strongly for the application of a comprehensive neuropsychological test battery by a qualified neuropsychologist.

Well-conceptualized and validated neuropsychological test batteries exist. Due to conceptual and practical considerations, however, these batteries may be more appropriate for use with children with known brain damage. The Luria-Nebraska Children's Battery, for instance, may identify too many false positives (diagnosing brain damage when none exists) in clinical application with children experiencing learning problems (Snow, Hynd, & Hartlage, in press).

Behavioral and neuropsychological paradigms may not be theoretically inconsistent if one views neuropsychological test data as a hypothetical construct. Data from both types of assessment thus are appropriate for evaluation of the dyslexic child. The neuropsychological test data, furthermore, may be able to focus behaviorally based intervention on available cognitive and behavioral strengths, thus maximizing the potential for academic intervention.

An information processing model provides an excellent conceptual framework for developing a neuropsychological test battery. Assessment of the sensation and sensory recognition, perception, motor, psycholinguistic, academic (reading), and cognitive-intellectual domains is warranted.

Professional standards for ensuring competency of examiners or neuropsychologists need to be heeded so that potential pitfalls in the application of the perspective outlined in this volume may be avoided.

Finally, neuropsychological reports for use in the academic setting should avoid the use of jargon and labels, should attempt to emphasize deficits or strengths in cognitive-intellectual processing skills rather than localize cortical dysfunction, and should point the way for further refinement of recommended strategies for intervention. The following case reports will serve to illustrate these points.

CASE STUDIES*

Auditory-Linguistic Dyslexia

Reason for Referral

David, a nine-year-old male Caucasian, was referred for a reevaluation because of inadequate academic progress in his regular classroom and in his resource-room program. His resource-room teacher observed that David was unable to profit from

---

*The following cases are presented for illustrative purposes only. The reader should note that the reports have been written from a neuropsychological perspective, jargon has been avoided, and the recommendations direct instructional efforts toward areas of relative cognitive strength. The first case has been adapted from Obrzut, A. A neuropsychological case report of a child with auditory-linguistic dyslexia. *School Psychology Review*, 1981, *10*, 356–361, with permission. The second case describes a typical visual-spatial dyslexic seen by the authors.

a regular classroom setting and the limited amount of remedial services amounting to 45 minutes a day. The school's multidisciplinary team felt that a complete neuropsychological assessment would provide additional insight into David's particular needs.

Developmental/Medical History

David's developmental and medical history revealed some significant findings. His mother reported a normal prenatal period and his birth and delivery were uneventful; however, he consistently lost weight for the first six weeks until his feeding schedule was stabilized. At age one year he was coughing up blood and was hospitalized with dehydration and intestinal flu for a two-week period. David had five ear infections during his first year of life.

Motor development for David appeared essentially within normal limits. In contrast, his language development was quite delayed. His early attempts to speak were almost unintelligible and a single-word vocabulary was not recognizable until 2.5 to 3 years of age. At 3.5 to 4 years of age he was able to combine words into single sentences, yet his speech was still unclear.

Physically, David is near age appropriate in both height and weight, being at the 40th percentile and 60th percentile, respectively. Visual screening indicates that both near- and far-point vision are normal. Audiological screening (puretone), including a tympanogram, was also normal.

Behavioral Observations

Classroom observation and a report by the teacher suggest that David is poorly motivated, inattentive, and an active student who performs inconsistently. He readily established rapport in the testing situation. David frequently requested repetition of directions and seemed to give up quite easily on most tasks. He responded most favorably to highly structured tasks that provided immediate feedback. The bell and buzzer differentially reinforcing responses on the Category Test, for example, appeared to have a marked affect on his performance as does his impulsiveness; and, extraneous motor activity ceased and he became highly motivated. Although his attention and concentration fluctuated, the following test results are thought to be valid and to adequately reflect his performance (Table 7-3).

Components of Evaluation

Wechsler Intelligence Scale for Children–Revised (WISC-R)
Peabody Picture Vocabulary Test (PPVT)
Category Test
Aphasia Screening Test
Illinois Test of Psycholinguistic Ability (ITPA)
Trail Making Test
Auditory Attention Span for Unrelated Words
Structured Photographic Language Test
Seashore Rhythm Test
Speech Sounds Perception Test

Dichotic Listening Test
Lateral Dominance Examination
Miles ABC Test of Ocular Dominance
Bender Visual Motor Gestalt Test
Key Math Diagnostic Test
Wide Range Achievement Test
Woodcock Reading Test
Tactile Form Recognition
Tactile Finger Recognition
Tactile Performance Test
Manual Finger Tapping

Interpretation of Results

David's performance on the WISC-R places him in the average range of intellectual functioning: Full Scale IQ = 95. David had a 41-point discrepancy, however, between his Verbal-Scale IQ (77) and Performance-Scale IQ (118), reflecting an overall strength in his ability to solve problems involving spatial relationships, visual perception, and motor coordination. Nonetheless, his usually poor performance on tasks involving verbal response suggests a weakness in the ability to process language.

Other language measures supported David's difficulty in verbal processing. His receptive language, for example, as measured by the PPVT, was delayed 2.5 years. His ability to formulate ideas from auditory input and to utilize correct morphological structures was delayed, as evidenced by the ITPA. A significant deficit in auditory reception, analysis, short-term memory and conceptualization were apparent, as evidenced on his performance on the Digit Span test and the Auditory Attention Span for Unrelated Words test. Furthermore, his expressive language abilities were two standard deviations below the mean for his age. His performance was significantly poor on the Structured Photographic Language Test.

A number of symptoms typical of the auditory-linguistic dyslexic were also noted on the Reitan-Indiana Aphasia Screening Test. David was able to name various objects and reproduce drawings, ruling out anomia and constructional apraxia. He had, however, an extremely difficult time reading, spelling, and computing arithmetic problems. David was initially asked to read single letters and he demonstrated some confusion. When presented a simple sentence, "See the black dog," David read the letters of each word individually. He demonstrated extreme difficulty associating the appropriate sound with the symbol, applying phonetic principles and blending to spell words common to his receptive and speaking vocabulary. Some of his misspellings included *screr* for *square*, *ecx* for *cross*, and *trago* for *triangle*. These characteristic misspellings are also commonly found in the auditory-linguistic dyslexic.

David, as previously noted, had consistent difficulty with most aspects of auditory perception, despite normal hearing. He had difficulty with tasks involving auditory discrimination, auditory-memory, acoustic sequencing, and auditory-verbal comprehension. With regard to visual-spatial perception, David was able to rec-

Table 7-3
Summary of David's Neuropsychological Test Results

WISC-R (Full Scale IQ = 95)

Verbal IQ = 77	Scaled Score	Performance IQ = 118	Scaled Score
Information	2	Picture Completion	14
Similarities	1	Picture Arrangement	15
Arithmetic	6	Block Design	14
Vocabulary	9	Object Assembly	13
Comprehension	13	Coding	7
Digit Span	6	Mazes	13

Peabody Picture Vocabulary Test

C.A. = 9−0
M.A. = 6−6

Halstead-Reitan Neuropsychological Test

Trial Making Test
Part A: 73 seconds; 0 errors (1st percentile)
Part B: 153 seconds; 0 errors (1st percentile)

Miles ABC Test of Ocular Dominance

Right eye: 0
Left eye: 10

Lateral Dominance Examination

Right hand/right preferred (12/12 times)

Dichotic Listening CVs

Right ear: 23 percent
Left ear: 47 percent
Score = percent correct

Tactile Form Recognition

Preferred hand: 11.7 seconds, 2 errors
Nonpreferred hand: 9.7 seconds, 0 errors

Tactile Finger Recognition

Right: 2 errors
Left: 0 errors

Tactile Performance Test

Dominant hand	1'50'' (96th percentile)
Nondominant hand	1'36'' (87th percentile)
Both hands	29'' (97th percentile)
Total time	3'58'' (98th percentile)
Memory	6
Localization	5

Manual Finger Tapping

Preferred hand: $\overline{X} = 19.8$
Nonpreferred hand: $\overline{X} = 25.0$

Speech Sound Perception Test

17 errors

Seashore Rhythm Test

Raw Score: 26
Ranked Score: 5

Category Test

26 errors (86th percentile)

Auditory Attention Span for Unrelated Words

C.A. = 9.0
M.A. = 6.3

ITPA (selected subtests)

Auitory Association
  C.A. = 9−0; M.A. = 8−3
Grammatic Closure
  C.A. = 9−0; M.A. = 5−8

Structured Photographic Language Test

2 standard deviations below the mean for a child 8−11 years of age

Bender Visual Motor Gestalt Test

C.A. = 9.0
P.A. = 8.5

Key Math Diagnostic Test

2.2 grade equivalent

Woodcock Reading Test

Word Identification: 1.2 grade equivalent
Passage Comprehension: 1.5 grade equivalent

Wide Range Achievement Test

Reading (Word Recognition): 2.1 grade equivalent
Spelling: 2.2 grade equivalent
Arithmetic: 2.5 grade equivalent

Medical Screening

Visual: Far Point: (R) 20/20, (L) 20/20; Near Point: normal; Titmus Fly: normal
Audio: Puretone: (R) normal, (L) normal; Tympanogram: normal
Height: 40th percentile
Weight: 60th percentile

Data from Obrzut, A. A neuropsychological case report of a child with auditory-linguistic dyslexia. *School Psychology Review,* 1981, *10,* 356−361. With permission.

ognize visual-spatial forms to reproduce drawings, to solve visual-spatial problems, and to utilize visual memory. These abilities are a relative strength for David and were evidenced on the Performance Scale subtests of the WISC-R, the Tactile Performance Test, and the Bender Gestalt. He did, however, experience some difficulty with visual sequencing, as demonstrated on the Coding subtest of the WISC-R and Trails A & B. On tests measuring tactile-form recognition, finger localization, and tactile sensitivity, David performed adequately. Directional confusion was noted in some of his writing, as he wrote from right to left. Motor speed and accuracy were adequate with the nonpreferred hand although they were somewhat depressed with the preferred (right) hand.

One of the most striking features of David's test performance involves the consistent discrepancies noted between his performance on tasks primarily associated with lateralized processing strategies. The processing of analytical, sequential, and linguistic stimuli, for example, seems to present more difficulty than the processing of visual-spatial, nonverbal, rhythmic, and gestalt stimuli. Another very distinctive comparison involves David's very poor performance on the Similarities subtest (scaled score = 1) and his exceptional performance on the Halstead Category Test (26 errors = 86th percentile). The Category Test taps a child's ability to incorporate inductive and deductive reasoning with spatial tasks. Furthermore, his strong performance on Block Design (scaled score = 14) is supportive of his conceptual superiority on nonverbal measures. His depressed performance on the Similarities subtest nonetheless reflects a weakness in his abilities to differentiate and integrate verbal concepts.

Other comparisons involving motor and tactile performances revealed discrepancies. David had a very depressed fingertapping rate with the preferred hand (right $\bar{X}$ = 19.8), for example, in comparison to his nonpreferred hand (left $\bar{X}$ = 25.0). David made two errors on the right hand on Tactile Finger Recognition and performed more slowly and inaccurately with his right hand on the Tactile Form Recognition (stereognosis), while his left-hand performance remained normal.

Discrepancies were also noted in his auditory processing of information. He did poorly on the Speech Sounds Perception Test, for example, yet scored within normal limits on the Seashore Rhythm Test, reflecting a marked difference in ability to analyze and process verbal linguistic information versus his ability to discriminate rhythmic nonverbal auditory patterns. On the dichotic listening test, he reported 23 percent correct stimuli from the right ear and 47 percent correct from the left ear. This is consistent with the poor linguistic processing abilities demonstrated on other verbal tests administered to David.

Formal achievement testing revealed a discrepancy between his estimated ability level and reading performance (see Table 7-3). David had a very limited sight vocabulary and was unable to apply phonetic principles to decode familiar or new words. He read better in context and guessed from the visual configuration or from a single familiar letter in a word. His comprehension skills were limited by poor reading ability. In brief, his deficits constitute an auditory-linguistic form of dyslexia in that he is lacking phonetic concepts, has inadequate word analysis, and is unable to sound out or blend letter or syllables in words.

David's performance on the Keymath Diagnostic Test revealed difficulty with processes dependent on automatic retrieval of facts (division, multiplication, mental computation) and with problems involving verbal concepts. His development of mathematic skills is, in general, better developed than are his reading abilities. His superior spatial abilities, despite weaknesses in language areas, most likely enable him to succeed in this area.

Summary and Recommendations

David is a ten-year-old boy experiencing a significant reading disability characteristic of children with auditory-linguistic dyslexia. Although he appears to have average intelligence, his auditory-linguistic skills appear to be severely depressed when compared with his visual-spatial abilities. The following recommendations should be considered in developing his individual educational plan.

David would benefit from a highly structured environment with clearly defined expectations and consistent positive reinforcement. Behavior modification techniques might be useful in shaping attention-concentration skills and enhancing motivation.

His learning environment should be void of unnecessary distraction. Particular attention should be given to acoustical variables, and whenever possible a quiet place, free of competing background noise, should be provided. Others should make sure David is attending before verbal directions are given. For example, it might be helpful to touch him, to establish eye contact, and then to verbalize directions. David should be seated near the source of sound (teacher, record player). If he appears distracted, ear plugs or headphones to muffle background noise might be useful during seatwork time. When David has difficulty with auditory presentations, visual or graphic representations should be incorporated.

A speech/language specialist should provide therapy to help increase David's receptive and expressive language skills, as well as to provide support in the auditory processing areas. Auditory memory and listening skills might be enhanced by teaching memory techniques such as rehearsal, association, visual imagery, recognition of critical elements, and chunking.

David would benefit from intense remedial-reading instruction from a learning-disabilities specialist in a self-contained setting. The Fernald methods (Visual, Auditory, Kinesthetic, and Tactile [VAKT]) may be useful in establishing a basic sight vocabulary. A sequenced linguistic approach to reading with frequent repetition and a controlled vocabulary should be used. The Schmerler Instruction sequence would involve this and might be useful because David may be able to utilize his conceptual ability to understand the structure of language despite his auditory deficits. Engleman's SRA corrective reading could be a useful complement to the Schmerler program as it is very well sequenced and is highly motivating.

Visual-Spatial Dyslexia

Reason for Referral

Bob, an 8-year, 10-month-old boy, was referred for a complete neuropsychological evaluation by the multidisciplinary team in his school. Since Bob has already been placed in a Title I Reading Program and has made no progress over the past year, a neuropsychological evaluation was deemed appropriate so that a more complete picture of his current functioning could be obtained. Specifically, Bob's teacher noted that he still had difficulty following oral directions; reversed many letters, words, and numbers; often seemed inattentive and overly sensitive; and had great difficulty in producing legible handwriting. Bob is presently repeating second grade, and his teacher wonders if he is capable of third-grade work.

Developmental/Medical History

Bob is the oldest of three children. Prenatal history was apparently normal, but labor was induced due to toxemia. At birth Bob weighed 7 lbs. 13 oz., and he experienced no difficulty in establishing a regular feeding schedule. Most developmental milestones relative to language were reached early. He repeated syllables (*mama, dada*) at six months and said his first word at ten months. Complete toilet training was established by his third birthday. Motor development was somewhat delayed when compared with his language acquisition. He did not walk until he was 15 months old and has never, according to his mother, been well-coordinated. At the present time, Bob is age-appropriate in appearance for both weight and height.

Significantly, a history of reading problems is noted on his paternal side of the family. Both Bob's father and an uncle were "slow" in learning to read and neither considers himself a proficient reader today. His mother, a housewife, experienced no difficulties in school and reads for entertainment on a regular basis. His father did finish high school with the help of his teachers and works with the Department of Transportation.

No major illnesses were reported. Bob does suffer some mild allergies, for which he takes weekly shots. He wears glasses and his vision is corrected to normal limits. Audiological screening revealed normal (puretone) hearing in both ears.

Behavioral Observations

Bob appeared for his evaluation wearing new clothes. He seemed quite proud of his clothes and said he had to be careful not to soil them at recess. He was quite concerned over his appearances and played with his vest zipper throughout the two evaluation sessions. Classroom observation suggested that Bob was disorganized in his use of time, had difficulty in planning his work, and resisted paper and pencil tasks. Similar behaviors were noted during the evaluation sessions. He seemed quite verbal and would rather carry on a conversation than complete a spelling or reading task. Orientation still seemed to be difficult for Bob as he frequently mixed left and right. Fine motor skills seemed delayed and weak; his pencil grasp was awkward (his thumb was wrapped over his index finger), as was his manipulation of test materials. Although Bob clearly preferred to verbally interact with the examiner, his level of motivation and cooperation suggest that the present evaluation results are valid and reliable indicators of his current level of functioning.

Components of Evaluation

Wechsler Intelligence Scale for Children-Revised (WISC-R)
Peabody Picture Vocabulary Test-Revised (PPVT-R)
Category Test
Aphasia Screening Test

Slosson Intelligence Test (SIT)
Boder Reading Spelling Pattern Test
Wepman Auditory Discrimination Test
Keystone Visual Survey Tests
Key Math Diagnostic Arithmetic Test
Morrison-McCall Spelling Scale
Wide Range Achievement Test (WRAT)
Woodcock Reading Mastery Tests
Dolch Service Word List
Informal Reading Inventory
Bender Visual-Motor Gestalt Test
Finger Tapping (Oscilliation) Test
Tactile Finger Recognition
Tandem Walking
Rapid Alternating Movements
Grip Strength
Dichotic Listening Test

Interpretation of Results

On the Wechsler Intelligence Scale for Children-Revised (WISC-R) Bob demonstrated overall performance in the below-average range of functioning, as he obtained a Full-Scale IQ of 79. A very significant difference exists, however, between his Verbal-Scale IQ of 94, which is in the average range, and his Performance Scale IQ of 68. This estimate of performance abilities falls in the borderline range of functioning. An analysis of Bob's subtest scores indicates strong verbal-comprehension skills in that he has vocabulary and comprehension skills well within the average range for a boy his age. Linguistic reasoning abilities also seem adequate as do his receptive language skills as measured by the Peabody Picture Vocabulary Test-Revised. Of concern is Bob's very poor performance in perceptual-organizational tasks. He experienced great difficulty in perceiving gestalt relationships and conceptualizing ambiguous visual stimuli. This relative deficit was also noted on the Category Test, in which visual-spatial reasoning skills are required.

Further evaluation of Bob's perceptual-motor abilities likewise revealed areas of relative concern. Constructional praxis was poor for a boy his chronological age, as he achieved a developmental age of five years, six months on the Bender. His drawings from the Aphasia Screening Test, as well as his written numbers (1–20), are presented in Figure 7-1. His difficulty in perceptual-motor abilities also carried over to his performance on purely motor tasks. His bilateral performance on the Finger Tapping Test, for example, was approximately two standard deviations below age-appropriate expectations. Fine and gross motor performance seemed similarly delayed, as he experienced considerable difficulty on rapid alternating movements, tandem walking, and visual-tracking tasks. Grip Strength was bilaterally weak, most noticeably on the left side, and Tactile Finger Recognition tasks revealed a left-sided deficit commensurate with other visual-spatial deficits. Perceptual asymmetries also seemed poorly developed, and his normal right-ear score of 53 percent is offset by

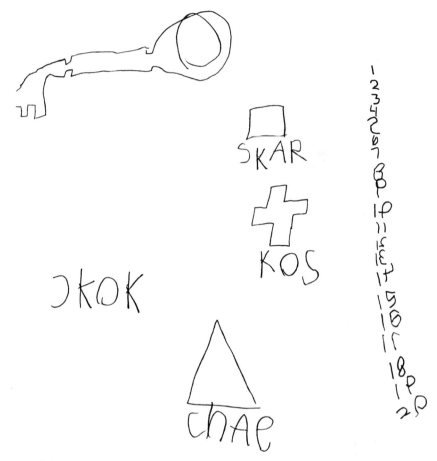

Fig. 7-1. Bob's drawings from the Aphasia Screening Test and his written numbers 1–20. On his written numbers note the increasing size and the reversed numbers.

an unusually low left-ear score (41 percent). This increase in the between-ear magnitude is not unusual among learning- and reading-disabled children who suffer visual-spatial processing deficits.

From an academic standpoint, Bob's achievement is as might be expected for a reading-disabled child demonstrating the characteristics of visual-spatial dyslexia. First, his overall reading performance, based on the Woodcock Reading Mastery Test, is equal to that of a normal child in the first grade, fourth month. Skills in word and letter recognition range from the low first grade level to the high first grade level. This discrepancy between his verbal skills and his actual reading achievement is especially significant when one considers he is now repeating a grade and is almost nine years old. Spelling errors were typical of a dyseidetic speller in that he demonstrated adequate phonetic skills but he failed to apply them correctly. For example, some of Bob's misspellings included *skar* for *square*, *mak* for *make*, *wel* for *will*, and *kut* for *cut*. Word-recognition performance similarily revealed a phonetic decoding strategy (Table 7-4)

Table 7-4
Summary of Bob's Neuropsychological Test Results

WISC-R (Full Scale IQ = 79)

Verbal IQ = 94	Scaled Score	Performance IQ = 68	Scaled Score
Information	8	Picture Completion	7
Similarities	8	Picture Arrangement	10
Arithmetic	7	Block Design	3
Vocabulary	10	Object Assembly	4
Comprehension	12	Coding	1
Digit Span	8		

Peabody Picture Vocabulary Test—Revised

Standard Score (IQ) = 97

Slossen Intelligence Test

Mental age = 7−4
IQ   = 83

Category Test

72nd percentile

Boder Reading Spelling Pattern Test

Classification: Dyseidetic

Aphasia Screening Test

Right-left orientation difficulty
Anomia
Dyslexia

Wepman Auditory Discrimination Test

No errors

Keystone Visual Survey Tests

Satisfactory

Key Math Diagnostic Arithmetic Test

Grade Score $\overline{X} = 2.5$
Poor Subtraction & Addition

(continued)

Table 7-4 (continued)

Morrison-McCall Spelling Scale

Score = 1.5

Wide Range Achievement Test

	Grade Level
Reading (Word Recognition)	1.3
Spelling	2.0
Arithmetic	2.1

Woodcock Reading Mastery Test

	Reading Level
Letter Identification	1.8
Word Identification	1.7
Word Attack	1.2
Word Comprehension	1.6
Passage Comprehension	1.2
Total Reading	1.4

Bender Visual Motor Gestalt Test

DA = 5−6
Errors = 10

Finger Tapping Test

Preferred hand (right) $\overline{X} = 28.00$
Non-preferred hand $\overline{X} = 26.00$

Tactile Finger Recognition

Right: 1 error
Left: 3 errors

Grip Strength

Right: 11.25 kg.
Left: 9.30 kg.

Dichotic Listening CVs

Right ear: 53 percent
Left ear: 41 percent

Summary and Recommendations

Overall, Bob would seem to possess adequate sequential verbal comprehension skills, as demonstrated on the Verbal Scale subtests of the WISC-R, on the PPVT-R, and by his attempted application of linguistic-phonetic analysis of known and unknown words. His borderline visual-spatial skills, however, seem to be providing considerable interference in acquiring more developed reading abilities. Neuropsychological deficit in this latter area is consistent with a diagnosis of visual-spatial dyslexia. Recommendations include the following.

Systematic instruction following the scope and sequence of a basal reading series should be eliminated. Individualized reading using a variety of materials, which may include basal reader stories, should be substituted. One-to-one or a small group setting would be optimal for instruction.

Bob's word-recognition skills can be enhanced significantly by using a word families approach. Due to Bob's relative strength in knowledge of vowel and consonant sounds, it is believed that this method may be successful when a few sight words with similar endings (i.e., ball, fall, call) have been learned to mastery. By substituting the initial consonant, he may be able to increase his sight vocabulary substantially. More advanced levels of reading proficiency may be obtained by using the Orton-Gillingham, or the Distar Programs, which rely on his more developed phonics skills.

Bob's classroom environment should be as free from distractions as is possible. A well-structured situation in which he clearly knows what is expected of him will greatly facilitate his ability to produce as expected. A desk organizer and timer may help him make better use of his school supplies and time. It is important to realize that Bob's deficits in the visual-spatial aspects of reading will continue to pose problems. A shift in instructional emphasis to a phonics approach, however, should contribute to greater levels of success than are presently evident.

Chapter 8

Remedial Approaches to Dyslexia

Within the last 150 years, the need to be a fluent reader has become crucial in terms of personal satisfaction and employment. Since the ability to read is so basic to everyday functioning, the major focus of our elementary schools is on the development of basic reading ability.

Those children who cannot learn to read present a special problem since, for some, the disability seems overwhelming and intractable. It can be said with some assurance that for the dyslexic child or for the reading disabled child who is severely affected, millions of dollars have been invested in terms of materials for remediation, special programs, and professional personnel to work with these children. In large part, the success of these efforts has been disappointing to say the least.

Reasons exist for these disappointing results, and it is the purpose of this chapter to briefly summarize programs that have been applied to the dyslexic child, to evaluate what the research says as to their effectiveness, to examine alternative perspectives based on our current knowledge of dyslexia, and to propose guidelines for future research in the remediation of the dyslexic child.

As new remedial approaches are offered (Valett, 1980), it is important to critically evaluate them from a theoretical perspective, since in many cases they are not new at all but are merely a rehash of old ideas long since proved worthless. Furthermore, those who argue that dyslexia is the result of cerebellar dysfunction and that it can be controlled through the use of anti–motion-sickness medication have failed to validate their claims to the scientific community (Levinson, 1980). A need exists, however, to continue to direct efforts into remedial programs, especially since subtypes of dyslexics have now been clearly identified. Past frustrations should not preclude continued effort but rather should encourage new and more refined research efforts. With these thoughts in mind, it is appropriate to consider the remediation approaches that are often used with dyslexic children.

HISTORICAL APPROACHES TO REMEDIATION

The early approaches to remediation of dyslexic children fall into one of two categories: those that focus on determining the "best method" of teaching all dyslexic readers, and those that stress the development of deficit or prerequisite skills. The intent of the first approach is obvious and includes the strategies of Orton-Gillingham (J. Orton, 1966) and Fernald (1943), to name a few. The basic theoretical contention underlying the second group is that inherent dysfunctions must be remediated before any academic training is given. Treatment within these approaches thus focuses on the need to provide opportunities to learn certain prerequisite or readiness skills that have not developed. Advocates of these approaches (Doman-Delacato, [Delacato, 1959]; Frostig, 1970; Kephart, 1971; Kirk & Kirk, 1971) contend that the dyslexic child lacks these prerequisite skills but does not lack the capacity to learn to read once these skills are developed.

The Orton-Gillingham Approach

One of the earliest programs of remediation for dyslexic children was developed by Gillingham (Gillingham & Stillman, 1970) based on the theoretical work of the neurologist J. Orton (S. Orton, 1937). On completion of a comprehensive clinical assessment that included a family and educational history and evaluation of hearing, vision, intelligence, achievement, and neurological status, J. Orton (1966) emphasized two basic principles for remediation. The first was simultaneous association of visual, auditory, and kinesthetic language stimuli. The second involved the fusing of small units into more complex wholes.

This system of remediation is based on the premise that children who do not develop the ability to read by group methods do so because group approaches rely too heavily on visual-receptive abilities. As a result, Gillingham's training program stresses auditory discrimination abilities with supplementary emphasis on kinesthetic and tactile modalities.

The child begins by learning basic sound production. Once this is mastered, phonograms are introduced (one letter or group of letters that represent a phonetic sound) on flash cards. Consonant and vowel sounds are printed on different color cards. After mastery of several phonograms, blending is begun with careful attention being given to this phase since many children have problems with auditory synthesis and sequencing. Several phonogram cards are placed side by side. Individual sounds are produced in succession and with increasing speed until a fluid rate is achieved. Once the blending procedure is underway, word analysis begins. Initially, this process is achieved on an auditory level with the teacher sounding the words and the child identifying the letters heard. In the next phase, the teacher says the word and the child repeats it, names the letters, and writes the letters while naming them. The child always works with phonetically pure words in this phase. When the child has learned to read and write three-letter words, they are then combined by the child into sentences and stories.

A major stipulation in the early part of this program is that the child is given no other printed material. If the child is able to be mainstreamed for part of his academic school day, all subject material must be presented audibly. In addition, books that the child uses must be carefully screened to ensure that all of the words included in the text are phonetic and are suitable for blending.

Research Findings with the Orton-Gillingham Approach

Childs (1965) reported on the academic progress made by several students who were instructed by this approach. In one case study, the author discussed the improvement of 14-year-old dyslexic male twins who were placed in different schools. One twin was in a public school classroom and showed a reading level gain of from 4.1 to 4.5 over a six-month period, while the other twin demonstrated a gain from 3.3 to 4.3 in his reading level over the same time period.*

Similarly, Kline and Kline (1975) reported on a follow-up study of 216 dyslexic children who were instructed with the Orton-Gillingham method. The authors stated that 96 percent of the cases demonstrated impressive gains in a relatively short period of time, while 49 percent of those not instructed in this method failed to show any significant progress. The authors concluded by saying that most children require two or more years of therapy for good results and recommend that the children continue to receive support, consultation, and on-going remediation in order to ensure success.

---

*The reader should be aware that several professional organizations (e.g., National Council on Measurement in Education, The International Reading Association) have argued against the use of grade-equivalent scores to demonstrate academic gains due to instruction. The reason for this is due to the manner in which grade-equivalent scores are derived. They do not, in reality, reflect a child's performance relative to grade level. Research that reports grade-equivalent–gain scores provides misleading data and should be questioned from a methodological standpoint.

Critics of this approach (Dechant, 1970; Gates, 1947) have expressed strong concern about the lack of meaningful material and activities incorporated into the program, as well as concern about the lack of emphasis given to comprehension, about the rigidity of the teaching procedures, and about the tendency to develop a labored reading style. In addition to these criticisms, it is the feeling of the authors as well as others (Boder, 1971; Johnson, 1978) that the strong emphasis placed on the auditory discrimination and sequencing abilities of the learner precludes the use of this method with subgroups of dyslexic children experiencing deficits in these abilities (e.g., Boder's [1973a] dysphonetic subgroup or Pirozzolo's [1981] auditory-linguistic subtype). While proponents of the Orton-Gillingham method could thus lead one to believe that this approach to reading remediation should be used with all dyslexic children, caution should be used when considering the use of this approach with children who exhibit deficits in auditory discrimination and sequencing abilities.

The Fernald Approach: Visual, Auditory, Kinesthetic, and Tactile (VAKT)

A second method of instruction for dyslexic readers was developed by Fernald (1943), who directed a clinic school at the University of California, Los Angeles, in the 1920s. Fernald was greatly concerned with the emotional components of reading failure and felt that all children who fail in school will always have an emotional problem. In order to avoid the development of a negative attitude toward learning and a poor self-concept, Fernald advocated a reconditioning method that directed the child's attention away from experiences that provoked unpleasant emotional reactions. To maintain a positive learning climate, the teacher must see to it that the following situations are avoided: emotionally laden situations, the use of methods that resulted in previous failure, embarrassing situations, and references to the child's specific problems.

Fernald developed the instructional aspect of her approach to remediation based on observation and work with Greek children who learned to read by finger-writing on a sand board. Many educators as a result refer to Fernald's method as a kinesthetic approach when, in fact, it is actually multisensory, involving four modalities simultaneously (i.e. VAKT).

The child begins remediation by story writing, initially about anything that interests the child and later, about content learned in school subjects. The child is instructed to ask for any unknown word. It is written for the child, learned by the child, and used immediately in the child's story. The completed story is then typed so that the child may read it while it is fresh in the mind.

The total process by which remediation takes place can be broken down into four stages. In stage I, when a child requests a word, the multisensory approach is employed to facilitate learning. First, the word is written for the child with black crayon on firm paper. Then the child traces over the word with a finger and says the word out loud while tracing it. The child repeats this process until able to write the word twice without looking at the sample. In order to increase the tactile-kinesthetic input, many teachers employ a clay tray made with permaplast clay and a lunchroom tray. The word is written in the clay with a stick and the child traces the indented letters with a finger. After the lesson, the words are filed alphabetically in the child's word box.

After a period of time (no fixed limit), the tactile component is discontinued and stage II is begun. In this phase, the child learns a new word by following the look-say-write steps of stage I (VAK). Stage III does away with the kinesthetic component, requiring the child to learn new words by looking at the samples and saying them out loud. Finally, stage IV is reached when the child is able to recognize new words by their similarity to words, or to parts of words, that have been already learned.

In addition to those already mentioned, Fernald holds several other cardinal principles: the child is never read to; the child never sounds out words, unless this is done while scanning a passage for new words prior to reading; and, material must be appropriate to the child's age and level of intelligence.

Research Findings with the Fernald Approach

The effectiveness of the Fernald approach relative to traditional group methods was evaluated by Talmadge, Davids, and Laufer (1963). The authors exposed groups of dyslexic children with and without cortical dysfunction to the respective approaches over a three-month period. Results indicated that with the Fernald method, the brain-damaged dyslexic group gained 1.04 years on a standard reading test, while the non-brain-damaged group demonstrated a gain of 0.62 years. Exposure to traditional methods resulted in gains of 0.45 years for both brain-damaged and non-brain-damaged dyslexic reading groups.

Roberts and Coleman (1958) attempted to validate several of Fernald's assumptions (1943) that underlie the use of her method with disabled readers. These assumptions are as follows: children with reading failure are deficient in visual perception; these children are less efficient than normal readers in learning new material when only visual cues are used; and children with reading failure are more efficient in learning new material when kinesthetic cues are added to the visual cues.

In order to test these hypotheses, Roberts and Coleman (1958) compared a group of 27 male retarded readers (with average reading levels of 2.9 years below expectancy) matched for age, sex, IQ, and socioeconomic status (SES) with a group of 29 normal readers. The groups were required to learn nonsense syllables written in black crayon under two conditions: visual presentation alone, and visual and tactile-kinesthetic presentation. No auditory cues were given with either presentation. Results indicated that, as a group, the retarded readers were less efficient than normal readers were when learning new material by means of visual cues only. The retarded readers, in addition, were better able to learn new material if tactile-kinesthetic components were added, while the addition of these same cues did not aid normal readers. The authors concluded by stating that their results support the use of tactile-kinesthetic cues in remedial programs for children experiencing deficits in visual perception.

Ofman and Shaevitz (1963), after reviewing the Roberts and Coleman study (1958), felt that the essential variable of tactile-kinesthetic cueing was not adequately isolated, and pertinent attention cues were not adequately controlled. The authors, as a result, divided 30 male students from the Fernald Clinic into three groups of ten subjects, each matched for age, IQ, reading level, and length of time at the clinic. The groups were required to learn nonsense syllables under one of three treatment conditions: the child traced the syllable presented by visually following a moving point of light as it outlined the syllable; the child placed a finger on a slide of the syllable, was cautioned to press hard and trace the syllable with the finger, pronouncing the syllable as done by the experimenter; and, the child would simply read the syllable after the experimenter had pronounced it. Results indicated that both the eye-tracing and finger-tracing methods were more effective than simple reading, but the finger tracing was not more effective than eye tracing in the acquisition of new material. They concluded by speculating that the crucial variable provided by the finger-tracing method was not the tactile-kinesthetic input but rather that the method of finger tracing functions as an attention-holding device that compels the child to attend to the task at hand.

In summary, advocates of the Fernald approach (Roberts & Coleman, 1958; Talmadge et al., 1963) stress three major points in support of this method: a less-controlled presentation of vocabulary (i.e., student directed), the strong emphasis on success and student motivation, and that the added tactile-kinesthetic input provided by this method helps the child with visual-perceptual and visual-sequencing deficits.

Due to the fact that the studies cited here employed heterogeneous populations of dyslexic readers, it is difficult to conclusively state exactly for which subtype of dyslexic readers this method would be most appropriate. While proponents of this method advocate its use with children having visual-perceptual and visual-sequencing deficits (i.e., Boder's [1973a] dyseidetic subgroup or Pirozzolo's [1981] visual-spatial subtype), it is the author's opinion that this method could be extremely beneficial to the subgroup of dyslexic readers who have mixed auditory and visual deficits as well (i.e., Boder's [1973a] alexic subgroup).

The work of Ofman and Shaevitz (1963), in addition, indicate that this method would be extremely helpful to reading-disabled children who are suffering from an attention-deficit disorder characterized by distractibility, short attention span, and hyperactivity. Support for this contention comes from Harris (1970) who feels that the tactile-kinesthetic elements may be of minor importance. Harris believes that the tracing and writing helps the child remember the word because he must attend to all of the auditory and visual features.

A final caution must also be voiced if one is considering this approach with a "hyperactive" reading-disabled child. Assuming that hyperactivity may result from understimulation or overstimulation of the reticular activating system (Luria's [1980] arousal unit), it is highly possible that the multisensory input employed by this method will act in such a way as to overload the already over-aroused child, thus increasing his distractibility and hyperactivity. Support for this caution can, in fact, be found in Johnson and Myklebust's article (1967), which reports that some children do appear to become overloaded by multisensory stimulation. An evaluation of the nature of the child's attentional difficulties thus is extremely important prior to the implementation of any remedial system, especially when one considers the interaction between attentional difficulties and subtypes of dyslexia.

The Doman-Delacato Neurological Organization Approach

According to the Doman-Delacato theory (Delacato, 1959, 1963, 1966), neurological development must proceed in a sequential fashion if a child is to attain normal psychomotor and linguistic skills. If, for any reason, the neurological development of a child does not proceed through the proper sequence of stages, Delacato believed that the child will demonstrate difficulties in mobility, in speech, and in the "essence of the human nervous system, reading" (Delacato, 1966, p. 44). Furthermore, Delacato proposed that ontogenetic neural development recapitulates the phylogenetic development of the human nervous system and develops in an upward fashion from the spinal cord to the medulla, to the pons, to the midbrain, and, finally, to the cortex.

More specifically, Doman and Delacato maintain that there are six major functional attainments of humans: motor skills, speech, writing, reading, understanding, and stereognosis (Reynolds, 1981). For these abilities to develop adequately, the child must progress, in an uninterrupted manner, to the point at which normal neurological organization is attained. Delacato (1959) postulated that, in man, the attainment of lateralized cerebral dominance was the pinnacle of neurological development. It is this development that gives man the capacity for communication and separates him from lower animals.

Doman and Delacato also proposed a diagnostic procedure that begins with an assessment of cerebral dominance and proceeds downward to the pons (Glass & Robbins, 1967), assessing neurological organization. At the highest level, neurological organization is diagnosed by observing whether the child has established a clear pattern of dominance on one side of the body in activities involving the feet, hands, and eyes. Mixed laterality (e.g., left-footed, right-handed, and left-eyed) is evidence of poor neurological organization. At the cortical level, neurological organization is evaluated by observing whether the child walks with good balance, smoothly and rhythmically, and in a cross-pattern manner (i.e., extending the right arm with the left leg). The smoothness of eye movements while visually tracking an object is also assessed. Examination at the level of the midbrain involves smooth and rhythmic cross-pattern creeping and smooth eye-movement while visually tracing an object held by the child. Finally, diagnosis at the level of the pons involves observing the child at sleep. At this level, a right-side dominance is related to the tendency to sleep on one's abdomen with the head turned to the left and with flexion in the left arm and leg. The left-dominant child sleeps in the exact opposite position.

Children who experience reading or other learning problems are assessed in this downward fashion until the lowest level of incomplete development is determined. Treatment of the child's learning problem centers around teaching the child to properly perform those activities that were failed during the assessment. This is accomplished within a developmental progression from lower-order to higher-order activities, with each particular level of neurological organization requiring specific remedial activities geared toward the development of specific objectives. In the event that the child is unable to perform the desired tasks on his own, passive manipulation of his body by the therapist or by a trained parent is done. The ultimate goal of treatment is thus to provide the child with the opportunity for the uninterrupted development of complete neurological organization, and to promote the attainment of lateralized cerebral dominance.

Research Findings with the Doman-Delacato Approach

The Doman–Delacato approach to remediation of reading and learning problems has received much criticism both theoretically and experimentally. Theoretically, evidence for cerebral dominance in other primates (Dewson, 1977; Gazzaniga, 1971; Warren & Nonneman, 1976) challenges Delacato's (1966) assertion that cerebral dominance sets man apart from lower animals. In addition, Doman and Delacato's notion that the highest level of neurological organization exists only when an individual has attained consistency of hand, eye, and foot preference is contradicted by Woo and Pearson (1972), who found no correlation between eye and hand preference in 7000 male subjects, and by numerous studies that indicate no clear relationship between handedness and cerebral dominance for language functions (Benton, 1955; Hardyck & Petrinovitch, 1977; Hardyck, Petrinovitch, &

Goldman, 1976; Milner, Branch, & Rasmussen, 1964; Reynolds, Hartlage, & Haak, 1980).

Research investigating the effectiveness of the Doman-Delacato method with dyslexic children has, at best, been highly critical. While Delacato (1959, 1963, 1966) cites 15 studies in support of the Doman-Delacato system of remediation for poor readers, Glass and Robbins (1967) reevaluated the methodology of these studies and raised serious doubts about their validity. Glass and Robbins found that 5 of the studies failed to control for regression effects, 14 of the studies neglected to randomly assign subjects to treatment groups, and all but 1 study failed to control for time and location of treatment, as well as for the teacher administering the treatment. Glass and Robbins (1967) concluded by stating that without exception, the empirical studies cited by Delacato as a "scientific appraisal" (p. 5) of his theory of neurological organization are shown to be of dubious value.

In another study, Robbins (1966) evaluated the effectiveness of the Doman-Delacato method in a group of normal second graders and a nonspecific treatment group matched for age, race, religion, SES, IQ, and laterality. On completion of pretesting with standardized measures of IQ, achievement, laterality, and creeping, the experimental group underwent a three-month program of cross-pattern creeping and walking consistent with the Doman-Delacato methods in addition to their regular curriculum. Subjects in the nonspecific group were subjected to three months of nonspecific activities unrelated to reading achievement in addition to their regular curriculum. Results failed to find significant gains in reading ability for the Doman-Delacato group as compared with the control and nonspecific treatment groups.

Finally, O'Donnell and Eisenson (1969) evaluated the effects of the Doman-Delacato program on the reading achievement and visual-motor integration of a group of disabled readers having crossed or uncertain lateral expression. Children were selected from the second through fourth grades, based on meeting the following criteria: Peabody Picture Vocabulary IQ $\geq$ 90; a total score on the Gray Oral Reading Test below 1.0, 2.7, and 3.4 for second, third, and fourth graders, respectively; uncertain lateral expression as measured by the Harris Test of Lateral Dominance; and visual acuity of 20/50 or better for both eyes. The children were then randomly placed in either one of two treatment groups or a control group. The treatment groups differed in time spent each day with the Doman-Delacato method (30 minutes versus 15 minutes). Pretest and posttest analysis after 20 weeks revealed no significant gains in reading (as measured by the Gray Oral Reading Test) or in visual-motor integration (as measured by the Developmental Test of Visual-Motor Integration) for either treatment group as compared with that of the controls.

In conclusion, the results of the research studies presented here as well as the articles cited in contradiction to the Doman-Delacato theory seriously question the validity of this treatment approach in the remediation of reading disabilities or of any other learning disability.

The Illinois Test of Psycholinguistic Ability (ITPA) Psycholinguistic Approach

Psycholinguistics deals with the systematic study of the psychological functions and interactions involved in communication (Hammill & Larsen, 1974). While many models of psycholinguistic functioning exist, the model proposed by Osgood (1957) has had the greatest impact on the development of remedial programs for special-education children.

Simply stated, Osgood's model encompasses two dimensions of language: language processes and levels of organization. The process dimension is comprised of decoding (i.e., receiving and perceiving of stimuli), association (i.e., the ability to infer relationships from what is seen or heard), and encoding (i.e., the expression of thought). These processes are mediated through three levels of neurological organization. The most basic level, that of projection, relates receptor and muscle events to the brain. The second level, integration, allows for the sequencing and integration of information, both incoming and outgoing. Finally, the highest level of organization, the representational, is involved with the more sophisticated mediation processes necessary for meaningful symbolization (Hammill & Larsen, 1974).

According to Hammill and Larsen (1974):

> Psycholinguistic training is based upon the assumption that discrete elements of language behavior are identifiable and measurable, that they provide the underpinning for learning, and that if defective they can be remediated. When using this approach, an additional assumption is made that the cause of the child's learning failure is within himself and that strengthening weak areas will result in improved classroom learning. (pp. 5–6)

Given these underlying assumptions, a number of psycholinguistically oriented remedial programs have been developed (Bush & Giles, 1969; Kirk & Kirk, 1971; Minskoff, Wiseman, & Minskoff, 1972) that are based on the theoretical principles of Osgood (1957) and of the ITPA, a diagnostic instrument designed by Kirk, McCarthy, and Kirk (1968) to delineate specific psycholinguistic abilities and disabilities for subsequent remediation. The test is composed of 12 subtests based on the model of communication described by Osgood (1957). Each subtest is thought to measure a specific communication function with six subtests at the representational level and with six at the automatic level. The composite of all the subtests is believed to represent all of the basic communication skills required for success in the major academic areas.

The ITPA model of remediation developed by Kirk and Kirk (1971) assumes that a poor performance on a given subtest of the ITPA requires direct remediation at the level of that particular subtest. This remedial approach has been chosen for review in the following section for two reasons. First, this approach has been widely used in the public schools as a remedial program for reading-disabled children for many years; and, second, the research done with this model is more extensive than with the others previously mentioned.

Research Findings with the ITPA
Psycholinguistic Approach

Hammill and Larsen (1974) comprehensively reviewed 38 studies that evaluated the effectiveness of training children in psycholinguistic skills that employed the ITPA or portions of it as the criterion for improvement. In order to facilitate this task, the authors grouped the studies by type of subject, type of teaching approach, and type of activities used by the teacher. Fifteen studies evaluated psycholinguistic training with mentally retarded children. Results indicated that there was not a single ITPA subtest for which a majority of the investigators reported that training was beneficial. Eighteen studies analyzed the efficacy of psycholinguistic training with disadvantaged children. Although some positive results were noted in the areas of verbal and auditory association as well as in the area of verbal expression, the majority of ITPA subtests failed to indicate a positive response to treatment. The effects of age on remediation of psycholinguistic skills was assessed by 15 studies at the preschool level and by 19 studies at the elementary level. Results indicated that, at both age levels, positive findings were limited to the representational subtests. Eight studies employed a prescriptive approach to remediation (i.e., an individualized program was designed for each child) based on areas of poor performance on the ITPA. This approach was found to be successful in stimulating visual association and expressive language abilities. The non-individualized approach to remediation (i.e., all the children were exposed to a set program) was evaluated in 30 studies and found to be minimally effective in teaching auditory association and verbal expression. Two types of curricula were employed: a selected activities approach was assessed in 13 studies and the Peabody Language Development Kit approach was assessed in 16 studies. The results of these studies indicated that the selective activities approach was successful in stimulating manual expression, while the Peabody Language Development Kit was successful in stimulating verbal expression. Based on these dismal results, Hammill and Larsen (1974) concluded that the effectiveness of psycholinguistic training has not been conclusively demonstrated, and therefore the rapid expansion of psycholinguistic training programs seems unwarranted.

The conclusions of Hammill and Larsen (1974) did not go unchallenged. Minskoff (1975) criticized Hammill and Larsen for lumping together many diverse studies without considering specific variables such as type of subjects, the nature of the treatment, and methodological flaws. Specifically, Minskoff argued that all of the studies investigated by Hammill and Larsen (1974) were done with mentally retarded, disadvantaged, or normal children, while none included reading- or learning-disabled children, for which this remedial approach was originally intended. Minskoff noted, in addition, that a majority of the studies contained methodological errors and assessed treatments that varied widely on such key factors as content, length of time, teacher competence, and group versus individual instruction. While accepting the fact that the research to date was not supportive of psycholinguistic training, Minskoff maintained that the efficacy of this approach still remained unresolved. As a result, she called for better controlled research in this area and outlined a series of guidelines for future research designed to explore the question of which remedial methods work best for what types of psycholinguistic disabilities and under what conditions.

Lund, Foster, and McCall-Perez (1978) reevaluated 24 of the original 38 studies cited by Hammill and Larsen (1974) and challenged Hammill and Larsen's conclusions. These authors noted that six of the originally cited studies showed positive gains in at least six of the ITPA subtests. In addition, Lund et al. (1978) pointed out that these six studies were among the most rigorous, employing long and structured treatment programs. The authors also claimed that Hammill and Larsen (1974) inaccurately reported the results of four studies, reached conclusions from two studies with insufficient data, and anticipated gains on all ITPA subtests when several studies intended to selectively remediate one or two of the 12 subtests.

In response to their critics, Hammill and Larsen (1978) stated that with the exception of one study that reported a 9-month and an 18-month posttest of treatment effectiveness (Hammill and Larsen only analyzed the 9-month results), they did not report or interpret data inaccurately. Hammill and Larsen countered by saying that Lund et al. (1978) tried to claim positive results when the data was clearly negative. Finally, Hammill and Larsen cited a study that was done after their original article (Sowell, 1975), that attempted to follow Minskoff's (1975) 15 guidelines for research in this area, and that used the Minskoff et al. (1972) treatment program. The results indicated that there were no significant differences between treatment and control groups in terms of psycholinguistic functioning. Hammill and Larsen, as a result, reiterated their original position that the effectiveness of psycholinguistic training is nonvalidated.

While there is a scarcity of research regarding the transfer of psycholinguistic training to reading ability, Newcomber and Hammill (1976) have reported that ITPA subtests fail to adequately correlate with achievement scores in reading, spelling, and arithmetic. Second, these authors found that none of the ITPA subtests can accurately discriminate between groups of children who were previously known to demonstrate different levels of reading ability.

In conclusion, the research data cited in this brief review appears to support Hammill and Larsen's (1974) conclusion that psycholinguistic training is nonvalidated. It is the opinion of the authors as a result that, like the Doman-Delacato method, psycholinguistic approaches to the remediation of dyslexia are unwarranted.

PERCEPTUAL TRAINING APPROACHES

Perceptual training programs have been widely employed in the public schools over the past two decades. Many special educators have strongly advocated their use in the development of visual-motor and readiness skills as well as in the development of reading ability. Due to the fact that the literature in this area contains a variety of definitions for the term, perception, it would be fruitful to explore the question of what exactly does the term, perception, or more specifically, visual perception, imply, prior to reviewing the literature in this area.

Hammill (1972), while reviewing the question of the trainability of the visual-motor process, located 33 definitions of perception in the literature. Finally, he settled on the following definition, which he summarized as follows:

> Visual perceptual processes are those brain operations which involve interpreting and organizing the physical elements of the visual stimulus rather than the symbolic aspects of the stimulus and are usually referred to a visual discrimination. (pp. 553–554)

Visual perception is thus differentiated from sensation (the reaction of the visual receptor cells) and cognition (the symbolic and abstract properties of the stimulus). It is this definition of perception that will be employed in the following review.

The Kephart Perceptual Training Approach

Kephart (1971), like Frostig (Frostig & Horne, 1964, to be discussed shortly), and the other perceptual-motor theorists, based his perceptual training program on two basic assumptions: that visual-motor abilities are essential to cognitive development and academic success and that these visual-motor processes are trainable.

Kephart (1971) contended that the higher forms of human behavior (e.g., reading) are dependent on lower forms. Concept formation is thus felt to be dependent on the manipulation of perceptual data that rests on the development of basic motor patterns. Subsequently, inadequate development of perceptual-motor skills prevents the child from effectively participating in educational programs requiring higher-order abstractions (e.g., reading).

According to Kephart's (1971) theory of neurological development, posture is the first of the basic motor patterns to emerge, followed by laterality (i.e., the initial awareness of the two sides of the body and their difference) and directionality (i.e., the projection of laterality into external space). These three operate to produce a generalized impression about one's body, called body image. Body image becomes the point of reference to which all spatial relations outside the body are compared.

As the child matures, he begins to investigate the world perceptually as well as motorically. Tactile, kinesthetic, visual, and auditory information received from the developing perceptual system are compared with existing motor information. The result is a synthesis of data, which Kephart calls the perceptual-motor match. The consistency of this match is directly related to the development of form perception, spatial discrimination, and ocular control, which are Kephart's three crucial perceptual skills. If the child fails to develop these skills, he will be unable to make proper perceptual-motor matches of his environment and, as a result, he will develop faulty intersensory integration abilities and concept formations.

In order to assess exactly where the breakdown is located within this developmental sequence, Kephart (1971) recommends the use of the Purdue Perceptual Survey Rating Scale (1966) for evaluating the child's motor and perceptual-motor abilities. For additional information about the child, Kephart recommends the use of the Wepman Auditory Discrimination Test (1958), the Frostig Developmental Test of Visual Perception (1964), and the Illinois Test of Psycholinguistic Ability (1968).

Finally, Kephart does not have a specialized training program that can be directly purchased. Instead, Kephart recommends a collection of activities for training each of the following skill areas: perceptual-motor training, perceptual-motor match, ocular control, chalkboard training, and form perception (Ebersole, Kephart, & Ebersole, 1968; Kephart, 1971).

Research Findings with the Kephart Perceptual Training Approach

A review of 42 studies in which the Kephart training techniques were utilized has been done by Goodman and Hammill (1973). Many of the studies unfortunately suffered from methodological problems such as small test groups, short training periods, and an absence of control groups. As a result, these authors concluded that the findings of these studies could not be accepted with confidence.

In order to make some statement about effectiveness, Hammill, Goodman, and Wiederholt (1974) analyzed the best of the previously reviewed studies according to the following minimal criteria: 20 or more experimental subjects, at least 12 weeks or 60 sessions of training, and utilization of an experimental control-group design. Sixteen of the original 42 studies were found to meet these minimal criteria and received further analysis.

Of the 16 studies, 11 dealt directly with the effects of visual-motor training on visual-motor performance. The results for the most part were unimpressive. Experimental groups performed better than control groups in only 4 studies, with the results of 1 of these 4 highly suspect due to significant differences in the teacher-pupil ratio (in favor of the experimental group).

Of the 16 studies, 8 examined the effects of visual-motor training on school readiness. Nine measures of readiness were employed. Results indicated that only 3 of the 8 studies reported significantly better readiness scores in favor of the perceptual training group. The authors noted, however, that 2 of these "positive" studies reported improvement in readiness skills with no concomitant improvement in visual-motor skills. This is a rather puzzling finding that points to the possibility of confounding treatment variables.

Finally, the effects of visual-motor training on intelligence, reading achievement, and language functioning were investigated in 10 of the 16 studies, which included 15 different posttest analyses. Results indicated that the experimental groups performed significantly better on only 6 of these 15 analyses.

Due to the fact that Hammill and his co-workers could only find one study that attempted to assess the efficacy of the Kephart training program with physically handicapped children (Hendry, 1970), a study was undertaken to accomplish this task (Goodman & Hammill, 1973). A test group of 44 preschool children with either neuromuscular disorders or skeletal deformities were randomly placed into a training or control group following pretesting. Training was done three times a week, for a period of five months, in small group format. Control children participated in their regular preschool program. Results indicated that the experimental subjects did not perform significantly better than the control subjects on any of the six standardized test instruments designed to assess different aspects of visual-motor functioning.

In conclusion, the research evidence strongly questions the usefulness of the Kephart perceptual training approach as a standard remedial reading technique in the schools. Not only has this approach been found ineffective in the remediation of reading disabilities and in the enhancement of readiness skills, it has not even been demonstrated effective in the development of the perceptual-motor performance, for which it was originally intended.

The Frostig-Horne Perceptual Training Approach

Marianne Frostig (Frostig, 1970; Frostig & Horne, 1964) was another perceptual-motor theorist who maintained that adequate perceptual functioning in young children is an important foundation on which later school success is dependent. More specifically, Frostig and Horne (1964) stated that the presence of perceptual problems increases the probability that a child will experience some degree of emotional disturbance and eventual academic failure. They believe that the debilitating influence of visual problems will be most apparent in the learning-to-read process.

Frostig contends, like Kephart, that visual perception is comprised of definable subskills that are both measurable and trainable. Together, these subskills (eye-hand coordination, figure-ground, form constancy, position in space, and spatial relations) form the underlying structure of both the Developmental Test of Visual Perception (Frostig, Maslow, Lefever, & Wittlesey, 1964) and the Developmental Program in Visual Perception (Frostig & Horne, 1964).

The Frostig-Horne training program, which was originally designed for kindergarten and first-graders, is comprised of 359 worksheets divided into sets that are analogous to the subskills listed above. Within each set, the worksheets are presented in an easy-to-difficult progression. It is recommended that training in sensory and language functions be integrated into the program and that the worksheets not be used in isolation. Frostig (1970) has additionally provided a set of exercises for children who might require more basic training in body image, gross and fine motor coordination, and ocular movement control.

Research Findings with the Frostig-Horne Perceptual Training Approach

The most extensive review of the Frostig-Horne approach has been done by Hammill, Goodman, and Wiederholt (1974). The authors examined 14 studies that evaluated the effects of the Frostig-Horne program on reading skill development. The results of this effort indicated that despite a wide variation among the studies in terms of statistical expertise, types and number of subjects, number of different trainers, evaluation instruments used, and overall quality, 13 of the 14 studies failed to demonstrate concomitant improvement in reading ability as a result of systematic use of the Frostig-Horne program. The single exception (Lewis, 1968) contained serious methodological weaknesses, and demonstrated significant reading improvement while failing to show significant improvement in visual perception. This is a puzzling result to say the least, especially when one considers the perceptual-motor theory.

Hammill, Goodman, et al. (1974) also reviewed seven studies that examined the effectiveness of the Frostig-Horne program on readiness-skill development. Four of the studies reviewed failed to indicate that perceptual training had any measurable effect on readiness attainment, while three studies supported the use of the procedure. Due to the conflicting nature of these findings, Hammill, Goodman, et al. (1974) were unable to make any definite statements regarding the efficacy of the Frostig-Horne program when used as a supplement to school readiness programs.

Finally, Wiederholt and Hammill (1971) studied 170 kindergarten and first grade children. The children were randomly selected and assigned to treatment and control groups. Pretest measures consisted of the Developmental Test of Visual Perception, the Slosson Intelligence Test, the Metropolitan Readiness Test, and the Metropolitan Achievement Test. The Developmental Test of Visual Perception, the Philadelphia Readiness Test, and the Philadelphia Reading and Arithmetic Tests comprised the posttest measures. The training sessions covered 16 weeks. Each child, on the average, completed 186 worksheets with no child being included in the study who completed less than 100 worksheets. Results indicated that the children trained in visual perception scored no higher on the academic and readiness tests than did the controls. The authors concluded by saying that the use of the Frostig-Horne program as a supplement to traditional readiness activities or as a method for facilitating the mastery of reading does not appear to be warranted.

In summary, the research evidence leads to the conclusion that the Frostig-Horne perceptual training approach does not appear to be a valid method of remediating reading disabilities of any type.

THE NEUROPSYCHOLOGICAL APPROACH

Despite the diversity of the remedial approaches presented thus far, not one has been truly validated as the single "best method" of teaching all dyslexic readers. The research evidence to date, in fact, appears to indicate that many of the approaches reviewed have even failed to produce results that would warrant their use as a remedial strategy with any type of reading disorder. One explanation for this finding may be uncovered if we explore the theoretical premise underlying these less fruitful approaches. As stated in the introduction of this chapter, these approaches all take the position of identifying and remediating areas of deficit in the dyslexic child. While this approach to treatment appears to make logical sense on the surface, research evidence in the areas of neurology and genetics (Adams & Victor, 1977;

Gaddes, 1980; Hartlage, 1975; Hartlage & Hartlage, 1973a, 1973b, 1978; Luria, 1966) has demonstrated a neurological and/or a genetic basis for the occurrence of many learning problems. From a neuropsychological point of view, deficit remediation is thus doomed to failure since it directs itself toward the training or retraining of damaged or dysfunctional areas of the brain (Hartlage & Reynolds, 1981; Reynolds, 1981).

A second explanation for the lack of positive findings with the deficit model of remediation lies in the lack of sophistication with respect to the diagnosis of dyslexia in children. One of the major points stated throughout this book is the notion that dyslexic children do not comprise a homogeneous diagnostic group. The research evidence presented in Chapter 6 has revealed that the population of dyslexic children is comprised of at least three distinct subgroups of disabled readers, each with its own characteristic diagnostic profile and complex of deficits. Based on these findings, it would be naive for one to expect positive trends in remediation studies that employ a deficit model or any model when the subjects employed in the study are actually heterogeneous in nature. Research efforts in the area of reading remediation, if they are to be effective, must heed the findings of the subgroup research and direct itself toward the matching of subtype with an appropriate treatment method.

Finally, a third reason for the lack of validation of the deficit model can be uncovered if one explores the emotional ramifications of this treatment method on the dyslexic reader (Hartlage & Reynolds, 1981). Assuming for the moment that, on the average, a dyslexic child spends two to three frustrating years, if not longer, in the regular classroom prior to being identified. Assume further that once diagnosed, the child is placed into a remedial program that stresses the activation and development of dysfunctional areas of the brain. The emotional stress, poor self-concept, and negative attitudes toward reading and school in general that develop in the dyslexic child as a result of this treatment approach would only serve to ensure failure. It is no wonder that emotional overlays are so prevalent in the dyslexic population and no wonder that many dyslexic children will be misdiagnosed as emotionally disturbed or as behavior disordered.

The neuropsychological approach to the remediation of dyslexic children, in contrast, is based on a different model of remediation. It considers each of the reasons for remedial failure discussed above and attempts to control for them.

The neuropsychological approach, theoretically, emphasizes the use of intact areas of neurological functioning in the development of remedial strategies. A concerted effort is thus made to match each child's cognitive neuropsychological strengths with an instructional method of presenting and acquiring information that relies most heavily on these cognitive strengths (Hartlage, 1981; Hartlage & Reynolds, 1981; Reynolds, 1981).

While there are several theoretical paradigms (Das et al., 1975; Hartlage, 1981; Kaufman, 1979; Luria, 1980) currently available that allow the neuropsychologist to analyze a child's test data for the purpose of developing remedial strategies, Luria's (1980) notion of the functional system is most useful here. A functional system (any higher mental process, such as reading), according to Luria, is a complex network of interconnected abilities that cannot be localized to any one particular area of the central nervous system. Each of the central nervous system acts may furthermore be part of several different functional systems. Each act may hence be important to the execution of several different kinds of behavior. The reader may recall the hypothesized functional system of reading as presented in Chapter 3 (see Fig. 3-2).

According to this schema, an insult to any of the component parts of a functional system is rarely accompanied by total loss of activity across the entire functional system. What usually results is instead a disorganization of the functional system and a characteristic abnormal performance of the activity. Recovery of function, which is often seen following injury, is attributed to a structural reorganization of the function into a new functional system, which is also widely dispersed throughout the central nervous system. In addition to the organization of the original functional system, an insult to the same component may also result in the disorganization of other functional systems that include this component in their chain. At the same time, all functional systems that do not include the disturbed component remain intact. Insults thus lead to particular qualitative changes in behavior, and insults to different components of a functional system are going to lead to different qualitative deficiencies in the performance of the behavior. It is the diagnosis of these qualitative changes that plays a central role in both Luria's method as well as in the neuropsychological model of remediation presented here.

More specifically, the first step in the neuropsychological approach to the remediation of dyslexia involves the assessment of each child's cognitive neuropsychological strengths and weaknesses. This can be accomplished in a qualitative manner if one is skilled in Luria's (1980) methods, or by a psychometric battery approach that requires both normative and ipsative test data interpretation (e.g., the Luria-Nebraska Neuropsychological Battery–Children's Revision, the Reitan-Indiana Neuropsychological Test Battery) or by the use of a common psychoeducational battery interpreted from a neuropsychological point of view (Hartlage, 1981; Kaufman, 1979). This was discussed in more detail in the previous chapter.

The next step in the neuropsychological approach is to match up the child's cognitive neuropsychological strengths with a remedial method that directs itself toward these strengths. Employing Luria's (1980) terminology, it is necessary to locate the intact components of the functional system that are capable of reorganization, and training them to moderate the learning processes that are necessary for acquiring the skill of reading. The dyslexic child thus is no longer viewed as a disabled reader who requires remediation in certain deficit areas. He is instead viewed as a disabled reader with certain neuropsychological deficits that cannot be significantly improved on and certain neuropsychological strengths that can be reorganized and developed to assume the learning processes necessary for reading at some level.

The final step in the neuropsychological approach involves motivational improvement and confidence building. As discussed earlier, it is very likely that the dyslexic child will come to the remedial setting (i.e., learning-disabilities classroom, reading specialist) after several years of frustration due to poor academic success in the regular classroom. The child's self-concept will be poor, he may be a behavior problem, and he may exhibit hyperactivity and/or an attention-deficit disorder. As a result, the child may require a reconditioning period, prior to the initiation of the remedial program, in which appropriate classroom behavior (i.e., staying on task, being able to follow directions, and attending to instruction for progressively longer periods of time) and self-concept are developed. In order to accomplish these goals as well as to maintain an optimum level of motivation throughout the training program, behavioral methods should be employed (Kazdin, 1977; O'Leary & O'Leary, 1976; Ulrich, Stachnik & Mabry, 1970, 1974).

Research Findings with the Neuropsychological Approach

The process of matching a child's neuropsychological strengths with a teaching strategy designed to exploit these strengths has received considerable case-study support from the subgroup research presented in Chapter 6. For example, Myklebust and Johnson (Johnson, 1978; Myklebust & Johnson, 1962) present case-study material in support of their neuropsychologically based method. The authors advocate the use of the Orton-Gillingham approach (Gillingham & Stillman, 1970) or other synthetic phonics methods with their visual dyslexics who have deficits in the areas of letter orientation, visual perception, and visual memory, and who have strengths in the area of auditory and phonetic processing. Johnson and Myklebust recommend a whole-word or look-say approach for their auditory dyslexic group. A good example might be the language-experience approach (Stauffer, 1970), in which the child is allowed to develop his own stories in his own language while the teacher writes them down. New words are written down by the child on index cards, which the child saves in his word box for later drill (i.e., flash card presentation and matching to pictures). Sight-word methods such as this capitalize on the auditory strengths of the dyslexic in visual processing and visual memory while downplaying their deficits in auditory and phonetic processing, auditory memory, and sound sequencing.

Boder (1971, 1973a, 1973b) has also advocated a neuropsychological approach to the remediation of her dyslexic subgroups. According to Boder, remediation for the dysphonetic reader should consist of whole-word approaches, such as the look-say or the language-experience approach (Stauffer, 1970), due to the reader's deficit in phonetic analysis. Boder feels, in addition, that reinforcement with tactile-kinesthetic cues may be required, in which case the Fernald method may be useful. Boder goes on to stress that the teaching of phonetic skills to the dysphonic child will not come easy and should only be attempted after the child has developed a significant sight-word vocabulary to provide an adequate foundation. For the dyseidetic reader, who has strengths in the area of phonetic analysis and deficits in the ability to perceive and remember whole words as gestalts, Boder recommends a remedial phonics approach such as the Orton-Gillingham method. For those dyseidetic readers who have not yet learned to recognize and write the letters of the alphabet, the tactile-kinesthetic techniques of Fernald are advocated as the initial method of choice. Finally, for the alexic reader who has the combined deficits of the dysphonetic and of the dyseidetic reader, the initial remedial approach of choice calls for the emphasis to be placed on the tactile-kinesthetic sensory channel. The Fernald approach is thus recommended.

Although Boder (1971, 1973a, 1973b) has not presented any data pertaining to outcome with these methods, she has discussed the prognosis for the three subgroups. According to her observations, Boder states that the dysphonetic child will approach normal proficiency in contextual reading since he can acquire a sight vocabulary at grade level. The dysphonetic child, however, will not develop good word-analysis skills and the child's spelling tends to remain poor. The dyseidetic reader tends to remain a slow reader and usually does not achieve a sight vocabulary commensurate with grade level. While the prognosis for reading in the dyseidetic group does not appear to be as good as that of the dysphonetic group, the prognosis for spelling is better. Finally, the prognosis for children in the alexic group is very guarded without intensive, long-term remediation. None of these children in her study had achieved proficiency in reading at the high school level.

Based on remedial experience in his hospital clinic, Mattis (1981) has also advocated a neuropsychologically based remedial approach with his independent dyslexic subgroups. The dyslexic child with a language-disorder syndrome presents a specific language disorder in which an anomia is viewed as the major factor. The child has intact visual and constructional skills and adequate graphomotor coordination. Blending of speech sounds is usually intact. The deficits in verbal learning and verbal retrieval, which underly the anomia, make the acquisition of a look-say vocabulary difficult because the child responds to sight words in a manner similar to his response to the naming of objects, of colors, and of body parts. Those children who are more severely impaired will also experience difficulty in learning letter names and sounds, because most basal reading series anchor the letter sound to the name of the letter. The child's anomia thus results in faulty letter-sound associations. According to Mattis, the overall treatment strategy with this subgroup is to capitalize on the child's soundblending skills and ability to make letter-sound associations while minimizing the need for verbal labeling of letters and whole words and paying scant attention to the meaning of a blended word. The first step is to teach the sounds to be associated with letters and letter groups without teaching letter names and without imbedding the sound referent in a word cue. Once a strong core of sound referents has been mastered, the child is ready to proceed into any synthetic phonic program, such as the SRA Basic Reading Series (Rasmussen & Goldberg, 1966). When the child has begun work on third and fourth grade material, the language-experience approach (Stauffer, 1970) should be introduced in an effort to stabilize word meaning, present more age-appropriate content, and augment comprehension.

The dyslexic child with an articulation and graphomotor dyscoordination syndrome presents with intact visual-spatial perception, language, and constructional skills. The child may exhibit an assortment of gross and fine motor coordination deficits, but the critical deficiencies are buccal-lingual dyspraxia with resultant poor speech and graphomotor dyscoordination. No child in this group has phonetic word-attack skills. For this reason, Mattis (1981) recommends that the initial treatment phase focus on the development of a sizable sight-word vocabulary via a whole-word look-say approach. The underlying idea is to capitalize on the child's intact visual-spatial perception and language skills while avoiding his deficits in articulation and sound blending. Once a third or fourth grade sight-word level has been attained, Mattis advocates the use of a linguistic or structural analysis approach (Chall, 1967) in order to help the child develop the word-attack skills necessary to comprehend unfamiliar words. The child thus is trained to analyze a new word according to its prefix, suffix, and root rather than by having to rely on his poor sound-blending abilities.

The third and final subgroup that Mattis (1981) has identified is the visual-perceptual syndrome group. The children in this subgroup present with intact language, graphomotor coordination, and speech-blending skills. Although constructional ability is poor, the primary deficit lies in the perception, storage, and retrieval of visual stimuli. Mattis initially recommends that letter recognition be learned by having the child select letters from his name and by asking him to describe them. This verbal description is used by the child as a mediator for graphic reproduction. For example, the letter T can be described as a line going up and down and a line going across. The letter is then removed, and the child is asked to draw what he has just said. Once the child can reliably draw a letter, its name and sound referent are introduced. Eventually the verbal description is faded out by having the child gradually decrease the amplitude of his vocalization when drawing. When the letters and their sound referents have been mastered, a phonetic program is begun. Mattis is quick to caution, however, that these children are easily flooded perceptually and a phonics approach that places a high stress on the visual nature of letters is not appropriate (e.g., the color phonics system, Bannatyne, 1966a).

There has only been one major study to date that, according to previous authors (Hartlage & Reynolds, 1981; Reynolds, 1981; Zarske, 1982), has attempted to validate the neuropsychological approach to remediation; and, that study was accomplished with normal children. The authors who report this study state that Hartlage and his colleagues (Hartlage, 1975; Hartlage & Lucas, 1973) screened 1132 first grade students on a group test battery that allowed the authors to place the children into subgroups based on their relative efficiency in the areas of visual sequencing, auditory sequencing, and perception of auditory and visual space. Following classification, the groups were matched with a special reading program for instructional purposes that was believed to capitalize on the child's identified neuropsychological strengths. Children performing best on visual sequencing, for example, were taught reading through the use of the initial teaching alphabet (ITA), which relies heavily on such skills. Children whose highest levels of performance were on the auditory sequencing tasks were instructed through a linguistics phonics approach. Children excelling in the areas of visual and auditory space were taught reading through the whole-word, look-say approach. Due to "logistical requirements of the school system," 684 of the 1132 children were randomly assigned to a reading method. The mean Metropolitan Readiness Test scores at the beginning of the school year were essentially the same for the control and experimental groups. At the end of the school year, after nearly a full year of reading instruction, the children were administered the reading subtest of the Wide Range Achievement Test (WRAT) and the teachers individually rated the global reading skills of each child. Results indicated that the mean standard score on the WRAT was 106 (standard score) for the control group, as compared with a mean standard score of 129 for the combined experimental group. In addition, the teacher's ratings of the global reading skills of the children were significantly correlated (p < .001) with their reading achievement test scores.

The results of this study, at first glance, would appear to lend support to those who advocate a neuropsychological approach to the remediation of dyslexic children even though the study was conducted with normal first grade children. On a thorough analysis of the articles reviewed by Reynolds

(1981), Hartlage and Reynolds (1981), and Zarske (1982), which are cited by these reviewers as containing a description of the study and the resulting data on which they reported, the authors found no such data available.

Hartlage (1975) makes a strong case in the first article for the use of neuropsychological test data as well as historical data relating to mental development in the diagnosis of a child's cognitive strengths and weaknesses; and, for the use of this data in predicting the outcome of remedial strategies with learning-disabled children. In the second article, Hartlage and Lucas (1973) discuss the development and validation of a group-screening procedure for reading disability in children beginning first grade. The authors evaluated 1132 beginning first graders on the Metropolitan Readiness Test. During the sixth week of class, the teachers administered the Group Reading Screening Test. Children were then "assigned more or less randomly to one of three methods of teaching initial reading skills, including phonetic, look-say, or special teaching alphabet" (Hartlage & Lucas, 1973, p. 50). On completion of the reading instruction ("during the second last week of first grade" [Hartlage & Lucas, 1973, p. 50]) the children were ranked within classes for reading skills by their respective teachers and were individually administered the Word Recognition section of the WRAT.

It does not take an astute reader to realize that the study described by Hartlage and Lucas (1973) is not the same study as described by the above-mentioned reviewers. Methodologically, the children were not matched with an appropriate instructional program in reading based on their diagnostic profile of strengths and weaknesses as the reviewers would have one believe. Instead, Hartlage and Lucas (1973) state that the subjects were "assigned more or less randomly to one of three methods of teaching initial reading skills," (p. 50). Furthermore, no control group was employed in the Hartlage and Lucas (1973) study, which is another methodological oversight on the part of the above-mentioned reviewers who incorrectly cite this article. The only methodological similarities that the current authors, in fact, can find between the two studies is the number of subjects (N = 1132) and the diagnostic instruments and teaching strategies used.

In summary, the research evidence presented here, as well as other case studies cited in the literature in support of this approach (Gaddes, 1980; Hartlage, 1981; Hartlage and Reynolds, 1981), leads the authors to conclude that although the neuropsychological approach to the remediation of dyslexic children appears to be theoretically sound, the empirical validation of this method remains to be accomplished before any claims as to its effectiveness can be made.

CONCLUSIONS

After reviewing the historical approaches to the remediation of dyslexic children, two significant findings are evident. First, it was found that although there were several remedial theorists who made the claim that theirs was "the best" treatment program for dyslexia, no one program has been verified as being effective with all dyslexic children. Second, the notion of remediating cognitive deficits in the child by exercising damaged or dysfunctional neurological tissue is fruitless and an emotionally damaging approach.

As a result of these findings, researchers have been forced to take a closer look at the syndrome of dyslexia. This re-analysis has resulted in a different perspective in the diagnosis and treatment of the dyslexic child. No longer is the diagnostic category of dyslexia viewed as a homogeneous entity with one underlying cause with one "best" method of treatment. The research presented in Chapter 6 has caused the medical and educational community to instead view the syndrome of dyslexia as a heterogeneous entity with multiple etiologies. It has more importantly led to the belief that each subgroup of dyslexia will require a unique treatment approach or combination of approaches based on the child's neurologically intact functional systems rather than on dysfunctional abilities.

The research literature on the neuropsychological approach to remediation is, at present, scant at best. The research literature has only been able to offer case-study material in support of this method, with no large-scale empirical study available at this time. As a result, validation of this theory and remedial method remains incomplete.

Finally, in order to help foster research efforts, the minimal research guidelines are offered. Because of the heterogeneity of the dyslexic population, it is imperative that researchers first identify the subjects under study according to one of the existing methods of subgrouping or, if deemed more fruitful, according to a new diagnostic subgrouping procedure.

As discussed in Chapter 1, it is also critical that researchers adequately define their dyslexic population so that replicable results may be obtained. The definitions developed by the World Federation of Neurology or the International Reading Association are exemplary and populations of dyslexic children should be defined according to the criteria noted in these definitions.

It should also be recognized that developmental age trends need to be controlled for as well. This can be accomplished by employing a longitudinal design or by selecting and grouping subjects within limited age spans.

The nature of the treatment must be adequately described so that replication is possible. The treatment must be designed so that it conforms to the requirements of the neuropsychological approach. To facilitate this ef-

Table 8-1
Dyslexia Subgroups

Treatment Method	Boder's Dysphonetic	Boder's Dyseidetic	Boder's Alexic	Mattis' Language Disorder Syndrome	Mattis' Graphomotor Syndrome	Mattis' Visual-Perception Syndrome
Orton-Gillingham or other phonics methods such as SRA or Distar	No	Yes	No	After letter recognition is established	No	After letter recognition is established
Fernald-VAKT	In some cases	No	Yes	No	No	No
Doman-Delacato	No	No	No	No	No	No
ITPA Psycholinguistic	No	No	No	No	No	No
Visual-Perceptual Kephart, Frostig	No	No	No	No	No	No
Look-Say or Language Experience	Yes	No	No	In later stages	Yes	No
Linguistic Structural Analysis	In later stages	No	No	No	In later stages	No

fort, Table 8-1 is offered. The treatment must be administered by professionals who are fully trained in these remedial methods. The method of training and practice in teaching methods should be spelled out in detail, again to aid in replication. The treatment must be administered over a time period that is felt to be adequate for change to take place. Three to six months of daily treatment is probably a minimum.

If a group design is employed, it would be most desirable if an attention placebo control group were used along with a normal control group in order to rule out the effects of special attention as a confounding variable. If a case-study design is used, adequate baseline data must be collected in order to rule out normal development as a confounding variable.

The neuropsychological perspective outlined in detail in this volume represents the current views of researchers from psychology, medicine, and education. Much of the basic research into the nature of dyslexia has provided rather compelling evidence as to the neurological basis of this severe reading disorder. The neuropsychological evidence has articulated the profiles of cognitive abilities associated with recognized subtypes of dyslexic children.

Much of the frustration over educational intervention with these children has arisen because the application of theory to practice is not an easy process. The Doman-Delacato approach, for example, makes great sense to a naive person but it has no logical neuroanatomical or neuropsychological basis. Simply because a history of frustration exists in attempts to apply neuropsychological knowledge to dyslexic children, there is no reason to abandon hope of ever treating these children from this perspective. Educators need to develop more refined programs that match materials to intact abilities, try the program out in large-scale research programs, and evaluate the success of intervention. As more advances are made in understanding basic brain-behavior relationships among dyslexic children, our efforts to apply knowledge should become equally more refined and precise. In this fashion, the multidisciplinary effort to help the dyslexic child to develop and to mature normally will have a higher probability of success.

Glossary

Agenesis. Developmental failure of tissue to mature.

Agnosia. An inability to recognize a sensory stimulation

Agraphia. An inability to learn to write

Alexia. A complete inability to learn to read

Anencephalic. Born without a substantial brain. Typically the brain stem is present in anencephalic babies but the cerebellum and cerebral hemispheres failed to develop.

Angiography. Practice of studying the circulatory system of the brain by injecting radiologic material into the arterial system

Angioma. A swelling or tumor due to proliferation of blood vessels

Angular Gyrus. A convolution at the juncture of the occipital, temporal, and parietal association cortex believed to be important in cross-modal integration necessary in fluent reading

Anomia. An inability to name a familiar object, usually due to damage in the left temporal lobe

Anterior. Toward the front

Aphasia. An inability to comprehend language or to express oneself verbally or in written form due to damage in those regions of the cortex responsible for language function

Apperceptive Visual Agnosia. An inability to recognize familiar objects because they are not perceived correctly

Apraxia. An inability to carry out motor acts normally, despite the fact that the patient can comprehend what is requested and has the motor skill to carry out the act

Archicerebellum. Oldest portion of the cerebellum important in keeping one oriented in space. Damage to this region of the cerebellum can result in staggering or swaying when walking

Articulatory and Graphomotor Dyscoordination Syndrome. According to Mattis et al. (1975), this syndrome is characterized by poor sound blending, poor graphomotor skills, and normal receptive language abilities

Association Visual Agnosia. An inability to copy or match an unfamiliar object

Associative Fibers. Neural fibers that transmit impulses between cortical points within a given hemisphere

Auditory-Linguistic Dyslexia. Pirozzolo (1981) characterizes this dyslexic subtype as having low verbal IQ relative to performance IQ, delayed language onset, expressive speech deficits, and a whole-word approach to reading. This subtype is roughly equivalent to Boder's (1971) dysphonetic dyslexic.

Backward Reader. Readers who achieve at the lowest possible level of the distribution of reading abilities, irrespective of ability

Bradykinesia. Slow movements

Broca's Area. A region of cortex usually found at the inferior juncture of the left motor strip. It is associated with verbal expression.

Callosal. Pertaining to the corpus callosum

Cerebral Asymmetries. Relating to asymmetrical or one-sided advantage in performance on a particular perceptual or cognitive task. The one-sided advantage is believed to reflect the development of specialized cortical regions for a particular task.

Cerebral Dominance. A one-sided advantage for a particular task. Most individuals evidence a left-sided cerebral dominance for language ability.

Closed-Head Injury. Damage to the brain resulting from a severe blow to the head. The skull is usually not fractured but the tissue is damaged by the concussion.

Color Agnosia. An inability to name colors despite normal color vision

Commissural Fibers. Neural fibers that transmit impulses between the two cerebral hemispheres

Contralateral. On the opposite side

Contrecoup Concussion. A concussion received by a blow to the opposite side of the head

Corpus Callosum. Long band of neural fibers that serve to interconnect the left and right cerebral hemispheres

Cortex. The outermost convoluted layer of the brain

Cortical. Relating to the cerebral cortex

Craniotomy. Usually refers to brain surgery; opening the cranium

CT Scan. A radiologic procedure also known as a CAT Scan (computed axial tomography) that uses a computer to develop an x-ray of a "slice" of brain tissue

Cytoarchitectonic. Pertaining to the mapping of the distribution of cell layers in the cerebral cortex

Dandy-Walker Syndrome. Agenesis of the vermis of the cerebellum leading to hydrocephalus in infants

Diaschisis. Disturbance of cortical function due to focal trauma in an area of the brain anatomically connected to, but distant to, the site of insult

Dichotic Listening. A technique for determining in which hemisphere language is localized. Paired stimuli are presented simultaneously. Most patients will correctly report more stimuli presented to the right ear if the stimuli are words.

Diencephalon. That region of the brain associated with the thalamus and the hypothalamus

Dysarthria. Slurred speech usually due to cerebellar dysfunction

Dyseidetic Dyslexia. Conceptualized by Boder (1970, 1971), this second most common form of dyslexia is marked by deficits in visual perception, phonetic misspellings, and a phonetic approach to word reading

Dysphonetic Dyslexia. As conceptualized by Boder (1970, 1971), this dyslexia is characterized by deficits in letter-sound integration, poor phonetic skills, misspellings of a nonphonetic nature, and semantic substitutions during reading. It is the most common form of dyslexia.

Dysplasia. Abnormal tissue development

Dystaxia. Incoordination of volitional motor movements

Ectopic. Aberrant or out of place

Edema. An accumulation of excessive fluid in cells and tissues

Electroencephalograph. A strip-chart recording of electrical activity from various regions of the brain. Usually referred to as an EEG.

Electrostimulation. Stimulation of the brain during brain surgery to localized cortical functions

Epilepsy. A condition characterized by seizures resulting from intense and abnormal electrical discharges in the brain

Exophthalmos. Prominence of the eyeball

Fissure. Deep fold between two gyri

Frontal Lobe. Cortex anterior to the central fissure

Genetic Dyslexic. As conceptualized by Bannatyne (1971), the genetic dyslexic represents the lower end of the normal continuum of verbal ability within the general population. The genetic dyslexic has difficulty with auditory discrimination, auditory sequencing, and association of sound-symbol relationships.

Gerstmann Syndrome. A constellation of symptoms usually associated with a lesion in the dominant parietal lobe. The four common symptoms include: agraphia, right-left disorientation, finger agnosia, and arithmetic disability or acalculia.

Graphesthesia. The ability to recognize letters or symbols drawn on the hand or fingers

Gyri. Raised cortical area or convolution

Hemianopia. Blindness in the left or right visual field

Hemiparesis. A partial paralysis on one side of the body

Hemiplegia. Paralysis of one side of the body

Hemispherectomy. An operation to remove one of the cerebral hemispheres

Heterogeneous. Consisting of parts having dissimilar properties

Hindbrain. Lowest clearly identifiable part of the brain consisting of the medulla, reticular activating system, and pons

Homogeneous. Consisting of a uniform composition

Hydrocephalus. Excessive accumulation of fluid in the cerebral ventricles that serve to dilate the ventricles causing the cortex to become thinner.

Hyperlexia. A rare condition sometimes associated with infantile autism or mental retardation in which there is superior word-calling ability with little or no comprehension

Hypothalamus. Portion of the brain associated with the diencephalon. Important in regulation (e.g., of appetite, sexual arousal, etc.).

Hypotonia. A floppiness of the extremities

Ideational Apraxia. Inability to show how to use some common and well-known object

Ideomotor Apraxia. An inability to pretend one is performing some manual task (e.g., saluting)

Inferior. Below some point of reference

Insula. Refers to cortex deep in the Sylvian fissure

Ipsilateral. Relating to the same side

Language Disorder Dyslexic. As conceptualized by Mattis et al. (1975), this dyslexic suffers disorders in comprehension, imitative speech, and anomia. He also has difficulty in speech sound discrimination.

Lesion. Any tissue that has been damaged or is abnormal due to developmental or congenital defects, infections, or other causes

Medulla.   Prolongation of the spinal cord into the brain. Lowest recognizable part of the brain responsible for life-sustaining functions (such as respiration, heart rate, etc.). It forms the floor of the fourth ventricle.

Minimal Neurological Dysfunction Dyslexia.   As conceptualized by Bannatyne (1971), this dyslexic suffers neurological deficits in visual-spatial and auditory perception, tactile recognition and integration, and concept formation

Minor Cerebral Hemisphere.   Usually refers to the right or nondominant hemisphere

Mixed Cerebral Dominance.   Refers to inconsistent hand, foot, or eye dominance or to a person who is left-handed, right-footed, etc.

Neocerebellum.   Most recently developed part of the cerebellum that acts as a central computer for the refinement of volitional motor movements

Neural Decussation.   Crossover of neural tracts from one side of the body to the other

Neuropsychology.   An applied specialization within psychology that focuses on the appraisal of human behavior as it relates to neurological functioning

Nystagmus.   Jerky eye movements usually associated with cerebellar dysfunction

Occipital Lobe.   Cortex posterior to the parietal and temporal lobes. Also thought of as the visual cortex.

Ontogenetic.   Relating to the development of the individual

Optic Agnosia.   A patient's inability to name an object even though the patient can still use it correctly or point to it when asked

Paleocerebellum.   Second oldest part of cerebellum responsible for "antigravity" posturing

Phylogenetic.   Relating to the development of the species

Planum Temporale.   Cortical area directly posterior to Heschl's gyrus in the superior portion of the temporal lobe

Polymicrogyria.   Many small, malformed gyria

Pons.   Structure between the medulla and the cerebral peduncles. In front of the cerebellum.

Posterior.   Toward the rear

Projection Fibers.   Neural fibers that transmit impulses between the cerebral cortex and lower neural centers

Prosopagnosia.   Difficulty in the recognition of familiar faces

Reticular Activating System (RAS).   Refers to many nerve centers or nuclei that are functionally related and found in the medulla. The RAS is important in cortical arousal.

Rostrum.   The anterior portion of the corpus callosum

Sinistral.   A person who exhibits dominance of the left hand

Splenium.   The most posterior portion of the corpus callosum

Stereognosis.   The ability to distinguish the shape of an object by touch alone

Strephosymbolia.   Twisted symbols as described by Orton (1928).

Subcortical.   Below the cerebral cortex

Subdural Hematoma.   A collection of blood in the space between the dura and the arachnoid tissue

Sulci.   Usually conceived of as a less-pronounced fissure

Superior.   Above some point of reference

Temporal Lobe.   The cortex inferior to the lateral or Sylvian fissure

Thalamus.   Largest portion of diencephalon. Acts as a waystation for all sensory data transmitted to the cortex.

Ventricle.   Spaces within the brain that are filled with fluid

Visual-Spatial Dyslexia.   Pirozzolo (1981) characterizes this dyslexic as average to above-average verbal-IQ, low performance-IQ, right-left disorientation, finger agnosia, phonetic spelling errors, faulty eye-movements, and spatial dysgraphia. It is roughly equivalent to Boder's (1971) dyseidetic dyslexic.

Visual-Spatial Perceptual Disorder.   As conceptualized by Mattis et al. (1975), the dyslexic suffering this syndrome evidences verbal IQ more than ten points above performance IQ, and also shows poor visual discrimination and memory

Wada Technique.   A medical technique for determining language dominance. Amytal is injected into the left carotid artery. If speech arrest occurs, it is then known that speech is localized in the left cerebral hemisphere. If speech arrest occurs when Amytal is injected into the right carotid artery, then it is known that speech is lateralized to the right hemisphere.

Wernicke's Area.   Cortical region usually in the left temporal lobe responsible for speech and language comprehension

References

Aaron, PG, Baxter, CF, & Lucenti, J. Developmental dyslexia and acquired alexia: Two sides of the same coin? *Brain and Language*, 1980, *11*, 1–11

Adams, RD, & Victor, M. *Principles of neurology*. New York: McGraw-Hill, 1977

Ahn, H, Prichep, L, John, GR, Baird, H, Trepetin, M, & Kaye, H. Developmental equations reflect brain dysfunction. *Science*, 1980, *210*, 1259–1262

Ajax, ET. Dyslexia without agraphia. *Archives of Neurology*, 1967, *17*, 645–652

Alajouanine, T, & Lhermitte, F. Acquired aphasia in children. *Brain*, 1965, *88*, 853–862

American Psychiatric Association. *Diagnostic and statistical manual of mental disorders (3rd ed.): DSM III*. Washington, DC: American Psychiatric Association, 1980

Anand, BK, & Brobeck, JR. Hypothalamic control of food intake. *Yale Journal of Biology and Medicine*, 1951, *24*, 123–140

Angelos, C. Dyslexia ruling against school seen as spark for more suits. *Seattle Times*, January 11, 1982

Annett, M. Hand preference and the laterality of cerebral speech. *Cortex*, 1975, *11*, 305–328

April, RS, & Han, M. Crossed aphasia in a right-handed bilingual Chinese man. *Archives of Neurology*, 1980, *37*, 342–346

Ayers, FW, & Torres, F. The incidence of EEG abnormalities in a dyslexic and a control group. *Journal of Clinical Psychology*, 1967, *23*, 334–336

Babinski, J. Contribution à l'é tude des troubles mentaux dans l'hémiplégie organique cérébale. *Review Neurology* (Paris), 1914, 27, 845

Bakker, DJ. Temporal order, meaningfulness, and reading ability. *Perceptual and Motor Skills*, 1967, *24*, 1027–1030

Bakker, DJ. *Temporal order in disturbed reading*. Rotterdam: University Press, 1972

Bakker, DJ. Hemispheric specialization and stages in the learning to read process. *Bulletin of the Orton Society*, 1973, *23*, 15–27

Bakker, DJ. Cognitive deficits and cerebral asymmetry. *Journal of Research and Development in Education*, 1981, *15*, 48–54

Bakker, DJ, Smink, T, & Reitsma, P. Ear dominance and reading ability. *Cortex*, 1973, *9*, 301–312

Bakker, DJ, Tuenissen, J & Bosch, J. Development of laterality—Reading patterns. In Knights,

RM, & Bakker, DJ. (Eds.), *The neuropsychology of learning disorders*. Baltimore: University Park Press, 1976

Ballard, PB. Sinstrality and speech. *Journal of Experimental Pedagogy*, 1912, *1*, 298–310

Bannatyne, AD. The etiology of dyslexia and the color phonics sytem. In Money J (Ed.), *The disabled reader: Education of the dyslexic child*. Baltimore: Johns Hopkins Press, 1966 (a)

Bannatyne, AD. *Psycholinguistic color system*. Urbana, Illinois: Learning Systems Press, 1966 (b)

Bannatyne, AD. *Language, reading, and learning disabilities*. Springfield: Charles C. Thomas, 1971

Bannatyne, AD. Diagnosis: A note on recategorization of the WISC scaled scores. *Journal of Learning Disabilities*, 1974, *7*, 272–274

Barbizet, J. *Human memory and its pathology*. San Francisco: W. H. Freeman and Company, 1970

Basso, A, Capitani, E, & Vignolo, LA. Influence of rehabilitation of language skills in aphasic patients. *Archives of Neurology*, 1979, *36*, 190–196

Bastian, HC. On the various forms of loss of speech in cerebral disease. *British and Foreign Medico-Surgical Review*, 1869, *43*, 470–492

Bastian, HC. *Aphasia and other speech defects*. London: H. K. Lewis, 1898

Bateman, B. *Interpretation of the 1961 Illinois Test of Psycholinguistic Abilities*. Seattle: Special Child Publications, 1968

Bauserman, DN, & Obrzut, J. Intrasensory integration abilities among average and subgroups of severely disabled readers. *Contemporary Educational Psychology* (in press)

Bay, E. Disturbances of visual perception and their examination. *Brain*, 1953, *76*, 515–550

Beck, A, & Mahoney, JJ. Schools of thought. *American Psychologist*, 1979, *34*, 93–98

Bender, LA. *Psychology of children with organic brain disorders*. Springfield: Charles C. Thomas, 1956

Bender, LA. Specific reading disabilities as a maturational lag. *Bulletin of the Orton Society*, 1957, *7*, 9–18

Bender, MB, & Feldman, M. The so-called "visual agnosias." *Brain*, 1972, *9*, 173–186

Benson, DF. Aphasia. In Heilman, KM, & Valenstein, E (Eds.), *Clinical neuropsychology*. New York: Oxford University Press, 1979

Benson, DF. Alexia and the neuroanatomical basis of reading. In Pirozzolo, FJ, & Wittrock, MC (Eds.), *Neuropsychological and cognitive process in reading*. New York: Academic Press, 1981

Benson, DF, & Geschwind, N. The alexias. In Vinken, PJ, & Bruyn, GW (Eds.), *Handbook of clinical neurology*. Amsterdam: North-Holland, 1969

Benton, AL. Right-left discrimination and finger localization in defective children. *Archives of Neurology and Psychiatry*, 1955, *74*, 583–589

Benton, AL. *Right-left discrimination and finger localization: Development and pathology*. New York: Hoebe, 1959

Benton, AL. The fiction of the Gerstmann syndrome. *Journal of Neurology, Neurosurgery, and Psychiatry*, 1961, *24*, 176–181

Benton, AL. Dyslexia in relation to form perception and directioral sense. In Money J (Ed.), *Reading disability: Progress and research needs in dyslexia*. Baltimore: Johns Hopkins Press, 1962

Benton, AL. Developmental aphasia and brain damage. *Cortex*, 1964, *1*, 40–52

Benton, AL. Developmental dyslexia: Neurological aspects. In Friedlander, WJ (Ed.), *Advances in neurology* (Vol. 7). New York: Raven Press, 1975

Benton, AL. Reflections on the Gerstmann syndrome. *Brain and Language*, 1977, *4*, 45–62

Benton, AL. Visuoperceptive, visuospatial and visuoconstructive disorders. In Heilman, KM, & Valenstein, E (Eds.), *Clinical neuropsychology*. New York: Oxford University Press, 1979

Benton, AL. Dyslexia: Evolution of a concept. *Bulletin of the Orton Society*, 1980, *30*, 10–26

Berent, S. Lateralization of brain function. In Filskov, SB, & Boll, TJ (Eds.), *Handbook of Clinical Neuropsychology*. New York: John Wiley and Sons, 1981

Berger, M, Yule, W, & Rutter, M. Attainment and adjustment in two geographical areas: II. The prevalence of specific reading retardation. *British Journal of Psychiatry*, 1975, *126*, 510–519

Berry, KE. *Developmental Test of Visual-Motor Integration*. New York: Psychological Corporation, 1974

Birch, HG. Dyslexia and maturation of visual function. In Money, J (Ed.), *Reading Disabilities: Progress and research needs in dyslexia*. Baltimore: Johns Hopkins Press, 1962

Birch, HG, & Belmont, L. Auditory-visual integration in normal and retarded readers. *American Journal of Orthopsychiatry*, 1964, *34*, 852–861

Birch, HG, & Belmont, L. Auditory-visual integration, intelligence, and reading ability in school children. *Perceptual and Motor Skills*, 1965, *20*, 295–305

Björklund, A, Segal, M, & Stenevi, U. Functional reinnervation of rat hippo campus by locus coeruleus implants. *Brain Research*, 1979, *170*, 409–426

Black, P, Jeffries, JJ, Blumer, D, Wellner, A, & Walker, AE. The posttraumatic syndrome in children: Characteristics and incidence. In Walker, AE, Caveness, WF, & Critchley, M (Eds.), *The late effects of head injury*. Springfield: Charles C. Thomas, 1969

Blank, M, & Bridger, W. Deficiencies in verbal labeling in retarded readers. *American Journal of Orthopsychiatry*, 1966, *36*, 840–847

Blank, M, Weider, S, & Bridger, W. Verbal deficiencies in abstract thinking in early reading retardation. *American Journal of Orthopsychiatry*, 1968, *38*, 823–834

Blinkov, JM, & Glezer, II. *The human brain in figures and tables*. New York: Plenum Press, 1968

Boder, E. Developmental dyslexia: A new diagnostic approach based on the identification of three subtypes. *Journal of School Health*, 1970, *40*, 289–290

Boder, E. Developmental dyslexia: Prevailing diagnostic concepts and a new diagnostic approach. In Myklebust, H (Ed.), *Progress in learning disabilities*. New York: Grune & Stratton, Inc., 1971

Boder, E. Developmental dyslexia: A diagnostic approach based on three atypical reading patterns. *Developmental Medicine and Child Neurology*, 1973, *15*, 663–687 (a)

Boder, E. Developmental dyslexia: A diagnostic screening procedure based on three characteristics patterns of reading and spelling. In Bateman, B (Ed.), *Learning Disorders*. Seattle: Special Child Publications, 1973 (b)

Bogen, JE. The other side of the brain: Part I. *Bulletin of the Los Angeles Neurological Society*, 1969, *34*, 73–105 (a)

Bogen, JE. The other side of the brain: Part II. An appositional mind. *Bulletin of the Los Angeles Neurological Society*, 1969, *34*, 135–162 (b)

Bogen, JE. Some educational aspects of hemispheric specialization. *UCLA Educator*, 1975, *17*, 24–32

Bogen, JE, & Vogel, PJ. Cerebral commissurotomy in man. Preliminary case report. *Bulletin of the Los Angeles Neurological Society*, 1962, *27*, 169–172

Boll, TJ. Behavioral correlates of cerebral damage in children aged 9 through 14. In Reitan, RM, & Davison, LA (Eds.), *Clinical neuropsychology: Current status and applications*. New York: John Wiley & Sons, 1974

Bond, MR. Assessment of the psychosocial outcome after severe head injury. In *Outcome of severe damage to the central nervous system*. CIBA Foundation Symposium 34. Oxford: Excerpta Medica, 1975

Bray, PF, Bale, JF, Anderson, RE, & Kern, ER. Progressive neurological disease associated with chronic cytomegalovirus infection. *Annals of Neurology*, 1981, *9*, 449–502

Bremer, F. Le corp calleux dans la dynamique cèrébrale. *Experientia*, 1966, *22*, 1–8

Brink, JD, Garrett, AL, Hale, WR, Woo-Sam, J, & Nickel, VL. Recovery of motor and intellectual function in children sustaining severe head injuries. *Developmental Medicine and Child Neurology*, 1970, *12*, 565–571

Broadbent, DE. Successive responses to simultaneous stimuli. *Journal of Experimental Psychology*, 1956, *8*, 145–152

Broadbent, W. Cerebral mechanisms of speech and thought. *Med.-Surg.* (Trans.) Royal Medical Society, 1872, *55*, 145–194

Broca, P. Nouvelle observation d'aphemie produite par une lesion de la moite posterieure des deuxieme et troisieme circonvolutions frontales. *Bulletin de la Society Anatomique de Paris*, 1861, *36*, 398–407

Brunner, WE. Congenital word-blindness. *Ophthalmology*, 1905, *1*, 189–195

Bryant, ND, & Friedlander, WJ. "14" and "6" in boys with specific reading disability. *Electroencephalography and Clinical Neurophysiology*, 1965, *19*, 318–322

Bryden, MP, & Allard, FA. Do auditory perceptual asymmetries develop? *Cortex*, 1981, *17*, 313–318

Bryden, MP, & Zurif, EB. Dichotic listening performance in a case of, agenesis of the corpus callosum. *Neuropsychologia*, 1970, *8*, 371–377

Burt, C. *The backward child*. New York: Appleton-Century, 1937

Bush, WJ, & Giles, MT. *Aids to psycholinguistic teaching*. Columbus, Ohio: Charles E. Merrill, 1969

Butfield, E, & Zangwill, OL. Re-education in aphasia: A review of 70 cases. *Neurology, Neurosurgery & Psychiatry*, 1945, *9*, 75–79

Butler, SR, & Norrsell, U. Vocalization possibly initiated by the minor hemisphere. *Nature*, 1968, *220*, 793–794

Buxbaum, E. The patient's role in etiology of learning disability. *Psychoanalytic Study of Children*, 1964, *19*, 421–477

Bykov, KM, & Speransky, AD. Observation upon dogs after section of the corpus callosum. *Collected Papers of the Physiology Labs of I. P. Pavlov*, 1924, *1*, 47–59

Carlsson, CA, Von Essen, C, & Löfgren, J. Factors affecting the clinical course of patients with severe head injury. *Journal of Neurosurgery*, 1968, *29*, 242–245

CELDIC Report. *One million children, a national study of Canadian children with emotional and learning disorders*. Toronto: Crainford, 1970

Centofanti, CC, & Smith, A. *The Single and Double Simultaneous (Face-hand) Stimulation Test*. Los Angeles: Western Psychological Service, 1978

Chadwick, O, Rutter, M, Shaffer, D, & Shrout, PE. A prospective study of children with head injuries: IV. Specific cognitive deficits. *Journal of Clinical Neuropsychology*, 1981, *3*, 101–120

Chadwick, O, Rutter, M, Thompson, J, & Shaffer, D. Intellectual performance and reading skills after localized head injury in childhood. *Journal of Child Psychology and Psychiatry*, 1981, *22*, 117–139

Chall, JS. *Learning to read: The great debate*. New York: McGraw-Hill, 1967

Charcot, JM. Sur un cas de cedite verbale. In *Lecons sur les maladies du systeme nerveux (Envres completes de JM Charcot)* (Vol. 3). Paris: Delahaye and Lecrosnier, 1877

Charcot, JM. On a case of sudden and isolated suppression of the mental vision of signs and objects (forms and colours). *Clinical lectures of diseases of the nervous system* (Vol. 3). London: The New Sydenham Society, 1889

Chi, JG, Dooling, EC, & Gilles, FH. Left-right asymmetries of the temporal speech areas of the human fetus. *Archives of Neurology*, 1977, *34*, 346–348

Chiarello, C. A house divided? Cognitive functioning with callosal agenesis. *Brain and Language*, 1980, *11*, 128–158

Child Neurology Society, Task force on nosology of disorders of higher cerebral function in children. *Proposed nosology of disorders of higher cerebral function in children.* Child Neurology Society, 1981

Childs, S. *Teaching the dyslexic child: Dyslexia in special education. Monograph* (Vol. 1). Pomfret, Connecticut: The Orton Society, 1965

Chusid, JG. *Correlative neuroanatomy and functional neurology.* Los Altos: Lange Medical Publications, 1970

Claiborne, JH. Types of congenital symbol amblyopia. *Journal of the American Medical Association*, 1906, *47*, 1813–1816

Clarke, E, & O'Malley, CD. *The human brain and spinal cord.* Berkeley: University of California Press, 1968

Cohn, R. Delayed acquisition of reading and writing abilities in children. *Archives of Neurology*, 1961, *4*, 153–164

Conrad, K. Beitrag zum problem der parietalen alexia. *Archives Psychologie*, 1948, *181*, 398–420

Corballis, MC. Laterality and myth. *American Psychologist*, 1980, *35*, 284–295

Corballis, MC, & Beale, IL. *The psychology of left and right.* Hillsdale: Erlbaum, 1976

Coren, S, Porac, C, & Duncan, P. A behaviorally validated self-report inventory to assess four types of lateral preference. *Journal of Clinical Neuropsychology*, 1979, *1*, 55–65

Craig, DL. Neuropsychological assessment in public psychiatric hospitals: The current state of practice. *Clinical Neuropsychology*, 1979, *1*, 1–7

Critchley, M. *The parietal lobes.* London: Edward Arnold, 1953

Critchley, M. *Developmental dyslexia.* London: William Heinemann Medical Books, Ltd., 1964

Critchley, M. *The dyslexic child.* London: William Heinemann Medical Books, Ltd., 1970

Critchley, M, & Critchley, EA. *Dyslexia defined.* London: William Heinemann Medical Books, Ltd., 1978

Culton, G. Spontaneous recovery from aphasia. *Journal of Speech and Hearing Research*, 1969, *12*, 825–832

Cummings, L, Benson, DF, Walsh, MJ, & Levine, HC. Left-to-right transfer of language dominance: A case study. *Neurology*, 1979, *29*, 1547–1550

Cutts, NE. (Ed.), *School psychologists at mid-century.* Washington: American Psychological Association, 1955

Dalby, JT, & Gibson, D. Functional cerebral lateralization in subtypes of disabled readers. *Brain and Language*, 1981, *14*, 34–48

Damasio, A. The frontal lobes. In Heilman, KM, & Velenstein, E (Eds.), *Clinical neuropsychology.* New York: Oxford University Press, 1979

Darby, R. *Ear asymmetry phenomenon in dyslexic and normal children.* Unpublished master's thesis. University of Florida, 1974

Das, JP, Kirby, JR, & Jarman, RF. Simultaneous and successive syntheses: An alternative model for cognitive abilities. *Psychological Bulletin*, 1975, *82*, 87–103

Dean, RS. Cerebral lateralization and reading dysfunction. *Journal of School Psychology*, 1980, *18*, 324–332

Dean, RS, Schwartz, NH, & Smith, LS. Lateral preference patterns as a discriminator of learning difficulties. *Journal of Consulting and Clinical Psychology*, 1981, *49*, 227–235

Dearborn, WF. The etiology of congenital word blindness. *Harvard Monographs in Education*, 1925, *1*, 50–76

Dechant, EV. *Improving the teaching of reading.* Englewood Cliffs: Prentice-Hall, 1970

Decker, SN, & DeFries, JC. Cognitive ability profiles in families of reading-disabled children. *Developmental Medicine and Child Neurology*, 1981, *23*, 217–227

deHirsch, K, Jansky, J, & Langford, W. *Predicting reading failure.* New York: Harper and Row, 1966

Dejerine, J. Contribution a petude anatamopathologique et clinique des differentes varieties de cecite verbale. *Mem. Soc. Biol.*, 1892, *4*, 61

Dejerine, J. *Semiologie des affections du systeme nerveaux*. Paris: Masson, 1914

Delacato, CH. *The treatment and prevention of reading problems: The neuropsychological approach*. Springfield, Illinois: Charles C. Thomas, 1959

Delacato, CH. *The diagnosis and treatment of speech and reading problems*. Springfield, Illinois: Charles C. Thomas, 1963

Delacato, CH. *Neurological organization and reading*. Springfield, Illinois: Charles C. Thomas, 1966

DeMyer, W. *Technique of the neurological examination: A programmed text* (2nd ed.). New York: McGraw-Hill, 1974

Denckla, MB, & Bowen, FP. Dyslexia after left occipitotemporal lobectomy: A case report. *Cortex*, 1973, *9*, 321–328

Dennis, M. Language in a congenitally acallosal brain. *Brain and Language*, 1981, *12*, 33–53

Dewson, JH. Preliminary evidence of hemispheric asymmetry of auditory function in monkeys. In Harnad, S, Doty, R, Goldstein, L, Jaynes, J, & Krauthamer, G (Eds.), *Lateralization in the nervous sytem*. New York: Academic Press, 1977

Diller, L, Ben-Yishay, Y, Gerstmann, LJ, Goodkin, R, Gordon, W, & Weinberg, J. *Studies in cognition and rehabilitation in hemiplegia*. New York: New York University Medical Center Institute of Rehabilitation, 1974

Dimond, SJ, & Beaumont, JG. Experimental studies of hemisphere function in the human brain. In Dimond, SJ, & Beaumont, JG (Eds.), *Hemisphere function in the human brain*. New York: Wiley, 1974

Dimond, SJ, & Blizard, DA (Eds.). *Evolution and lateralization of the brain*. New York: New York Academy of Sciences, 1977

Dogan, K, Dogan, S, & Lovrencic, M. Agenesis of the corpus callosum in two brothers. *Lijecnicki Vjesnik*, 1967, *89*, 377–386

Downs, MP. The expanding imperatives of early identification. In Bess, FH (Ed.), *Childhood deafness*. New York: Grune & Stratton, 1977

Drake, WE. Clinical and pathological findings in a child with a developmental learning disability. *Journal of Learning Disabilities*, 1968, *1*, 486–502

Dreifuss, FP. The pathology of central communicative disorders in children. In Tower, DB (Ed.), *The nervous system: Human communication and its disorders, Vol. 3*. New York: Raven Press, 1975

Drew, AL. A neurological appraisal of familial congenital word-blindness. *Brain*, 1956, *79*, 440–460

Duane, DD. Toward a definition of dyslexia: A summary of views. *Bulletin of the Orton Society*, 1979, *29*, 56–64

Duffy, FH. Topographic mapping in childhood developmental dyslexia: A reply. *Annals of Neurology* (letter), 1980, *7*, 643

Duffy, FH. Brain electrical activity mapping (BEAM): Computerized access to complex brain function. *International Journal of Neuroscience*, 1981, *13*, 55–65

Duffy, FH, Burchfiel, JL, & Lombroso, CT. Brain electrical activity mapping (BEAM): A method for extending the clinical utility of EEG and evoked potential data. *Annals of Neurology*, 1979, *5*, 309–321

Duffy, FH, Denckla, MB, Bartels, PH, & Sandini, G. Dyslexia: Regional differences in brain electrical activity by topographic mapping. *Annals of Neurology*, 1980, *7*, 412–420

Duffy, FH, Denckla, MD, Bartels, PH, Sandini, G, & Kiessling, LS. Dyslexia: Automated diagnosis by computerized classification of brain electrical activity. *Annals of Neurology*, 1980, *7*, 421–428

Dykman, RA, Wallis, RC, Suzuki, T, Ackerman, PT, & Peters, JE. Children with learning disabilities: Conditioning differentiation and the effect of distraction. *American Journal of Orthopsychiatry*, 1970, *40*, 766–782

Dykman, RA, Wallis, RC, Suzuki, T, Ackerman, PT, & Peters, JE. Children with learning disabilities: As attentional deficit syndrome. In Myklebust, HR (Ed.), *Progress in learning disabilities* (Vol. 3). New York: Grune & Stratton, Inc., 1971

Ebersole, M, Kephart, NC, & Ebersole, JB. *Steps to achievement for the slow learner.* Columbus, Ohio: Charles E. Merrill, 1968

Eccles, JC. Evolution of the brain in relation to the development of the selfconscious mind. In Dimond, SJ & Blizard, DA (Eds.), Evolution and lateralization of the brain. *Annals of the New York Academy of Science,* 1977, *299*, 161–279

Eidelberg, DS, & Galaburda, AM. Symmetry and asymmetry in the human posterior thalamus: I. Cytoarchitectonic analysis in normal persons. *Archives of Neurology,* 1982, *39*, 325–332

Eisenberg, L. Reading retardation: I. Psychiatric and sociologic aspects. *Pediatrics,* 1966, *37*, 352–365

Ellis, A. On Joseph Wolpe's espousal of cognitive-behavioral therapy. *American Psychologist,* 1979, *34*, 98–99

Ettlinger, G, Blakemore, CB, Milner, AD, & Wilson, J. Agenesis of the corpus callosum: A behavioral investigation. *Brain,* 1972, *95*, 327–346

Ettlinger, G, Blakemore, GB, Milner, AD, & Wilson, J. Agenesis of the corpus callosum: A further behavioral investigation. *Brain,* 1974, *97*, 225–234

Federal Register. *Education of handicapped children and incentive grants programs.* Bethesda: U. S. Department of Health, Education, and Welfare, 1976, *41*, 46977

Fedio, P, & Mirsky, AF. Selective intellectual impairment in children with temporal lobe or centrencephalic epilepsy. *Neuropsychologia,* 1969, 7, 287–300

Fernald, G. *Remedial techniques in basic school subjects.* New York: McGraw-Hill, 1943

Fildes, LG. A psychological inquiry into the nature of the condition known as congenital word-blindness. *Brain,* 1922, *4*, 286–307

Filskov, SB, Grimm, BH, & Lewis, JA. Brain-behavior relationships. In Filskov, SB, Boll, TJ (Eds.), *Handbook of clinical neuropsychology.* New York: John Wiley and Sons, 1981

Fischer, WF, Libeman, IV, & Shankweiler, D. Reading reversals and developmental dyslexia: A further study. *Cortex,* 1978, *14*, 496–510

Fisher, JH. Case of congenital word-blindness (inability to learn to read). *Ophthalmic Review,* 1905, *24*, 315–318

Foerster, R. Beiträge zur pathologie des lesens und schreibens (congenitale wort-blindheit bei einen schwachsirnigen). *Neurol. Centralbl.,* 1905, *24*, 235–236

Ford, EB. Polymorphism and taxonomy. In Huxley, J (Ed.), *The new systematic.* Oxford: Claredon Press, 1940

Ford, EB. *Ecological genetics.* New York: John Wiley and Sons, 1964

Franz, SI. Studies in re-education: The aphasias. *Comparative Psychology,* 1918, *4*, 349–429

French, JD. The reticular formation. In McGaugh, JL, Weinberger, NM, & Whalen, RE (Eds.), *Psychobiology: The biological basis of behavior.* San Francisco: W. H. Freeman, 1966

Freud, S. *Zur auffassung der aphasien.* Deuticke: Leipzig and Wien, 1891. Translation by Stengel, E. New York: International Universities Press, 1953

Fried, I, Tanguay, PE, Boder, E, Doubleday, C, & Greensite, M. Developmental dyslexia: Electrophysiological evidence of clinical subgroups. *Brain and Language,* 1981, *12*, 14–22

Frisch, GR, & Handler, LA. A neuropsychological investigation of "functional disorders of speech articulation." *Journal of Speech and Hearing Research,* 1974, *17*, 432–445

Fromkin, W, Krashens, CS, Rigler, D, & Rigler, M. The development of language acquisition beyond the "critical period." *Brain and Language,* 1974, *1*, 81–93

Frostig, M. *Frostig Developmental Tests of Visual Perception.* Palo Alto, California: Consulting Psychologists Press, 1964

Frostig, M. *Movement education: Theory and practice.* Chicago: Follett Publishing Co., 1970

Frostig, M, & Horne, D. *The Frostig Program for the Development of Visual Perception.* Chicago: Follett Publishing Co., 1964

Frostig, M, Maslow, P, Lefever, D, & Wittlesey, JRB. *The Marianne Frostig Development Test of Visual Perception*. Palo Alto, California: Consulting Psychologists, 1964

Fuster, JM, & Jervey, JP. Inferotemporal neurons distinguish and retain behaviorally relevant features of visual stimuli. *Science*, 1981, *212*, 952–955

Gaddes, WH. Prevalence estimates and the need for definition of learning disabilities. In Knights, RM, & Bakker, DJ (Eds.), *The neuropsychology of learning disorders: Theoretical approaches*. Baltimore: University Park Press, 1976

Gaddes, WH. *Learning disabilities and brain function: A neuropsychological approach*. New York: Springer-Verlag, 1980

Galaburda, AM, & Eidelberg, D. Symmetry and asymmetry in the human posterior thalamus: II. Thalamic lesions in a case of developmental dyslexia. *Archives of Neurology*, 1982, *39*, 333–336

Galaburda, AM, & Kemper, TL. Cytoarchitectonic abnormalities in developmental dyslexia: A case study. *Annals of Neurology*, 1979, *6*, 94–100

Galambos, R, Norton, TT, & Frommer, GP. Optic tract lesions sparing pattern vision in cats. *Experimental Neurology*, 1967, *18*, 8–25

Gardner, E. *Fundamentals of neurology*. Philadelphia: W. B. Saunders, 1975

Gardner, H, Denes, G, & Zurif, E. Critical reading at the sentence level in aphasia. *Cortex*, 1975, *11*, 60–72

Gardner, H, & Zurif, E. Bee but not be: Oral reading of single words in aphasia and alexia. *Neuropsychologia*, 1975, *13*, 181–190

Garron, DC, & Cheifetz, DI. Comment of "Bender Gestalt discernment of organic pathology." *Psychological Bulletin*, 1965, *63*, 197–200

Gates, AI. *The improvement of reading* (3rd ed.). New York: Macmillan, 1947

Gazzaniga, MS. Changing hemisphere dominance by changing reward probabilities in split-brain monkeys. *Experimental Neurology*, 1971, *33*, 412–419

Gazzaniga, MS. Recent research on hemispheric lateralization of the human brain: Review of the split-brain. *UCLA Educator*, 1975, *17*, 9–12

Gerstmann, J. Fingeragnosie: Ene unschriebene störung der orientierung am eigerst korper. *Wein Klin. Wchnschr.*, 1924, *37*, 1010–1012

Gerstmann, J. Zur Symptomatologie der Hirnlasionen im Uebergangsgebiet der unteren parietal und mitteleren occipitalwindung. *Nervenarzt*, 1930, *3*, 691–695

Gerstmann, J. Some notes on the Gerstmann syndrome. *Neurology*, 1957, 7, 866–869

Geschwind, N. The anatomy of acquired disorders of reading. In Money, J (Ed.), *Reading disability*. Baltimore: Johns Hopkins Press, 1962

Geschwind, N. Language disturbances in cerebrovascular disease. In Benton, AL (Ed.), *Behavioral change in cerebrovascular disease*. New York: Harper & Row, 1970

Geschwind, N. Disconnection syndromes in animals and man. *Brain*, 1972, *88*, 237–294, 585–644

Geschwind, N. The development of the brain and the evolution of language. In Geschwind, N, *Selected papers on language and the brain*. Dordrecht-Holland: D. Reidel Publishing Company, 1974 (a)

Geschwind, N. Disorders of higher cortical function in children. In Geschwind, N, *Selected papers on language and the brain*. Dordrecht-Holland: D. Reidel Publishing Company, 1974 (b)

Geschwind, N. Anatomical foundations of language and dominance. In Ludlow, CL, & Doran-Quine, ME (Eds.), *The neurological bases of language disorders in children: Methods and directions for research*. Bethesda: U. S. Department of Health, Education, and Welfare (NIH Publication No. 79-440), 1979

Geschwind, N, & Levitsky, W. Human brain: Left-right asymmetries in temporal speech region. *Science*, 1968, *161*, 186–187

Gillingham, A, & Stillman, B. *Remedial training for children with specific disability in reading, spelling, and penmanship*. Cambridge, Massachusetts: Educators Published Service, 1970

Glass, GV, & Robbins, MP. A critique of experiments on the role of neurological organization in reading performance. *Reading Research Quarterly*, 1967, *3*, 5–52

Goh, DS, Teslow, CJ, & Fuller, GB. *The practice of psychological assessment among school psychologists.* Paper presented at the Twelfth Annual Convention of the National Association of School Psychologists. Washington, DC, April, 1980

Golden, CJ. The Luria-Nebraska Children's Battery: Theory and initial formulation. In Hynd, GW, & Obrzut, JE (Eds.), *Neuropsychological assessment and the school-age child: Issues and procedures.* New York: Grune & Stratton, 1981

Goldstein, K. Die lokalisation in der Grosshirnrinde. In Bethe, A (Ed.), *Handbuch der normalen und pathologischen physiologie* (Vol. 10), Berlin: Springer, 1927

Goldstein, K. *After effects of brain injuries in war.* New York: Grune & Stratton, 1942

Goldstein, K. *Language and language disturbances.* New York: Grune & Stratton, 1948

Goodglass, H, & Quadfasel, FA. Language laterality in left-handed aphasics. *Brain*, 1954, 77, 521–548

Goodman, L, & Hammill, D. The effectiveness of Kephart-Getman activities in developing conceptual-motor and cognitive skills. *Focus on Exceptional Children*, 1973, *4*, 1–9

Gott, PS. Cognitive abilities following right and left hemispherectomy. *Cortex*, 1973, *9*, 266–274.

Gott, PS, & Saul, RE. Agenesis of the corpus callosum: Limits of functional compensation. *Neurology*, 1978, *28*, 1272–1279.

Groenendaal, HA, & Bakker, DJ. The part played by mediation processes in the retention of temporal sequences by two reading groups. *Human Development*, 1971, *14*, 62–70

Gross, CG, & Weiskrantz, L. Some changes in behavior produced by lateral frontal lesions in the macaque. In Warren, JM, & Akert, K (Eds.), *The frontal granular cortex and behavior.* New York: McGraw-Hill, 1964

Guilford, JP. *The nature of human intelligence.* New York: McGraw-Hill, 1967

Hallahan, DP, & Cruickshank, WM. *Psychoeducational foundations of learning disabilities.* Englewood Cliffs: Prentice-Hall, 1973.

Hallgren, B. Specific dyslexia ("congenital word-blindness"): A clinical and genetic study. *Acta Psychiat. Scand. Supp.*, 1950, *65*

Halstead, WC. *Brain and intelligence: A quanitative study of the frontal lobes.* Chicago: University of Chicago Press, 1947

Halstead WC, & Wepman, JM. The Halstead-Wepman aphasia screening test. *Journal of Speech and Hearing Disorders*, 1949, *14*, 9–13

Hammil, D. Training visual perceptual processes. *Journal of Learning Disabilities*, 1972, *5*, 552–558

Hammill, D, Goodman, L, & Wiederholt, JL. Visual-motor processes: Can we train them? *The Reading Teacher*, 1974, 27, 470–479

Hammill, DD, & Larsen, SC. The effectiveness of psycholinguistic training. *Exceptional Children*, 1974, *41*, 5–14

Hammill, DD, & Larsen, SC. The effectiveness of psycholinguistic training: A reaffirmation of position. *Exceptional Children*, 1978, *44*, 402–414

Hammill, DD, Leigh, JE, McNutt, G, & Larsen, SC. A new definition of learning disabilities. *Learning Disability Quarterly*, 1981, *4*, 336–342

Hanley, J & Sklar, B. Electroencephalographic correlates of developmental reading dyslexias: Computer analysis of recordings from normal and dyslexic children. In Leisman, G (Ed.), *Basic visual processes and learning disability.* Springfield: Thomas, 1976

Hardyck, C, & Petrinovich, LF. Left-handedness. *Psychological Bulletin*, 1977, *84:*385–400

Hardyck, C, Petrinovitch, CF, & Goldman, R. Lefthandedness and cognitive deficit. *Cortex*, 1976, *12*, 266–278

Harnad, S, Doty, R, Goldstein, J, Jaynes, J, & Krauthamer, G (Eds.). *Lateralization in the nervous system.* New York: Academic Press, 1977

Harris, A. *How to increase reading ability* (5th ed.). New York: David McKay, 1970

Harris, TL, & Hodges, RE (Eds.). *A dictionary of reading and related terms*. Newark: International Reading Association, 1981

Hartlage, LC. Neuropsychological approaches to predicting outcome of remedial educational strategies for learning disabled children. *Pediatric Psychology*, 1975, *3*, 23–28

Hartlage, LC. Neuropsychological assessment techniques. In Reynolds, CR, & Gutkin, TB (Eds.), *The handbook of school psychology*. New York: John Wiley, 1981

Hartlage, PL, & Hartlage, LC. Comparison of hyperlexic and dyslexic children. *Neurology*, 1973, *23*, 436–437 (a)

Hartlage, PL, & Hartlage, LC. *Dermatoglyphic markers in dyslexia*. Paper presented to the annual meeting of the Child Neurology Society, 1973 (b)

Hartlage, LC, & Hartlage, PL. Clinical consultation to pediatric neurology and developmental pediatrics. *Journal of Clinical Child Psychology*, 1978, *7*, 52–53

Hartlage, LC, & Lucas, DG. Group screening for reading disability in first grade children. *Journal of Learning Disabilities*, 1973, *6*, 48–52

Hartlage, LC, & Reynolds, CR. Neuropsychological assessment and the individualization of instruction. In Hynd, GW, & Obrzut, JE (Eds.), *Neuropsychological assessment and the school-age child: Issues and procedures*. New York: Grune & Stratton, Inc., 1981

Haslam, RH, Dalby, JT, Johns, RD, & Rademaker, AW. Cerebral asymmetry in developmental dyslexia. *Archives of Neurology*, 1981, *38*, 679–682

Hatta, T. Lateral recognition of abstract and concrete kanji in Japanese. *Perceptual and Motor Skills*, 1977, *45*, 731–734

Head, H. *Aphasia and kindred disorders of speech*. Cambridge: Cambridge University Press, 1926

Healy, JM. The enigma of hyperlexia. *Reading Research Quarterly*, 1982, *17*, 319–338

Hebb, DO. Man's frontal lobes: A critical review. *Archives of Neurology and Psychiatry*, 1945, *54*, 10–24

Hebb, DO, & Penfield, W. Human behavior after extensive bilateral removals from the frontal lobes. *Archives of Neurology and Psychiatry*, 1940, *44*, 421–438

Hécaen, H, & Piercy, M. Paroxysmal dysphasia and the problem of cerebral dominance. *Journal of Neurology, Neurosurgery, and Psychiatry*, 1956, *19*, 194–201

Heilman, KM, & Valenstein, E. (Eds.). *Clinical neuropsychology*. New York: Oxford University Press, 1979

Heiskanen, O, & Sipponen, P. Prognosis of severe head injury. *Acta Neurologica Scandinavica*, 1970, *46*, 343

Hendry, BC. The effects of gross-motor movements on the perceptual-motor development of primary age multiply handicapped children, abstracted. *Dissertation Abstracts*, 1970, *31*, 5231

Henschen, SE. *Klinische und anatomische bertrage zur pathologie der gehirns*. Stockholm: Almquist und Wiksell, 1922

Hermann, K. *Reading disability: A medical study of world-blindness and related handicaps*. Copenhagen: Munksgaar, 1959

Hermann, K. Specific reading disability. *Danish Medical Bulletin*, 1964, *11*, 34–40

Herron, J (Ed.), *Neuropsychology of left-handedness*. New York: Academic Press, 1980

Hersher, L. Minimal brain dysfunction and otitis media. *Perceptual and Motor Skills*, 1978, *47*, 723

Hewison, J. The current status of remedial intervention for children with reading problems. *Developmental Medicine and Child Neurology*, 1982, *24*, 183–186

Hewitt, W. The development of the human corpus callosum. *Journal of Anatomy*, 1962, *96*, 355–358

Hier, DB. Sex differences in hemisphere specialization: Hypothesis for the excess of dyslexia in boys. *Bulletin of the Orton Society*, 1979, *29*, 74–83

Hier, DB, LeMay, M, Rosenberger, PB, & Perlo, VP. Developmental dyslexia: Evidence for a subgroup with a reversal of cerebral asymmetry. *Archives of Neurology*, 1978, *35*, 90–92

Hieronymus, AN, & Lindquist, FF. *Manual for administrators, supervisors, and counselors: ITBS*. Boston: Houghton Mifflin, 1974

Hincks, EM. Disability in reading in relation to personality. *Harvard Monographs in Education*, 1926, *1*, 1–92

Hinshelwood, J. Word-blindness and visual memory. *Lancet*, 1895, *2*, 1564–1570

Hinshelwood, J. Congenital word-blindness. *Lancet*, 1900, *1*, 1506–1508

Hinshelwood, J. Congenital word-blindness, with reports of two cases. *Ophthalmic Review*, 1902, *21*, 91–99

Hinshelwood, J. Four cases of congenital word-blindness occurring in the same family. *British Medical Journal*, 1909, *2*, 1229–1232

Hirschenfang, SA. A comparison of Bender Gestalt reproductions of right and left hemiplegic patients. *Journal of Clinical Psychology*, 1960, *16*, 439

Hobbs, N. *The futures of children*. San Francisco: Jossey-Bass, 1975

Horton, AM Jr. Behavioral neuropsychology in the schools. *School Psychology Review*, 1981, *10*, 367–372

Howie, VM. Acute and recurrent otitis media. In Jaffe, B (Ed.), *Hearing loss in children*, Baltimore: University Park Press, 1977

Hughes, JR. Electroencephalography and learning disabilities. In Myklebust, HR. (Ed.), *Progress in learning disabilities*. New York: Grune & Stratton, 1968

Hughes, JR, & Denckla, MB. Outline of a pilot study of electroencephalographic correlates of dyslexia. In Benton, AL, & Pearl, D (Eds.), *Dyslexia: An appraisal of current knowledge*. New York: Oxford University Press, 1978

Hughes, JR, Leander, R, & Ketchum, G. Electroencephalographic study of specific reading disabilities. *Electroencephalography and Clinical Neurophysiology*, 1949, *1*, 377–378

Humphrey, ME, & Zangwill, OL. Dysphasia in left-handed patients with unilateral brain lesions. *Journal of Neurology, Neurosurgery, and Psychiatry*, 1952, *15*, 184–193

Hynd, GW. Rebuttal to the critical commentary on neuropsychology in the schools. *School Psychology Review*, 1981, *10*, 389–393

Hynd, GW. *Neuropsychological considerations in educational intervention*. Paper presented at the Annual Convention of the American Psychological Association, Washington, D.C., August, 1982

Hynd, GW, Cannon, SB, & Haussmann, SE. The exceptional child. In Hynd, GW (Ed.), *The school psychologist: An introduction*. Syracuse: Syracuse University Press, 1983

Hynd, GW, & Obrzut, JE. The effects of grade level and sex on the magnitude of the dichotic ear advantage. *Neuropsychologia*, 1977, *15*, 689–692

Hynd, GW, & Obrzut, JE. Reconceptualizing cerebral dominance: Implications for reading and learning disabled children. *Journal of Special Education*, 1981, *15*, 447–457

Hynd, GW, Obrzut, JE, & Obrzut, A. Are lateral and perceptual asymmetries related to WISC-R and achievement test performance in normal and learning disabled children? *Journal of Consulting and Clinical Psychology*, 1981, *49*, 977–979

Hynd, GW, Obrzut, JE, Weed, W, & Hynd, CR. Development of cerebral dominance: Dichotic listening asymmetry in normal and learning disabled children. *Journal of Experimental Child Psychology*, 1979, *28*, 445–454

Hynd, GW, Quackenbush, R, & Obrzut, JE. Training school psychologists in neuropsychological assessment: Current practices and trends. *Journal of School Psychology*, 1980, *18*, 148–153

Hynd, GW, & Teeter, A. *Callosal agenesis in infancy: Two case studies*. Paper presented at the First Annual Conference of the National Academy of Neuropsychologists, Orlando, Florida, October, 1981

Inglis, J, & Lawson, JS. Sex differences in the effects of unilateral brain damage on intelligence. *Science*, 1981, *212*, 693–695

Ingram, TS, Mason, AW, & Blackburn, I. A retrospective study of 82 children with reading disability. *Developmental Medicine and Child Neurology*, 1970, *12*, 271–281

Isserlin, M. Die pathologie physiologie der sprache. *Eigeben Physiologie*, 1929, *29*, 129–249

Isserlin, M. Die pathologie physiologie der sprache. *Eigeben Physiologie*, 1931, *33*, 1–202

Isserlin, M. Die pathologie physiologie der sprache. *Eigeben Physiologie*, 1932, *34*, 1065–1144

Jackson, E. Developmental alexia (congenital word-blindness). *American Journal of Medical Science*, 1906, *131*, 843–849

Jackson, JH. On the nature of the duality of the brain. *Medical Press Circulator*, 1874, *1*, 19, 41, 63

Jackson, JH. Case of large cerebral tumor without optic neuritis and with left hemiplegia and imperception. *Review Ophthalmology Hospital Report*, 1876, *8*, 434

Jacobsen, CF. Studies of cerebral function in primates: I. The functions of the frontal association areas in monkeys. *Comparative Psychology Monographs*, 1936, *13*, 3–60

Jacobson, S. Neuroembryology. In Curtis, BA, Jacobson, S, & Marcus, EM (Eds.), *An introduction to the neurosciences*. Philadelphia: W. B. Saunders 1972

James, W. *Talks to teachers on psychology*. New York: Holt, 1900

Jansky, JJ. Specificity and parameters in defining dyslexia. *Bulletin of the Orton Society*, 1979, *29*, 31–38

Jansky, J, & de Hirsch, K. *Preventing reading failure—prediction, diagnosis, and intervention*. New York: Harper and Row, 1972

Jasper, HH. The ten-twenty electrode system of the International Federation. *Electroencephalography and Clinical Neurology*, 1958, *10*, 371–375

Jerison, HJ. Quantitative analysis of evolution of the brain in mammals. *Science*, 1961, *133*, 1012–1014

Johnson, DJ. Remedial approaches to dyslexia. In Benton, AL, & Pearl, D (Eds.), *Dyslexia: An appraisal of current knowledge*. New York: Oxford University Press, 1978

Johnson, DJ, & Myklebust, HR. *Learning disabilities, educational principles and practices*. New York: Grune & Stratton, 1967

Joynt, RJ, & Goldstein, MN. Minor cerebral hemisphere. In Friedlander, WJ (Ed.), *Advances in neurology*. New York: Raven Press, 1975

Kahn, P. Time orientation and reading achievement. *Perceptual and Motor Skills*, 1963, *21*, 157–158

Kamphaus, RW, Kaufman, AS, & Kaufman, NL. *A cross-validation study of sequential-simultaneous processing at ages 2½–12½ using the Kaufman Assessment Battery for Children (KABC)*. Paper presented at the Annual Convention of the American Psychological Association, Washington, D.C., August, 1982

Kapur, N, & Perl, NT. Recognition reading (time course) related to disorder in paralexia. *Cortex*, 1978, *14*, 439–443

Katz, J. The effects of conductive hearing loss on auditory function. *Journal of the American Speech and Hearing Association*, 1978, *20*, 879

Kaufman, AS. *Intelligent testing with the WISC-R*. New York: Wiley Interscience, 1979

Kaufman, NL, & Kaufman, AS. Remedial intervention in education. In Hynd, GW (Ed.), *The school psychologist: An introduction*. Syracuse: Syracuse University Press, 1983

Kaufman, AS, Kaufman, NL, Kamphaus, RW, & Naglieri, JA. Sequential and simultaneous factors at ages 3–12½: Developmental changes in neuropsychological dimensions. *Clinical Neuropsychology*, 1982, *4*, 74–81

Kaufman, AS, Zalma, R, & Kaufman, WL. The relationship of hand dominance to the motor coordination, mental ability, and right-left awareness of young normal children. *Child Development*, 1978, *49*, 885–888

Kazdin, AE. *The token economy*. New York: Plenum Press, 1977

Keefe, B, & Swinney, D. On the relationship of hemispheric specialization and developmental dyslexia. *Cortex*, 1979, *15*, 471–481

Kephart, NC. *The slow learner in the classroom* (2nd ed). Columbus, Ohio: Charles E. Merrill, 1971

Kershner, JR. Cerebral dominance in disabled readers, good readers, and gifted readers. *Child Development*, 1977, *48*, 61–67

Kertesz, A, & McCabe, P. Recovery patterns and prognosis in aphasia. *Brain*, 1977, *100*, 1–18

Kimura, D. Cerebral dominance and the perception of verbal stimuli. *Canadian Psychologist*, 1961, *15*, 166–171

Kimura, D. Dual functional asymmetry of the brain in visual perception. *Neuropsychologia*, 1966, *4*, 275–285

Kimura, D. Functional asymmetry of the brain in dichotic listening. *Cortex*, 1967, *3*, 163–178

Kimura, D, & Durnford, M. Normal studies on the function of the right hemisphere in vision. In Diamond, SJ, & Beaumont, JG (Eds.), *Hemisphere function in the human brain*. London: Elek Science, 1974

Kinsbourne, M. Mechanisms of hemispheric interaction in man. In Kinsbourne, M, & Smith, WL (Eds.), *Hemispheric disconnection and cerebral function*. Springfield: Charles C. Thomas, 1974

Kinsbourne, M, & Hiscock, M. Cerebral lateralization and cognitive development: Conceptual and methodological issues. In Hynd, GW, & Obrzut, JE (Eds.), *Neuropsychological assessment and the school-age child: Issues and procedures*. New York: Grune & Stratton, Inc., 1981

Kinsbourne, M, & Warrington, E. Developmental factors in reading and writing backwardness. *British Journal of Psychology*, 1963, *54*, 145–156

Kirk, S. *Educating exceptional children*. Boston: Houghton-Mifflin Company, 1972

Kirk, SA, & Kirk, WD. *Psycholinguistic learning disabilities: Diagnosis and remediation*. Urbana, Illinois: University of Illinois Press, 1971

Kirk, SA, McCarthy, JJ, & Kirk, WD. *Examiner's manual: Illinois Test of Psycholinguistic Abilities* (rev. ed.). Urbana, Illinois: University of Illinois Press, 1968

Kirshner, HS, & Kistler, KH. Aphasia after right thalamic hemorrhage. *Archives of Neurology*, 1982, *39*, 667–669

Kline, C, & Kline, C. Follow-up study of 216 dyslexic children. *Bulletin of the Orton Society*, 1975, *25*, 127–144

Klonoff, H, & Low, MD. Disordered brain function in young children and early adolescents: Neuropsychological and electroencephalographic correlates In Reitan, RM, & Davison, LA (Eds.), *Clinical neuropsychology: Current status and applications*. New York: John Wiley and Sons, 1974

Klonoff, H, Low, MD, & Clark, C. Head injuries in children: A prospective five year follow-up. *Journal of Neurology, Neurosurgery, and Psychiatry*, 1977, *40*, 1211–1219

Knights, RM, & Norwood, JA. *A neuropsychological test battery for children*. Ottawa, Canada: Psychological Consultants, 1979

Kolata, G. Grafts correct brain damage. *Science*, 1982, *217*, 342–344

Kolb, D, & Whishaw, IQ. *Fundamentals of human neuropsychology*. San Francisco: W. H. Freeman and Company, 1980

Kolstoe, OP. Programs for the mildly retarded: A reply to the critics. *Exceptional Children*, 1972, *39*, 51–56

Koppitz, EM. *The Bender Gestalt Test for Young Children*. New York: Grune & Stratton, Inc., 1963

Kromer, LF, Björklund, A, & Stenevi, U. Utilization of embryonic hippocampal implants to promote regeneration of the cholinergic input to the hippocampus in the adult rat, abstracted. *Neuroscience Abstracts*, 1978, *8*, 532

Kurachi, M, Yamaguchi, N, Inasaka, T, & Torii, H. Recovery from alexia without agraphia: Report of an autopsy. *Cortex*, 1979, *15*, 297–312

Kussmaul, A. Disturbance of speech. *Cyclopedia of Practical Medicine*, 1877, *14*, 581–875

Lashley, KS. *Brain mechanisms and intelligence*. Chicago: University of Chicago Press, 1929

Lashley, KS. Factors limiting recovery after central nervous lesions. *Journal of Nervous and Mental Diseases*, 1938, *88*, 733–755

Lassonde, MC, Lortie, J, Ptito, M, & Geoffroy, G. Hemispheric asymmetry in callosal agenesis as revealed by dichotic listening performance. *Neuropsychologia*, 1981, *19*, 455–458

Lazarus, AA. A matter of emphasis. *American Psychologist*, 1979, *34*, 100

Leischner, A. *Die Storungen der schriftspracke (agraphie und alexie)*. Stuttgart: Georg Thieme Verlag, 1957

LeMay, M. Are there radiological changes in the brains of individuals with dyslexia? *Bulletin of the Orton Society*, 1981, *31*, 135–141

LeMay, M, & Culebras, A. Human brain: Morphological differences in the hemispheres demonstrable by carotid arteriography. *New England Journal of Medicine*, 1972, *287*, 168–170

Lenneberg, EH. *Biological foundations of language*. New York: John Wiley and Sons, 1967

Leong, CK. Lateralization in severely disabled readers in relation to functional cerebral development and synthesis of information. In Knights, RM, & Bakker, DJ (Eds.), *Neuropsychology of learning disorders: Theoretical approaches*. Baltimore: University Park Press, 1976

Levine, DN, Hier, DB, & Calvanio, R. Acquired learning disability for reading after left temporal lobe damage in childhood. *Neurology*, 1981, *31*, 257–264

Levinson, HN. *A solution to the riddle dyslexia*. New York: Springer-Verlag, 1980

Lewis, JN. The improvement of reading ability through a developmental program in visual perception. *Journal of Learning Disabilities*, 1968, *1*, 652–653

Lewitter, FI, DeFries, JC, & Elston, RC. Genetic models of reading disability. *Behavior Genetics*, 1980, *10*, 9–30

Lezak, MD. *Neuropsychological assessment*. New York: Oxford University Press, 1976

Liebeman, IY, Shankweiler, D, Orlando, L, Harris, KS, & Bertt, FB. Letter confusion and reversals of sequence in the beginning reader: Implications for Orton's theory of developmental dyslexia. *Cortex*, 1971, 7, 127–142

Lichtheim, L. On aphasia. *Brain*, 1885, 7, 433–484

Lieberman, AD. The right not to read controversy. *Pediatrics*, 1979, *64*, 976

Lindgren, SD. Finger localization and the prediction of reading disability. *Cortex*, 1978, *14*, 87–101

Lovell, K, Shapton, D, & Warren, NS. A study of some cognitive and other disabilities in backward readers of average intelligence as assessed by a non-verbal test. *British Journal of Educational Psychology*, 1964, *34*, 58–64

Lund, KA, Foster, GE, & McCall-Perez, FC. The effectiveness of psycholinguistic training, a re-evaluation. *Exceptional Children*, 1978, *44*, 310–319

Lund, RD. *Development and plasticity of the brain: An introduction*. New York: Oxford University Press, 1978

Luria, AR. Disorders of simultaneous perception in a case of bilateral occipitoparietal brain injury. *Brain*, 1959, *82*, 437–449

Luria, AR. *Higher cortical functions in man*. New York: Basic Books, 1980

Luria, AR. Frontal lobe syndromes. In Vicken, PJ & Bruyn, GW (Eds.), *Handbook of clinical neurology* (Vol. 2). Amsterdam: North Holland Publishing Company, 1969

Luria, AR. *Traumatic aphasia: Its syndromes, psychology and treatment*. The Hague: Mouton, 1970

Luria, AR. *The man with a shattered world*. New York: Basic Books, 1972

Luria, AR. *The working brain*. New York: Basic Books, 1973

Lyle, JG. Reading retardation and reversal tendency: A factorial study. *Child Development*, 1969, *40*, 833–843

Lyle, JG, & Goyen, J. Visual recognition, developmental lag and strephosymbolia in reading retardation. *Journal of Abnormal Psychology*, 1968, *73*, 25–29

Lyle, JG, & Goyen, J. Effects of speed of exposure and difficulty of discrimination on visual recognition of retarded readers. *Journal of Abnormal Psychology*, 1975, *8*, 613–616

Lynn, RB, Buchanan, DC, Fenichel, GM, & Freeman, FR. Agenesis of the corpus callosum. *Archives of Neurology*, 1980, *37*, 444–445

Maccoby, EE, & Jacklin, CN. *The psychology of sex differences*. Stanford: Stanford University Press, 1974

Mackie, RD. *Special education in the United States: Statistics 1946–1966.* New York: Teacher's college, 1969

Mahl, GF, Rothenberg, A, Delgado, JM, & Hamlin, H. Psychological responses in the human to intracerebral electrical stimulation. *Psychosomatic Medicine,* 1964, *26,* 337–368

Mahut, H, & Zola, S. Ontogenetic time-table for the development of three functions in infant macaques and the effects of early hippocampal damage upon them, abstracted. *Neuroscience Abstracts,* 1977, *3,* 428

Makita, K. The rarity of reading disability in Japanese children. *American Journal of Orthopsychiatry,* 1968, *38,* 599–614

Marcel, T, Katz, K, & Smith, M. Laterality and reading proficiency. *Neuropsychologia,* 1974, *12,* 131–139

Marcel, T, & Rajan, P. Lateral specialization of recognition of words and faces in good and poor readers. *Neuropsychologia,* 1975, *13,* 489–497

Marcus, EM. Cerebral cortex. In Curtis, BA, Jacobson, S, & Marcus, EM (Eds.), *An introduction to the neurosciences.* Philadelphia: W. B. Saunders, 1972

Marie, P. Revision de la question de l'aphasie: Le 3^{e} circonvolution frontale gauche ne jove aucum role speciale dans la fonction du language. *Semaine Medicale,* May 23, 1906, 241–247

Marx, JL. Transplants as guides to brain development. *Science,* 1982, *217,* 340–342

Mattis, S. Dyslexia syndromes: A working hypothesis that works. In Benton, AL, & Pearl, D (Eds.), *Dyslexia: An appraisal of current knowledge.* New York: Oxford University Press, 1978

Mattis, S. Dyslexia syndromes in children: Toward the development of syndrome-specific treatment programs. In Pirozzolo, FJ, & Witrock, MC (Eds.), *Neuropsychological and cognitive process in reading.* New York: Academic Press, 1981

Mattis, S, French, JH, & Rapin, I. Dyslexia in children and young adults: Three independent neuropsychological syndromes. *Developmental Medicine and Child Neurology,* 1975, *17,* 150–163

McCulloch, MS. Functional organization of the cerebral cortex. *Psychological Review,* 1944, *23,* 390–407

McFie, J. Psychological testing in clinical neurology. *Journal of Nervous and Mental Disease,* 1960, *131,* 383–393

McFie, J. Intellectual impairment in children with localized post-infantile cerebral lesions. *Journal of Neurology, Neurosurgery, and Psychiatry,* 1961, *24,* 361–365

McFie, J. *Assessment of organic impairment.* London: Academic Press, 1975

McKeever, WF, & Huling, MD. Lateral dominance in tachistoscopic word recognition of children at two levels of ability. *Quarterly Journal of Experimental Psychology,* 1970, *22,* 600–604

McKeever, WF, & Van Deventer, AD. Dyslexic adolescents: Evidence of impaired visual and auditory language processing. *Cortex,* 1975, *11,* 361–378

Meader, CC, & Muyskens, JH. *Handbook of biolinguistics.* Toledo: H.C. Weller, 1962

Meier, MJ. Education for competency assurance in human neuropsychology: Antecedents, models, and directions. In Filskov, SB & Boll, TJ (Eds.), *Handbook of clinical neuropsychology.* New York: John Wiley and Sons, 1981

Menkes, JH, Philippart, M, & Clark, DB. Hereditary partial agenesis of the corpus callosum. *Archives of Neurology,* 1964, *11,* 198–208

Meyer, V, & Yates, AJ. Intellectual changes following temporal lobectomy for psychomotor epilepsy. *Journal of Neurology, Neurosurgery, and Psychiatry,* 1955, *18,* 44–52

Meyner, T. *Der Bau der Grosshirnrinde.* Leipzig, 1867

Milner, B. Psychological deficits produced by temporal lobe excision. *Research Publications of the Association for Research on Nervous and Mental Disease,* 1958, *36,* 244–257

Milner, B. Laterality effects in audition. In Mountcastle, VB (Ed.), *Interhemispheric relations and cerebral dominance.* Baltimore: Johns Hopkins Press, 1962

Milner, B. Brain mechanisms suggested by studies of the temporal lobes. In Millikan, CH & Darley, FL (Eds.), *Brain mechanisms underlying speech and language.* New York: Grune & Stratton, 1967

Milner, B. Hemispheric specialization: Scope and limits. In Schmitt, FO, & Worden, FS (Eds.), *The neurosciences: Third study program.* Cambridge: The MIT Press, 1974

Milner, B. Psychological aspects of focal epilepsy and its neurosurgical management. *Advances in Neurology,* 1975, *8,* 299–321

Milner, B, Branch, C, & Rasmussen, T. Observations on cerebral dominance. In DeRuck, ABS, & O'Connor, M (Eds.), *CIBA Foundation symposium on disorders of language.* London: Churchill, 1964

Milner, PM. *Physiological psychology.* New York: Holt, Rinehart, and Winston, 1970

Mingazzini, G. Der balken. *Monographien aus dem Gesamt-gebiete der psychiatrie* (Vol. 28), 1922

Minskoff, E. Research on psycholinguistic training: Critique and guidelines. *Exceptional Children,* 1975, *42,* 136–144

Minskoff, E, Wiseman, DE, & Minskoff, JG. *The MWM program for developing language abilities.* Ridgefield, New Jersey: Educational Performance Associates, 1972

Mohr, JP. Rapid amelioration of motor aphasia. *Archives of Neurology,* 1973, *28,* 77–82

Molfese, DC, & Molfese, VJ. Hemisphere and stimulus differences as reflected in the cortical responses of newborn infants to speech stimulus. *Developmental Psychology,* 1979, *15,* 505–511

Molfese, DL, & Molfese, VJ. Cortical responses of preterm infants to phonetic and nonphonetic speech stimuli. *Developmental Psychology,* 1980, *16,* 574–581

Money, J. The law of constancy and learning to read. In *International approach to learning disabilities of children and youth.* Tulsa: Association for Children with Learning Disabilities, San Rafael: Academic Therapy Press, 1966

Moore, T. Language and intelligence: A longitudinal study of the first eight years. *Human Development,* 1967, *10,* 88–106

Morely, ME. *The development and disorders of speech in childhood.* Edinburgh: Livingstone, 1965

Morgan, WP. A case of congential word-blindness. *British Medical Journal,* 1896, *2,* 1378

Muehl, S, Knott, JR, & Benton, AL. EEG abnormality and psychological test performance in reading disability. *Cortex,* 1965, *1,* 434–440

Munk, H. Weitere mittheilungen zur physiologie der gross-hirnrinde. *Archives fur Anatomie und Physiologie,* 1878, *2,* 161–178

Munk, H. *Ueber die funktionen der grosshirnrinde. Gesammelte milleilunger aus den jahren.* Berlin: August Hershwald, 1881

Myklebust, HR, & Boshes, B. *Final report, minimal brain damage in children.* Bethesda: U. S. Department of Health, Education, and Welfare, 1969

Myklebust, HR, & Johnson, DJ. Dyslexia in Children. *Exceptional Children,* 1962, *29,* 14–25

Naeser, MA, Alexander, MP, Helm-Estabrooks, N, Levine, HL, Laughlin, SA, & Geschwind, N. Aphasia with predominantly subcortical lesion sites: Description of three capsular/putaminal aphasia syndromes. *Archives of Neurology,* 1982, *39,* 2–14

Nathan, P, & Smith, M. Effects of two unilateral cordotomies on the mobility of the lower limbs. *Brain,* 1973, *96,* 471–494

Needleman, H. Effects of hearing loss from early recurrent otitis media on speech and language development. In Jaffe, B (Ed.), *Hearing loss in children.* Baltimore: University Park Press, 1977

Nettleship, E. Cases of congenital word-blindness (inability to learn to read). *Ophthalmic Review,* 1901, *20,* 61–67

Neville, AC. *Animal asymmetry.* London: Edward Arnot'd, 1976

Newcombe, F. *Missle wounds of the brain.* New York: Oxford University Press, 1969

Newcombe, F, & Marshall, JC. Stages in recovery from dyslexia following a left cerebral abscess. *Cortex,* 1973, *9,* 329–332

Newcombe, F, Marshall, JC, Carrivick, PH, & Hiorns, RW. Recovery curves in acquired dyslexia. *Journal of the Neurological Sciences*, 1974, *24*, 127–133

✓Newcomber, PL, & Hammill, DD. *Psycholinguistics in the schools.* Columbus, Ohio: Charles E. Merrill, 1976

✓Nielson, H, & Binge, K. Visuo-perceptual and visuo-motor performance of children with reading disabilities. *Scandinavian Journal of Psychology*, 1969, *10*, 225–237

Obrzut, A. A neuropsychological case report of a child with auditory-linguistic dyslexia. *School Psychology Review*, 1981, *10*, 356–361

Obrzut, JE. Dichotic listening and bisensory memory skills in qualitatively diverse dyslexic readers. *Journal of Learning Disabilities*, 1979, *12*, 304–314

Obrzut, JE. Neuropsychological assessment in the schools. *School Psychology Review*, 1981, *10*, 331–342(a)

Obrzut, JE. Neuropsychological procedures with school-age children. In Hynd, GW, & Obrzut, JE (Eds.), *Neuropsychological assessment and the school-age child: Issues and procedures.* New York: Grune & Stratton, 1981(b)

Obrzut, JE, & Hynd, GW. Development of cerebral dominance in learning-disabled children. In Gottlieb, MI, & Bradford, LJ (Eds.), *Learning disabilities: An audio journal for continuing education.* New York: Grune & Stratton, Inc., 1979

O'Donnell, DA, & Eisenson, J. Delacato training for reading achievement and visual-motor integration. *Journal of Learning Disabilities*, 1969, *2*:441–447

Ofman, W, & Shaevitz, M. The kinesthetic method in remedial reading. *The Journal of Experimental Education*, 1963, *31*, 317–320

Oldendorf, WH. Nuclear medicine in clinical neurology: An update. *Annals of Neurology*, 1981, *10*, 207–213

Oldfield, RC. The assessment and analysis of handedness: The Edinburgh Handedness Inventory. *Neuropsychologia*, 1971, *9*, 97–113

O'Leary, SG, & O'Leary, KD. Behavior modification in the schools. In Leitenberg, H (Ed.), *Handbook of behavior modification and behavior therapy.* Englewood Cliffs: Prentice-Hall, 1976

Oppé, TE. The neurological examination. In Rose, FC (Ed.), *Paediatric Neurology.* Oxford: Blackwell Scientific Publications, 1979

Orton, J. The Orton-Gillingham approach. In Money, J, & Shiffman, G (Eds.), *The disabled reader.* Baltimore: Johns Hopkins Press, 1966

Orton, ST. "World-blindness" in school children. *Archives of Neurology and Psychiatry*, 1925, *14*, 581–615

Orton, ST. Specific reading disability-strephosymbolia. *Journal of the American Medical Association*, 1928, *90*, 1095–1099

Orton, ST. *Reading, writing, and speech problems in children.* New York: Norton, 1937

Orzeck, AZ. *The Orzeck Aphasia Evaluation.* Los Angeles: Western Psychological Services, 1966

Osgood, CE. Motivational dynamics of language behavior. In Jones, M (Ed.), *Nebraska Symposium on Motivation.* Lincoln: University of Nebraska Press, 1957

Paterson, J, & Bramwell, B. Two cases of word-blindness. *Medical Press*, 1905, *13*, 507–508

Penfield, W. The interpretive cortex. *Science*, 1959, *129*, 1719–1725

Penfield, W, & Jasper, H. *Epilepsy and the functional anatomy of the human brain.* Boston: Little Brown, 1954

Penfield, W, & Perot, P. The brain's record of auditory and visual experience. *Brain*, 1963, *86*, 595–696

Penfield, W, & Rasmussen, T. *The cerebral cortex of man.* New York: Macmillan, 1955

Penfield, W, & Roberts, L. *Speech and brain mechanisms.* Princeton: Princeton University Press, 1959

Peters, A. Ueber kongenitale woertblindheit. *Münchener Med. Wschr.*, 1908, *55*, 1116–1119

Pick, A. *Beiträge zur pathologie und pathologischen anatomie des central nerven systems mas bemerkungen zur normalen anatomie desselben.* Berlin: Karger, 1898

Pirozzolo, FJ. Cerebral asymmetries and reading acquisition. *Academic Therapy*, 1978, *13*, 261–266

Pirozzolo, FJ. *The neuropsychology of developmental reading disorders.* New York: Praeger Press, 1979

Pirozzolo, FJ. Language and brain: Neuropsychological aspects of developmental reading disability. *School Psychology Review*, 1981, *10*, 350–355

Pirozzolo, FJ, & Hansch, EC. The neurobiology of developmental reading disorders. In Malatesha, RN, & Aaron, PG (Eds.), *Neuropsychological and neurolinguistic aspects of reading disorders.* New York: Academic Press, 1982

Pirozzolo, FJ, & Hess, DW. A neuropsychological analysis of the ITPA. *New York State Orton Society Annual Convention Proceedings* (pamphlet), 1976

Pirozzolo, FJ, & Horner, FA. Auditory-memory and linguistic deficits in left temporal lobe agenesis: Evidence for linguistic specialization of the left hemisphere. *Brain and Language* (in press)

Pirozzolo, FJ, & Kerr, K. Recovery from alexia: Factors influencing restoration of function after focal cerebral damage. In Pirozzolo, FJ, & Witrock, MC (Eds.), *Neuropsychological and cognitive processes in reading.* New York: Academic Press, 1981

Pirozzolo, FJ, Pirozzolo, PH, & Ziman, RB. Neuropsychological assessment of callosal agenesis. *Clinical Neuropsychology*, 1979, *1*, 13–16

Pirozzolo, FJ, & Rayner, K. Cerebral organization and reading disability. *Neuropsychologia*, 1979, *17*, 485–491

Rabinovitch, RD. Reading and learning disabilities. In Arieti, S (Ed.), *American Handbook of Psychiatry* (Vol. 1). New York: Basic Books, 1959

Rakic, P, & Yakovlev, PI. Development of the corpus callosum and cavum septi in man. *Journal of Comparative Neurology*, 1968, *132*, 45–72

Rasmussen, D, & Goldberg, L. *SRA Basic Reading Series.* Chicago: Science Research Associates, 1966

Rasmussen, T, & Milner, B. Clinical and surgical studies of the cerebral speech areas in man. In Zulch, KJ, Creutzfeldt, O, & Galbraith, G (Eds.), *Otfrid Foerster symposium on cerebral localization.* Heidelberg: Springer-Verlag, 1975

Rasmussen, T, & Milner, B. The role of early left brain injury in determining lateralization of cerebral speech functions. *Annals of the New York Academy of Sciences*, 1977, *229*, 335–369

Reed, HBC. Pediatric neuropsychology. *Journal of Pediatric Psychology*, 1976, *1*, 5–7

Reitan, RM. Certain differential effects of left and right cerebral lesions in human adults. *Journal of Comparative and Physiological Psychology*, 1955, *48*, 474–477

Reitan, RM. Investigation of relationships between "psychometric" and "biological" intelligence. *Journal of Nervous and Mental Disease*, 1956, *123*, 536–541

Reitan, RM. Qualitative versus quantitative mental changes following brain damage. *Journal of Psychology*, 1958, *46*, 339–346

Reschly, D. *Neuropsychological versus behavioral models: A debate.* Presentation at the Annual Conference of the North Carolina Association of School Psychologists. Wilmington, North Carolina, September, 1982

Reynolds, CR. Neuropsychological assessment and the habilitation of learning: Considerations in the search for the aptitude x treatment interaction. *School Psychology Review*, 1981, *10*, 343–349

Reynolds, CR, Hartlage, LC, & Haak, R. *Lateral preference as determined by neuropsychological performance and aptitude/achievement discrepancies.* Paper presented to the Annual Meeting of the American Psychological Association, Montreal, Canada, September 1980

Richman, LC, & Kitchell, MM. Hyperlexia as a variant of developmental language disorder. *Brain and Language*, 1981, *12*, 203–212

Robbins, MP. A study of the validity of Delacato's theory of neurological organization. *Exceptional Children*, 1966, *32*, 517–523

Roberts, RW, & Coleman, JC. An investigation of the role of visual and kinesthetic factors in reading failure. *Journal of Educational Research*, 1958, *51*, 445–451

Robinson, RG. The temporal lobe agenesis syndrome. *Brain*, 1964, *83*, 87–100

Rosenberger, PB, & Hier, DB. Cerebral asymmetry and verbal intellectual deficits. *Annals of Neurology*, 1980, *8*, 300–304

Rosner, BB. Recovery of function and localization of function in historical perspective. In Stein, DG, Rosen, JJ, & Butters, N (Eds.), *Plasticity and recovery of function in the central nervous system*. New York: Academic Press, 1974

Ross, AO. *Psychological aspects of learning disabilities and reading disorders*. New York: McGraw-Hill, 1976

Ross, DM, & Ross, SA. *Hyperactivity, research, theory, action*. New York: John Wiley and Sons, 1976

Ross, ED. Disorders of higher cortical functions: Diagnosis and treatment. In Rosenberg, RN (Ed.), *Neurology*. New York: Grune & Stratton, Inc., 1980

Rossi, GF, & Rosadini, G. Experimental analysis of cerebral dominance in man. In Millikan, CF, & Darley, FL (Eds.), *Brain mechanisms underlying speech and language*. New York: Grune & Stratton, Inc., 1967

Rourke, BD. Issues in the neuropsychological assessment of children with learning disabilities. *Canadian Psychological Review*, 1976, *17*, 89–102

√Rourke, BP, Young, GC, & Flewelling, RW. The relationships between WISC verbal-performance discrepancies and selected verbal, auditory-perceptual, visual-perceptual, and problem solving abilities in children with learning disabilities. *Journal of Clinical Psychology*, 1971, *27*, 475–479

Rubens, AB. Agnosia. In Heilman, KM, & Valenstein, E (Eds.), *Clinical neuropsychology*. New York: Oxford University Press, 1979

Rudel, RG. Neuroplasticity: Implications for development and education. In Chall, JS, & Mirsky, AF (Eds.), *Education and the brain*. Chicago: University of Chicago Press, 1978

√Rudnick, M, Sterritt, GM, & Flax, M. Auditory and visual rhythm perception and reading ability. *Child Development*, 1967, *37*, 581–587

Rugel, RP. WISC subtest scores of disabled readers: A review with respect to Bannatyne's recategorization. *Journal of Learning Disabilities*, 1974, *7*, 48–55

Rutter, M, Graham, P, & Yule, W. *A neuropsychiatric study in childhood*. Philadelphia: Lippincott, 1970

Rutter, M, Tizard, J, & Whitmore, K (Eds.). *Education, health, and behavior*. London: Longmans, 1970

Rutter, M, & Yule, W. The concept of specific reading retardation. *Journal of Child Psychology and Psychiatry*, 1975, *16*, 161–197

Rylander, G. *Personality changes after operations on the frontal lobes*. London: Oxford University Press, 1939

Sadick, TL, & Ginsburg, BE. The development of the lateral functions and reading ability. *Cortex*, 1978, *14*, 3–11

Sandoval, J, & Haapanen, RM. A critical commentary on neuropsychology in the schools: Are we ready? *School Psychology Review*, 1981, *10*, 381–388

Sarno, J, Sarno, M, & Levita, E. Evaluating language improvement after completed stroke. *Archives of Physical Medicine and Rehabilitation*, 1971, *52*, 73–78

Satz, P. Cerebral dominance and reading disability. In Knights, RM, & Bakker, DJ (Eds.), *Neuropsychology of learning disorders: Theoretical approaches*. Baltimore: University Park Press, 1976

Satz, P, & Friel, J. Some predictive antecedents of specific learning disability: A preliminary one year follow-up. In Satz, P & Ross, J (Eds.), *The disabled learner*. Rotterdam: Rotterdam University Press, 1973

Satz, P, & Friel, J. Some predictive antecedents of specific reading disability: A preliminary two year follow-up. *Journal of Learning Disabilities*, 1974, *7*, 437–444

Satz, P, Friel, J, & Rudegeair, F. Differential changes in the acquisition of developmental skills in children who later became dyslexic. In Stein, DG, Rosen, JJ, and Butters, N (Eds.), *Plasticity and recovery of function in the central nervous system.* New York: Academic Press, 1974

Satz, P, Friel, J, & Rudegeair, F. Some predictive antecedents of specific reading disability: A two-, three-, and four-year follow-up. In Guthrie, JT (Ed.), *Aspects of reading acquisition.* Baltimore: Johns Hopkins Press, 1976

Satz, P, & Morris, R. Learning disability subtypes: A review. In Pirozzolo, FJ, & Wittrock MC (Eds.), *Neuropsychological and cognitive processes in reading.* New York: Academic Press, 1981

Satz, P. Rardin, D, & Ross, J. An evaluation of a theory of specific developmental dyslexia. *Child Development,* 1971, *42,* 2009–2021

Satz, P, & Sparrow, S. Specific developmental dyslexia: A theoretical reformation. In Bakker, DJ, & Satz, P (Eds.), *Specific reading disability: Advances in theory and method.* Rotterdam: University of Rotterdam Press, 1970

Sauerwin, HC, Lassonde, MC, Cardu, B, & Geoffroy, G. Interhemispheric integration of sensory and motor functions in agenesis of the corpus callosum. *Neuropsychologia,* 1981, *19,* 445–454

Saul, RE, & Sperry, RW. Absence of commissurotomy symptoms with agenesis of the corpus callosum. *Neurology,* 1968, *18,* 307–315

Schaltenbrand, G, & Woolsey, CN. *Cerebral localization and organization.* Madison: University of Wisconsin Press, 1964

Schepers, GWH. The corpus structure in the South African Negro brain. *American Journal of Physical Anthropology,* 1938, *24,* 161–184

Schneider, GE. Is it really better to have your brain lesion early? A revision of the "Kennard Principle." *Neuropsychologia,* 1979, *17,* 557–584

Schurr, PH. Head injuries. In Rose, FC, (Ed.), *Paediatric neurology.* Oxford: Blackwell Scientific Publishers, 1979

Sears, ES, & Franklin, GM. Diseases of the cranial nerves. In Rosenberg, RN (Ed.), *Neurology.* New York: Grune & Stratton, 1980

Selnes, OA. The corpus callosum: Some anatomical and functional considerations with special reference to language. *Brain and Language,* 1974, *1,* 111–140.

Selz, M. Halstead-Reitan Neuropsychological Test Batteries For Children. In Hynd, GW, & Obrzut, JE (Eds.), *Neuropsychological assessment and the school-age child: Issues and procedures.* New York: Grune & Stratton, 1981

Senf, GM. Development of immediate memory for bisensory stimuli in normal children, and children with learning disabilities. *Developmental Psychology,* 1969, *6,* 28–32

Senf, GM, & Feshback, S. Development of bisensory memory in culturally deprived dyslexic and normal readers. *Journal of Education Psychology,* 1970, *61,* 461–470

Senf, GM, & Freundl, PC. Memory and attention factors in specific learning disabilities. *Journal of Learning Disabilities,* 1971, *4,* 94–106

Scholl, DA. *The organization of the cerebral cortex.* London: Methuen, 1956

Shoumura, K, Ando, T, & Kato, K. Structural organization of "callosal" OB in human corpus callosum agenesis. *Brain Research,* 1975, *93,* 241–252

Silberberg, NE, Iversen, IA, & Goins, JT. Which remedial method works best? *Journal of Learning Disabilities,* 1973, *6,* 547–557

Silver, A, & Hagen, R. Memory and attention factors in specific learnings disabilities. *Journal of Learning Disabilities,* 1971, *4,* 94–106

Silverberg, R, & Gordon, HW. Differential aphasia in two bilingual individuals. *Neurology,* 1979, *29,* 51–55

Skinner, BF. *The behavior of organisms.* New York: Appleton-Century, 1938

Sladen, BK. Inheritance of dyslexia. *Bulletin of the Orton Society,* 1970, *20,* 30–40

Smith, A. Principles underlying human brain functions in neuropsychological sequelae of different neuropathological processes. In Filskov, SB, & Boll, TJ (Eds.), *Handbook of clinical neuropsychology*. New York: John Wiley and Sons, 1981

Smith, F. *Understanding reading* (3rd ed.). New York: Holt, Rinehart, & Winston, 1982

Smith, MD, Coleman, JM, Dokecki, PR, & Davis, EE. Recategorized WISC-R scores of learning disabled children. *Journal of Learning Disabilities*, 1977, *10*, 444–449

Snow, JH, Hynd, GW, & Hartlage, LC. Differences between mildly and more severely learning disabled children on the Luria-Nebraska Neuropsychological Battery—Children's Revision. *Journal of Psychoeducational Assessment* (in press)

Snyder, RD. The right not to read. *Pediatrics*, 1979, *63*, 791–794 (a)

Snyder, RD. The right not to read controversy. *Pediatrics*, 1979, *64*, 977–978 (b)

Snyder, RD. Topographic mapping in childhood developmental dyslexia. *Annals of Neurology*, 1980, 7, 642–643

Sowell, VM. *The efficacy of psycholinguistic training through the MWM Program*. Unpublished Doctoral dissertation, Austin, University of Texas, 1975

Spache, GD. *Diagnosing and correcting reading disabilities*. Boston: Allyn & Bacon, 1976

Sperry, RW. Cerebral organization and behavior. *Science*, 1961, *133*, 1749–1757

Sperry, RW. The great cerebral commissure. *Scientific American*, 1964, *210*, 240–250

Sperry, RW. Cerebral dominance in perception. In Young, FA, & Lindsley, DB (Eds.), *Early experience in visual information processing in perceptual reading disorders*. Washington, DC: National Academy of Science, 1970

Sperry, RW. Lateral specialization of cerebral function in the surgically separated hemispheres. In McGuigan, F (Ed.), *The psychophysiology of thinking*. New York: Academic Press, 1973

Sperry, RW. Lateral specialization in the surgically separated hemispheres. In Schmitt, FO, & Worden, FG (Eds.), *The neurosciences third study program*. Cambridge: MIT Press, 1974

Sperry, RW, Gazzaniga, MS, & Bogen, JH. Interhemispheric relationships: The neocortical commissures; syndromes of hemisphere disconnection. In Vinken, PJ, & Bruyn, GW (Eds.), *Handbook of clinical psychology* (Vol. 4). New York: John Wiley and Sons, 1969

Spitzka, EA. Report of a study of the brains of six eminent scientists and scholars belonging to the American Anthropometric Society; together with a brief description of the skull by one of them. *American Journal of Anatomy*, 1905, *4*(3)

Stark, R. An investigation of unilateral cerebral pathology with equated verbal and visual-spatial tasks. *Journal of Abnormal and Social Psychology*, 1961, *62*, 282–287

Stauffer, RG. *The language experience approach to the teaching of reading*. New York: Harper & Row, 1970

Stedman's medical dictionary. Baltimore: The Williams & Wilkins Company, 1972

Stephenson, S. Six cases of congenital word-blindness affecting three generations of one family. *Ophthalmoscope*, 1907, *5*, 482–484

Sterritt, GM, & Rudnick, M. Auditory and visual rhythm perception in relation to reading ability in fourth grade boys. *Perceptual and Motor Skills*, 1966, *22*, 859–864

Stoch, MB, & Smythe, PM. Undernutrition during infancy, and subsequent brain growth and intellectual development. In Scrimshaw, NS, & Gordon, JE (Eds.), *Malnutrition, Learning, and Behavior*. Cambridge: MIT Press, 1968

Stumpf, SE. *Socrates to Sartre: A history of philosophy*. New York: McGraw-Hill, 1966

Swiercinsky, DP. Factorial pattern description and comparison of functional abilities in neuropsychological assessment. *Perceptual and Motor Skills*, 1979, *48*, 231–241

Talmadge, M, Davids, A, & Laufer, M. A study of experimental methods for teaching emotionally disturbed, brain damaged, retarded readers. *Journal of Educational Research*, 1963, *56*(2)

Teeter, A, & Hynd, GW. Agenesis of the corpus callosum: A developmental study during infancy. *Clinical Neuropsychology*, 1981, *3*, 29–32

Teitelbaum, P, & Epstein, AA. The lateral hypothalamic syndrome: Recovery of feeding and drinking after lateral hypothalamic lesions. *Psychological Preview*, 1962, *69*, 74–90

Teitelbaum, P, & Stellar, E. Recovery from the failure to eat produced by hypothalamic lesions. *Science*, 1954, *120*, 893–895

Thomas, CJ. Congenital "word-blindness" and its treatment. *Ophthalmoscope*, 1905, *3*, 380–385

Tindall, R. School psychology: The development of a profession. In Phye, G & Reschly, D (Eds.), *School psychology: Perspectives and issues*. New York: Academic Press, 1979

Tobin, D, & Pumfrey, PD. Some long-term effects of the remedial teaching of reading. *Educational Review*, 1976, *29*, 1–12

Tomasch, J. Size, distribution, and number of fibers in the human corpus callosum. *Anatomical Record*, 1954, *119*, 119–135

Torrance, EP, Reynolds, CR, Ball, OE, & Riegel, T. *Norms-Technical Manual for Your Style of Learning and Thinking* (Revised). Athens: University of Georgia, Department of Educational Psychology, 1978

Twitchell, TE. The automatic grasping response in infants. *Neuropsychologia*, 1965, *3*, 247–259

Ukhtomskii. *Essays on the Physiology of the Nervous System*, Collected works, (Vol. 4). Leningrad, 1945

Ullman, DG. Children's lateral preference patterns: Frequency and relationships with achievement and intelligence. *Journal of School Psychology*, 1977, *15*, 36–43

Ulrich, R, Stachnik, T, & Mabry, J. *Control of human behavior* (Vol. 2). New York, Scott Foresman, 1970

Ulrich, R, Stachnik, T, & Mabry, J. *Control of human behavior* (Vol. 3). New York, Scott Foresman, 1974

Valett, RE. *Dyslexia: A neuropsychological approach to educating children with severe reading disorders*. Belmont: Fearon Pitman Publishers, Inc., 1980

Vande Voort, L, & Senf, GM. Audiovisual integration in retarded readers. *Journal of Learning Disabilities*, 1973, *6*, 170–179

Vande Voort, L, Senf, GM, Benton, AL. Development of audiovisual integration in normal and retarded readers. *Child Development*, 1972, *43*, 1260–1272

Variot, G, & Lecomte, A. Un cas de typholexia congenitale (cécité congénitale verbale). *Bulletins et Memoires de la Société-Medicale des Hopitaux des Paris*, 1906, *23*, 995–1001

✓Vellutino, FF. Toward an understanding of dyslexia: Psychological factors in specific reading disabilities. In Benton, AL, & Pearl, D. (Eds.), *Dyslexia: An appraisal of current knowledge*. New York: Oxford University Press, 1978

✓Vellutino, FF, Smith, H, Steger, JA, & Kaman, M. Reading disability: Age differences and the perceptual deficit hypothesis. *Child Development*, 1975, *46*, 487–493

Vellutino, FF, Steger, JA, Kaman, M., & Desetto, L. Visual form perception in deficient and normal readers. *Cortex*, 1975, *11*, 22–30

✓Vellutino, FF, Steger, JA, & Kandel, G. Reading disability: An investigation of the perceptual deficit hypothesis. *Cortex*, 1972, *8*, 106–118

Vellutino, FF, Steger, JA, & Pruzek, K. Inter vs. intrasensory deficit in paired associate learning in poor and normal readers. *Canadian Journal of Behavioral Sciences*, 1973, 111–123

Vignolo, LA. Evolution of aphasia and language rehabilitation: A retrospective exploratory study. *Cortex*, 1964, *1*, 344–367

Villaverde, JM. De la terminaison des fibres du corps calleux dans le cerveau. *Revue Neurologique*, 1931, *38*, 518–519

Von Bonin, G. Anatomical asymmetries of the cerebral hemispheres. In Mountcastle, VB (Ed.), *Interhemispheric relations and cerebral dominance*. Baltimore: Johns Hopkins Press, 1962

Von Bonin, G, & Bailey, P. Pattern of the cerebral isocortex. In Hofer, H, Schultz, AH, & Starck, D (Eds.), *Primatologia*. Basel, Karger, 1961

Von Monakow, CV. Lokalization der hirnfunktionen. *Journal für Psychologie und Neurologie*, 1911, *17*, 185–200

Voss, G. Ueber die assoziationsprüfung bei kindern nebst einen beitrag zur frage der "wort-blindheit." *Z. Neurol.*, 1914, *26*, 340–351

Wada, JA, Clarke, R, & Hamm, A. Cerebral hemisphere asymmetry in humans: Cortical speech zones in 100 adult and 100 infant brains. *Archives of Neurology*, 1975, *32*, 239–246

Walzer, S, & Richmond, JB. The epidemiology of learning disorders. *Pediatric Clinics of North America*, 1973, *20*, 549–565

Warburg, F. Ueber die angeborene wortblindheit und die bedeatung ihrer kenntnis für der unterricht. *Z. Kinder-Forschung*, 1911, *16*, 97–113

Warren, JM, & Nonneman, AJ. The search for cerebral dominance in monkeys. *Annals of the New York Academy of Science*, 1976, *280*, 732–744

Webster's third new international dictionary (unabridged). Chicago: Encyclopedia Britannica. Inc., 1966

Wechsler, A. Transient left hemialexia: A clinical and angiographic study. *Neurology*, 1972, *22*, 628–633

Wechsler, A, Weinstein, EA, & Antin, SP. Alexia without agraphia. *Bulletin of the Los Angeles Neurological Society*, 1972, *37*, 1–11

Weiderholt, JA, & Hammill, DD. Use of the Frostig-Horne Perception Program in the urban school. *Psychology in the Schools*, 1971, *8*, 268–274

Weinshank, AB. The right not to read controversy. *Pediatrics*, 1979, *64*, 976–977

Weisenburg, TS, & McBride, KC. *Aphasia: A clinical and psychological study.* New York: Commonwealth Fund, 1935

Weisenburg, TS, & McBride, KC. *Aphasia.* New York: Hafner, 1964

Wepman, JM. *Recovery from aphasia.* New York: Ronald Press, 1951

Wepman, JM. *Auditory discrimination test.* Chicago: Language Research Associates, 1958

Wernicke, C. *Der aphasiche symptomenkomplex.* Breslau: Cohn and Weigert, 1874

Whitaker, HA. Neurobiology of language. In Carterette, ER, & Friedman, MP (Eds.), *Handbook of perception* (Vol. 7). New York: Academic Press, 1976

Whitaker, HA. *Electrical stimulation studies of the language regions of the brain.* Presentation to the GRECC Clinical Conference, V. A. Medical Center, Minneapolis, May, 1981

Whitty, CWM, & Zangwill, OL. Traumatic amnesia. In Whitty, CWM, & Zangwill, OL (Eds.), *Amnesia.* London: Butterworths, 1966

Wilde, W. *Practical observations on aural surgery.* London: J. Churchill, 1853

Wilkie, OL. The right not to read controversy. *Pediatrics* (letter), 1979, *64*, 977

Wilson, RM. *Diagnostic and remedial reading: For classroom and clinic* (4th ed.). Columbus: Charles E. Merrill, 1981

Wilson, SAK. *Aphasia.* London: Kegan Paul, 1926

Witelson, SF. Abnormal right hemisphere specialization in developmental dyslexia. In Knights, RM, & Bakker, DJ (Eds.), *Neuropsychology of learning disorders: Theoretical approaches.* Baltimore: University Park Press, 1976

Witelson, SF. Developmental dyslexia: Two right hemispheres and none left. *Science*, 1977, *195*, 309–311

Witelson, SF, & Pallie, W. Left hemisphere specialization for language in the newborn: Neuroanatomical evidence of asymmetry. *Brain*, 1973, *96*, 671–646

Witelson, SF, & Rabinovitch, MS. Hemispheric speech lateralization in children with auditory-linguistic deficits. *Cortex*, 1972, *8*, 412–426

Witherspoon, YT. Brain weight and behavior. *Human Biology*, 1960, *32*, 366–369

Woertz, RT, Collins, MJ, Brookshire, R, Friden, T, Kurtzke, J, Pierce, J, & Weiss, D. *The Veterans Administration cooperative study on aphasia.* Paper presented to the Academy of Aphasia, Chicago, 1978

Wolpe, J. Cognition and causation in human behavior and its therapy. *American Psychologist*, 1978, *33*, 437–446

Woo, TL, & Pearson, K. Dextrality and sinistrality of hand and eye. *Biometrica*, 1972, *19*, 165–169

Woods, BT, & Teuber, HC. Early onset of complementary specialization of cerebral hemispheres in man. *Transactions of the American Neurological Association*, 1973, *98*, 113–117

Yakovlev, PI, & Lecours, AR. The myelogenetic cycles of regional maturation in the brain. In Minkowski, A (Ed.), *Regional development of the brain in early life*. Oxford: Blackwell, 1967

Yeni-Komshian, GH, Isenberg, P, & Goldstein, H. Cerebral dominance and reading disability: Left visual-field deficit in poor readers. *Neuropsychologia*, 1975, *13*, 83–94

Young, WM. Poverty, intelligence, and life in the inner city. *Mental Retardation*, 1969, *7*, 24–33

Yule, W. Differential prognosis of reading backwardness and specific reading retardation. *British Journal of Educational Psychology*, 1973, *43*, 244–248

Yule, W, & Rutter, M. Epidemiology and social implications of specific reading retardation. In Knights, RM, & Bakker, DJ (Eds.), *The neuropsychology of learning disorders: Theoretical approaches*. Baltimore: University Park Press, 1976

Zaidel, S. Auditory vocabulary of the right hemisphere following brain bisection or hemidecortication. *Cortex*, 1976, *12*, 191–211

Zaidel, E. The split and half brains as models of congenital language disability. In Ludlow, CL, & Doran-Quine, ME (Eds.), *The neurological bases of language disorders in children: Methods and directions for research*. NIH Publication No. 79-440, Washington, DC: U. S. Government Printing Office, 1979

Zarske, J. Neuropsychological intervention approaches for handicapped children. *Journal of Research and Development in Education*, 1982, *15*, 66–75

Zinkus, PW, Gottlieb, Mi, & Shapiro, M. Developmental and psychoeducational sequelae of chronic otitis media. *American Journal of Disease of Childhood*, 1978, *132*, 1110–1117

Zurif, EB, & Carson, G. Dyslexia in relation to cerebral dominance and temporal analysis. *Neuropsychologia*, 1970, *8*, 351–361

Index

Absence seizures, *see* Seizures, petit mal
Academic achievement, 175, 184–186
  formal batteries for, 175, 185–186
  informal evaluation of, 175, 184–186
Agenesis, 55, 60–69, 95
  case study literature on, 63–69
  of corpus callosum, 61–62
  definition of, 60–61
  of left temporal lobe, 66–69
  of vermis of cerebellum, 64
Agnosia, 44–45, 137, 144–145, 173
  theories of, 45
  types of, 45–46
Agrammatism, 145
Agraphia, 76–77. *See also* Dysgraphia
Alexia, 11, 74, 76–82, 92, 140–141. *See also*
  Subgroups of Dyslexia
  recovery from, 76–82
  types of, 76
Alpha activity, 87, 88
American Psychological Association, 13, 191
American Speech and Hearing Association,
  10
Amnesia, 75, 96
Amygdala, 48
Angiography, 67
Angular gyrus, 12–13, 47, 51, 57–60, 76–77,
  87–88, 91–92, 95, 137
  reading process and, 57–60
  uniqueness of, 59

Anomia, 29, 76, 142–145, 172, 227
Anterior lobe, *see* Frontal lobe
Antilocalizationists, 29. *See also* Equipoten-
  tiality
Aphasia, 29, 71, 74, 76–79, 89, 116, 137, 172,
  182–183
  recovery from, 76–79
  types of, 76
Aphasia Screening Test, 174, 179, 181, 194,
  200
Aphemia, 29
Apraxia, 31, 46–47. *See also* Dyspraxia
  dressing, 31
  ideational, 46–47
  ideomotor, 46–47
Arachnoid cysts, 66
Archicerebellum, 37
Arcurate fasciculus, 57, 59–60, 77
Association cortex, *see* Cerebral cortex, asso-
  ciation areas of
Association fibers, 39, 59
Association for Children and Adults with
  Learning Disabilities, 10
Asymmetry, ear, 123. *See also* Cerebral asym-
  metry; Dichotic listening; Right ear ad-
  vantage
Attention, 37, 50, 108, 112, 211–212, 225
  deficits of, 37, 50, 211–212, 225
Auditory nerve, 117. *See also* Cranial nerves
Auditory pathway, 117

Autopsy on dyslexics' brains, *see* Cytoarchitectonic studies of dyslexics' brains
Axon, 33–39

Backward readers, 18–19
  prognosis of, 19
BEAM, *see* Brain electrical activity mapping
Beery VMI, *see* Developmental Test of Visual Motor Integration
Bender Visual-Motor Gestalt Test, 101, 174, 176–178, 191, 195, 201
Benton Test of Visual Retention, 142–143, 174
Bisensory memory task, *see* Memory, bisensory
Boder Diagnostic Reading-Spelling Test, 175, 186, 201
Boston Diagnostic Aphasia Examination, 175, 179, 182
Bradykinesia, 50
Brain, 26–52, 60–82, 90–95, 213. *See also* Trauma to brain
  cytoarchitectonic studies of, 90–95
  development of, 32–35
  disordered function of, 60–82
  functional organization of, 26–52, 93, 187
  hierarchical organization of, 30, 213
  weight of, 32
Brain–behavior relationships, 26, 28, 31, 51, 55, 167, 169–170, 176
  in children, 70
  methods to study, 31
Brain damage, *see* Trauma to brain
Brain electrical activity mapping, 16, 86–87, 89–90, 92, 112
Brain injury, *see* Trauma to brain
Brain stem, 28, 35–37, 51, 164, 179
Broca's area, 49, 56–57, 59–60, 77, 88
Bulb, *see* Medulla

Category Test, 175, 188, 194, 200
Central fissure, *see* Central sulcus
Central nervous system, 9–10, 32–35, 73, 162, 164, 166, 224
  development of, 32–35
  learning disabilities and, 9–10
Central sulcus, 36, 42–43, 49
Cerebellum, 36–37, 51, 64, 91–92, 163–164, 178–179, 206
  agenesis of vermis of, 64

functions of, 163, 178–179
  hemorrhage of, 91–92
  motor deficits and, 37
  zones of, 37
Cerebral asymmetry, 4, 14, 16, 23, 47, 51, 56, 66, 82–86, 90, 93, 96, 126
  central and peripheral measures of, 14
  neurodevelopmental, in dyslexics, 82–86, 96
Cerebral cortex, 35–37, 39–51, 57–59, 69, 88, 95, 113, 117, 137, 173, 187, 212. *See also* names of lobes, cortex of
  association areas of, 42–43, 49, 57, 59, 88, 95, 113, 137
  electrostimulation of, 35–36, 40
  functional organization of, 40–51
  maturation of, 57–58
  primary projection zones of, 42–46, 49, 59, 113, 117
Cerebral dominance, 4, 13–14, 16, 65, 71, 82, 91, 97, 114–136, 146, 149, 212
  deficits in, 4, 13, 97
  delays in, 14, 97
  dyslexia and, 114–135
Cerebral function, tests of, 163
Cerebral hemisphere, 13, 23, 30–31, 39–42, 47, 62, 68, 70–71, 73, 76, 78, 82–83, 87–88, 93–94, 96, 111, 117–118, 120, 123–127, 130, 133–135, 147–149, 151, 153, 156–157, 176, 183, 189
  functions attributed to, 40–42
  left, 13, 23, 30, 40, 47, 70–71, 76, 87, 93–94, 111, 117–118, 120, 123–124, 126–127, 134–135, 147–149, 151, 153, 156–157, 176, 183
  right, 13, 30–31, 40, 78, 117–118, 120, 123, 127, 130, 133–134, 148, 151, 153, 156–157, 183, 189
Cerebral lateralization, 23, 65, 68, 70, 75, 82–83, 91, 93, 114–116, 122, 146–148, 152. *See also* Dichotic listening; Wada technique
Cerebral localization, 12, 28–32, 40, 51, 167–168, 185
  evidence against, 31
  theory of, 30–32
Cerebral palsy, 181
Cerebrum, *see* Telencephalon
Child guidance movement, 13
Child Neurology Society, 6, 143, 146
  Task Force on Nosology of Disorders of Higher Cerebral Functions in Children, 6

Cingulate gyrus, 94
Clinical interview, 175, 184
Closed head injury, *see* Trauma to brain
Cochlea, 117
Cognitive ability, 13, 28, 60–82, 136, 162, 163–164, 166, 168, 175–176, 178, 180–181, 186–190, 230
    assessment of, 13, 175, 186–190
    deficits in, associated with brain injury, 74–76
    disordered brain function and, 60–82
    functional differentiation of processes of, 28
Coma, 75
Commisural fibers, 39
Communication between professionals, lack of, 7–8
Computerized brain mapping techniques, 16
Computerized tomography, 67, 80, 83, 90, 163
Concussion, 70–71
Congenital word blindness, 5, 11–13, 20, 25
Contrecoup effect, 71, 74
Corpus callosum, 36, 39, 59, 61–66, 76–77, 92
    agenisis of, 61–66
    development of, 62
    regions of, 61–62
Corpus striatum, 29
Cortex, *see* Cerebral cortex
Council for Learning Disabilities, 10
Cranial nerves, 38, 163–164
Craniotomy, 40, 80–81
Cross-modal integration, 97, 103–112
    dysfunction in, 103–112
CT scan, *see* Computerized tomography
Culturally deprived children, 108
Cytoarchitectonic studies of dyslexics' brains, 90–95, 112. *See also* Cerebral localization
Cytomegalovirus, 62

Dandy-Walker syndrome, 64
Dendrite, 33–34
Developmental delay, 3–5, 14, 27, 58, 97, 115, 121–127, 177
    concept of, 121–127
    versus deficit, 3, 27, 58, 97, 115
Developmental Program in Visual Perception, 221
Developmental Test of Visual Motor Integration, 174, 177, 214

Developmental Test of Visual Perception, 101, 221–222
Diaschisis, 72
Dichotic listening, 31, 81, 86, 93–94, 117–127, 147, 149, 154, 163, 175, 181, 183, 195, 201
    research in, 117–127
Diencephalon, 32, 35, 38–39
    composition of, 38–39
Differential diagnosis, 157, 162, 181
Division for Children with Communication Disorders, 10
Dolch Word List, 185, 201
Doman-Delacato neurological organization remedial approach, 212–215, 231–232
    research findings with, 213–215
Dominant cerebral hemisphere, *see* Cerebral hemisphere, left
Duchenne's muscular dystrophy, 162
Durrell Analysis of Reading Difficulties, 175, 185
Dysarthria, 37, 174, 179
Dyseidetic dyslexia, *see* Subgroups of dyslexia
Dysgraphia, 89, 144–145
Dyslexia, 3–7, 9–26, 39, 82, 86–91, 94, 97–136, 142, 161, 166, 193–205, 223. *See also* Prevalence of, dyslexia; Reading failure; Remedial approaches to dyslexia; Subgroups of dyslexia; Treatment of dyslexia
    case studies of, 193–205
    causes of/explanations for, 9–10, 13, 39, 82, 97, 103, 136
    cerebral dominance and, 114–135
    concept of, 5, 25
    controversy over, 3, 25
    definitions of, 4–6, 9–11, 17, 142
    diagnosis of, 161, 166, 223
    electroencephalographic research in, 86–90
    epidemiology of, 16–25
    genetic transmission of, 11–12, 21–22, 25, 91, 94
    history of, 11–16
    incidence of, 6, 20, 22, 24–25
    male to female ratio in, 12, 19, 21–23, 25
    recent advances in research on, 15–16
    resistance to term of, 6–7, 25
    single factor research in, 98–113
Dysmetria, 179
Dysphonic dyslexia, *see* Subgroups of dyslexia

Dysplasia, 93–94
Dyspraxia, 227, *see also* Apraxia
Dystaxia, 37, 179

Ear asymmetry, *see* Asymmetry, ear
Edema, 72
Edinburgh inventory, 174, 180
EEG, *see* Electroencephalograph
Electroencephalograph, 31, 86–90, 92, 96,
    154, 163. *See also* Brain electrical activity
    mapping
    research with dyslexics, 86–90
Electrostimulation, 31, 35–36, 40
    of cerebral cortex, 35–36, 40
Epilepsy, *see* Seizures
Equipotentiality, 29, 31, 69. *See also* Plasticity
    of brain function; Recovery of function
ERP, *see* Event-related potential
Event-related potential, 153, 155
Evoked potential, 87–88, 163. *See also* Neural
    impulse
Exophthalmos, 66
Eyedness, 115

[18]FDG positron emission tomography, 16
Feral children, 71
Fernald remedial approach, 209–212, 226, 231,
    research findings with, 210–212
Finger Agnosia Test, 173–174, 180, 195, 201
Finger Oscillation Test, 174, 180, 195, 201
Finger Tapping Test, *see* Finger Oscillation
    Test
Finger-Tip Number Writing Task, 174, 178,
    180
Fissure of Rolando, *see* Central sulcus
Fluency Test, 175, 181–182
Footedness, 115
Forebrain, 38–39
    subdivisions of, 38
Frontal lobe, 28–29, 37, 49–51, 56, 88–89,
    135, 187, 189
    cortex of, 49–50
    development of, 50
    effects of damage to, 29, 49–50, 88–89
    effects on reticular activating system, 37,
    135
Frostig-Horne Perceptual Training remedial
    approach, 221–222, 231
    research findings with, 221–222

Functional system, 167–168, 187, 224. *See also*
    Reading, functional system of

Gates-McGinite Reading Readiness Test, 124
Gates-McKillop Reading Diagnostic Test,
    175, 185
Gates Primary Reading Test, 106
Gerstmann syndrome, 46, 76, 137–138
Goodenough Draw-A-Person Test, 101
Graphesthesia, 46
Gray Oral Reading Tests, 102, 214
Grip Strength Test, 174, 180, 201
Group Reading Screening Test, 229
Gyri, 32, 91
    development of, 32

Halstead Neuropsychological Test Battery,
    166–168
Halstead-Reitan Lateral Dominance Exami-
    nation, 174, 180
Halstead-Wepman Aphasia Screening Test,
    182
Handedness, 14, 115–116
Hard neurological signs, 161
Harris Test of Lateral Dominance, 214
Hematoma, subdural, 66, 70
Hemianopsia, 76, 79
Hemiparesis, 79
Hemispherectomy, 66, 68, 71, 74
Hemispheric specialization, *see* Cerebral later-
    alization
Hemorrhage, intracranial, 91–92
Heschl's gyrus, 43, 47–48
    effects of damage to, 48
Hindbrain, 35–37
Hippocampus, 48
Hydrocephalus, 63
Hyperactivity, 36–37, 50, 87, 89, 212, 225
Hyperlexia, 91, 146
Hypothalamus, 35–36, 39
    results of lesions of, 39
Hypotonia, 37, 174, 179

Illinois Test of Psycholinguistic Ability, 47,
    138, 143–144, 175, 182, 194, 215–219,
    231
    remedial approach based on, 215–218, 231
    research findings with remedial approach of,
    216–218

Inferior colliculus, 117
Information processing, hierarchy of, 171, 174–176, 181, 192
Insula, 29, 94
Intellectual ability, *see* Cognitive ability
International Reading Association, 10, 208, 230
Task Force on Definition of Dyslexia, 10
Iowa Test of Basic Skills, 104
Isle of Wright studies, 18
Isotope brain scan, 67

Kaufman Assessment Battery for Children, 175, 189
Kephart Perceptual Training remedial approach, 218–21, 231
research findings with, 219–221

Labels, 8
Language, 30, 47–49, 55–96, 122, 126, 136–138, 142, 144, 181–183, 192, 215
comprehension of, 30, 47–48, 57, 66, 142
dimensions of, 215
expression of, 49, 57, 66
neurologic aspects of, 56–60
neuropsychology of, 55–96
process of reading and, 30
shift of functions of, 74
Lateral geniculate body, 128
Laterality, 13, 15, 21, 115–117, 180–181, 214. *See also* Cerebral lateralization
asymmetries in, 115–117
Lateralization, *see* Cerebral lateralization
Learning disability, 107–108, 118, 134, 161, 180, 215, 229
Learning modalities, 175, 185–186
Legal rights of handicapped children, 4, 9
Limbic system, 39, 48, 51, 60
Localization, *see* Cerebral localization
Luria-Nebraska Neuropsychological Battery—Children's Revision, 166–168, 193, 224

Mass action, *see* Equipotentiality
Maturational lag, *see* Developmental delay
McCarthy Scales of Children's Abilities, 175, 189
Medial geniculate body, 117
Medical model, 16–17, 26

Medulla, 32, 35–36, 212
development of, 32
Megaloencephalus, 64
Memory, 106–112, 136, 149–151, 181
bisensory, 106–110, 149–151
temporal order, 110–112, 136
Mental testing, *see* Cognitive ability, assessment of
Mentation, *see* Cognitive ability
Metropolitan Achievement Test, 105, 222
Metropolitan Readiness Test, 124, 222, 228–229
Micropolygria, 62
Midbrain, 32, 36–38, 117, 212–213
development of, 32
location of, 37
Mills Learning Methods Test, 175, 185
Mindblindness, *see* Agnosia
Mind versus soul conceptualization, 27–28
Minor cerebral hemisphere, *see* Cerebral hemisphere, right
Motoric evaluation, 174, 178–181
Motor strip, 43, 49
Multidisciplinary Team, 185
Myelinization, 33–34, 62

National Council on Measurement in Education, 208
National Foundation for Educational Research Reading Test, 129
National Joint Committee for Learning Disabilities, 9–10
definition of learning disabilities, 9
Neocerebellum, 37
Neural impulse, 33. *See also* Evoked potential
Neural regeneration, 73
Neural sprouting, 73
Neural tube, 32
Neurilemma, 33, 73
Neurodevelopmental anomaly, 4, 11, 25, 60, 62, 66, 69, 82, 168, 172
Neurological development, 32–35
Neurologic examination, 162–165, 192
focus of, 163
format of, 162–165
instruments used in, 163
reasons for referral for, 165, 192
Neurology, functional, *see* Brain, functional organization of
Neuron, 33–34, 92
composition of, 33

Neuron (continued)
ectopic, 92
number of, 33
size of, 33
Neurone Doctrine, 32–35
Neuropsychological evaluation, 16, 27, 67, 80, 142–143, 161–205
case study examples of, 193–205
conceptual framework of, 193–205
dyslexic children and, 161–205
integration of, with behavioral approaches, 169–170
perspectives on, 166–170
pitfalls of, 190–192
procedures in, 16, 142–143
purpose of, 168–169
test batteries for, 166–168, 174–175
Neuropsychological treatment approach, 222–230
research findings with, 225–230
Neuropsychologist, qualifications of, 190–192
Nuclear magnetic resonance imagery of the brain, 16
Nystagmus, 37, 174, 179–180

Occipital lobe, 44–45, 59, 76, 79, 95, 128, 189
cortex of, 44–45, 95, 128
Open head injury, see Trauma to the brain
Operculum, 56
Ophthalmology, 12
Optic chiasm, 128
Optic nerve, 128. See also Cranial nerves
Optic radiation, 128
Orton Dyslexia Society, 10
Orton-Gillingham remedial approach, 207–209, 225–226, 230–231
research findings with, 208–209
Orzeck Aphasia Evaluation, 175, 179, 182
Oscillopsia, 179
Otitis media, 173

Paleocerebellum, 37
Paraphasia, 182
Parietal lobe, 44–47, 56, 60, 87, 91, 95, 182, 187, 189
cortex of, 44–47, 60, 95
effects of damage to, 46–47, 176–178
Peabody Language Development Kit, 216
Peabody Picture Vocabulary Test, 123, 128, 194, 214

Peabody Picture Vocabulary Test—Revised, 175, 182, 200
Perceptual-deficit hypothesis, 97–103
controversy over, 99–102
problems with research on, 102–103
support for, 98–99
Perceptual processes, 174, 176–178
Peripheral nervous system, 73, 164
Personality, importance of evaluation of, 184. See also Reading failure, emotional components of
Petit mal seizures, see Seizures, petit mal
Philadelphia Arithmetic Test, 222
Philadelphia Readiness Test, 222
Philadelphia Reading Test, 222
Phrenology, 28, 31
Planum temporale, 47–48, 51, 83, 93
Plasticity of brain function, 68–74, 81, 96. See also Equipotentiality; Recovery of function
mechanism of, 72–74
Polymicrogyria, 93–94
Pons, 32, 35–37, 117, 179, 212–213
development of, 32
Postcentral gyrus, 43, 46
Prevalence of dyslexia, 4, 17–24
effects of language on, 20
effects of sex and inheritance on, 21–24
factors associated with, 19–24
Isle of Wight studies and, 18–19
Primary projection zones, see Cerebral cortex, primary projection zones of
Prosopagnosia, 45
Psycholinguistic functioning, 181–184
Purdue Perceptual Survey Rating Scale, 29

Raven's Coloured Progressive Matrices, 142–144, 152, 175, 188
Reading, 56–60, 69, 71, 89, 95, 100–104, 122, 125, 136, 139, 145, 172, 176, 182–183, 213
angular gyrus and, 57–60
conceptual paradigm for, 60
errors in, 100–102, 139, 145
functional system of, 69, 71, 89, 95, 172, 176, 182–183
neurologic aspects of, 56–60
visual scanning in, 100–103, 213
Reading ability, 105, 126, 129, 140, 157, 173, 212, 221

assessment of, 140, 173
predictors of, 105, 140
Reading failure, 55–96, 103, 165–166, 168–169, 171, 177, 188–189, 192, 209–210, 223
emotional components of, 209, 223
neuropsychology of, 55–96
Reading retarded individuals, 18–19, 93, 98, 105–106, 109, 123, 139, 142, 186
prognosis of, 19
Recovery of function, 55, 69–70, 72–81, 95–96, 224. *See also* Equipotentiality; Plasticity of brain function
Regional cerebral blood flow, 16
Reitan-Indiana Neuropsychological Test Battery for Children, 166–168, 224
Remedial approaches to dyslexia, 4, 14, 24, 27, 80, 139–141, 169–170, 182, 188, 192, 206–232. *See also* names of remedial approaches
failures of, 4, 169, 192
historical perspective on, 207–218
neuropsychological, 222–230
perceptual training, 218–222
Reticular activating system, 35–37, 135, 212
disorders in functioning of, 36
effects of stimulant medication on, 37
function of, 35
Reversals, letter and word, 14, 101–102, 115
Right-ear advantage, 121, 124, 146, 150, 183. *See also* Dichotic listening
Rostrum, 62

Scanning, *see* Reading, visual scanning in
Seashore Rhythm Test, 174, 176, 194
Seelenblindheit, *see* Agnosia
Seizures, 48, 63, 72, 80, 93, 162
petit mal, 162
temporal lobe, 48
Sensation, 172–174
Sensory recognition, 172–173
Sensory strip, *see* Postcentral gyrus
Single and Double Simultaneous (Face-Hand) Stimulation Test, 173–174
Sixth nerve palsy, 66
Skull fracture, 70
Slosson Intelligence Test, 201, 222
Slosson Oral Reading Test, 185
Soft neurological signs, 161, 164
Soma, 33
Speech, *see* Language, expression of

Spelling, 139–141, 145, 182, 226
assessment of, 140
Spinal cord, 32, 212
development of, 32
Splenium, 62, 66, 76
SRA Basic Reading Series, 227, 231
Stanford-Binet Intelligence Scale, 80, 92, 141, 188
Stereognosis, 46, 164, 212
Strephosymbolia, 14, 114
Subgroups of dyslexia, 4–6, 11, 16, 24, 81, 86–90, 93, 103, 119–120, 136–157, 162, 172, 178, 183, 186, 190, 207, 209, 211–212, 223, 225–227, 230–231
alexic, 140–141, 149–153, 155–156, 178, 186, 211, 226
dyseidetic, 140–141, 149–153, 155–156, 178, 186, 211, 226
dysphonetic, 140–141, 149–153, 155–156, 186, 209, 226
primary versus secondary, 11
Sulci, 32, 39
development of, 32
Supplemental motor area, 88
Supramarginal gyrus, 13
Sylvian fissure, 56
Synapse, 33–34

Tachistoscopic research, *see* Visual half-field, tachistoscopic research in
Tactile Form Recognition Test, 173–174, 177–178, 195
Tactile Performance Test, 174, 177, 195
Tandem walking, 174, 179, 201
Telencephalon, 32, 38–39
differentiation of, 32
Temporal gyrus, 29
Temporal lobe, 30, 43, 47–49, 51, 56–57, 66–69, 80–83, 88, 94–95, 182, 189
agenesis of, 66–69
cortex of, 47–49, 95
effects of damage to, 30, 48
uniqueness of in man, 46–57
Thalamus, 35–37, 39, 95
symptoms of lesions of, 39
Transverse convolution, 29
Trapezoid body, 117
Trauma to the brain, 55, 58, 60, 66, 69–82, 95–96, 168, 178, 188, 193
age effects and, 74, 76
in children, 69–82

Trauma to the brain (*continued*)
  cognitive deficits associated with, 74–76
  recovery from, 55, 95
Treatment of dyslexia, 3, 157, 178. *See also*
  names of remedial approaches; Remedial
  approaches to dyslexia
Truncus, 62

VAKT remedial approach, *see* Fernald reme-
  dial approach
Ventricles, 63–64, 83, 91
  dilation of, 64
Ventriculogram, 80
Verbal mediation, 111–112
Visual half-field, 31, 81, 86, 127–134, 147–
  148, 163, 175, 181, 183
  tachistoscopic research in, 127–134, 147–148
Visual pathway, 128
Visual tracking, *see* Reading, visual scanning
  in

Wada technique, 31, 68, 80–82, 86, 116, 118
Wechsler Adult Intelligence Scale, 81, 137,
  188
Wechsler Intelligence Scale for Children, 19,
  80–81, 137
Wechsler Intelligence Scale for Children—
  Revised, 67–68, 144, 167, 170, 175, 188–
  189, 194, 200
Wechsler Preschool and Primary Scale of In-
  telligence, 167, 175
Wepman Auditory Discrimination Test, 174,
  201, 219
Wernicke's area, 48, 57, 59–60, 77, 82, 88
Wide Range Achievement Test, 123, 133,
  141–142, 167, 175, 195, 201, 228–229
Woodcock Reading Mastery Tests, 175, 185,
  195, 201
Word amblyopia, 20
World Federation of Neurology, 9, 102, 134,
  230
  definition of dyslexia, 9

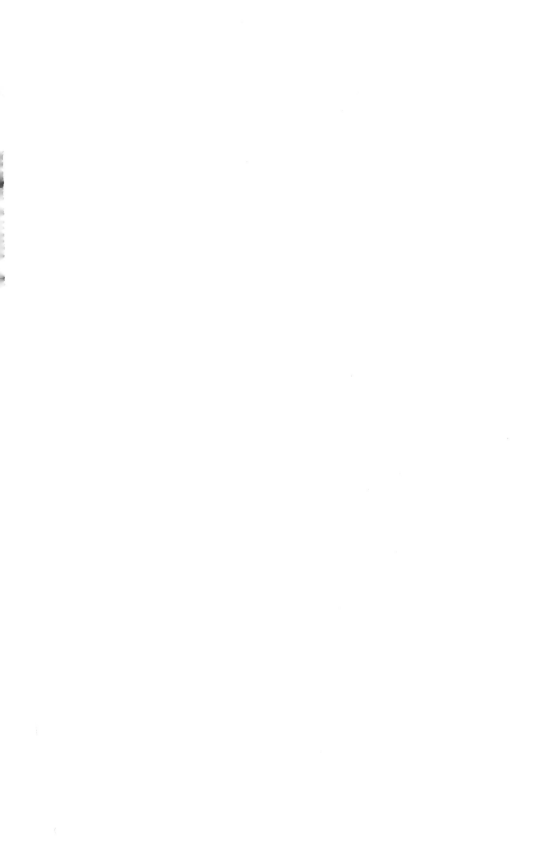